ADOLESCENCE
AND ITS
SOCIAL WORLDS

Adolescence
and its
Social Worlds

edited by

Sandy Jackson
University of Groningen
The Netherlands

and

Hector Rodriguez-Tomé
C.N.R.S., Paris
France

LEA LAWRENCE ERLBAUM ASSOCIATES, PUBLISHERS LEA
Hove (UK)   Hillsdale (USA)

Lawrence Erlbaum Associates Ltd., Publishers
27 Palmeira Mansions
Church Road
Hove
East Sussex, BN3 2FA
U.K.

British Library Cataloguing in Publication Data

A catalogue record for this book is available from the British Library

ISBN 0-86377-310-9 (Hbk)

Printed and bound by BPCC Wheatons Ltd., Exeter

Contents

List of Contributors

John Coleman, Trust for the Study of Adolescence, Brighton, U.K.
Nick Emler, University of Oxford, U.K.
Luc Goossens, University of Leuven, Belgium.
Terry Honess, University of Wales, Cardiff, U.K.
Sandy Jackson, University of Groningen, The Netherlands.
Erich Kirchler, University of Vienna, Austria.
Bärbel Kracke, University of Mannheim, Germany.
Alfons Marcoen, University of Leuven, Belgium.
Augusto Palmonari, University of Bologna, Italy.
Maria Luisa Pombeni, University of Bologna, Italy.
Margaret Robinson, University of Wales, Cardiff, U.K.
Hector Rodriguez-Tomé, C.N.R.S., Paris, France.
Inge Seiffge-Krenke, University of Bonn, Germany.
Shmuel Shulman, Bar Ilan University, Ramat-Gan, Israel.
Rainer K. Silbereisen, Penn State University, U.S.A.
Maria Tyszkowa, University of Poznan, Poland. [deceased]
Bruna Zani, University of Bologna, Italy.

Preface

The origins of this book can be traced back to a workshop on adolescence which took place in Paris in 1988. The workshop brought together some thirty researchers from different parts of Europe. Apart from their common interest in adolescence, all were keen to establish closer co-operative links with colleagues in other parts of Europe. Several factors contributed to this enthusiasm for European co-operation. One of these was the comparative isolation which the researcher on adolescence often experienced at University or even at national level. Even in the late eighties, not many people were engaged in research on adolescence and it was often difficult to make contact with others with similar interests. Europe offered a larger arena, with more prospects for fruitful contact.

A second factor was the increasing awareness in Europe that interesting work on adolescence was not necessarily confined to the other side of the Atlantic. During the 1980s, a variety of conference presentations and publications from different European centres served to establish this awareness. Attending to what was occurring in Europe was further stimulated by a third factor, the recognition that the linguistic and cultural variability of Europe might contribute to patterns of adolescent development which differed from those typically presented by the research literature. This idea may well have been stimulated by the decline in the idea that adolescence could best be seen as a period of storm and stress, and its replacement by a viewpoint which emphasised the constructive, adaptive characteristics of adolescent development.

One of the themes which emerged clearly from the Paris meeting concerned the ways in which progress through adolescence involves elaboration of various forms of social experience within the context of physical and intellectual change. This theme was again in evidence at the follow-up to the Paris meeting which took place in 1990 near Groningen in the Netherlands. On this occasion, a variety of papers emphasised the movement away from a view dominated by conflict with parents and pre-occupation with peers, to one in which attention was focused on issues concerning social adaptation, social strategies and the social construction of adolescence.

The two workshops were to lead to further concrete developments. One of these was the decision to form the European Association for Research on Adolescence and in doing so, to establish a forum for researchers from the different parts of Europe. The Association has already recruited an active and enthusiastic membership drawn from virtually all of the different European countries.

The second concrete development was the decision to publish a book which could serve to bring together some of the work currently taking place in Europe. The present volume is that book. Since social development in adolescence had been a prominent theme at the first two workshops, it was decided to centre the book upon that topic.

Despite the fact that it grew out of the workshops in Paris and Groningen, the book is not simply a set of conference proceedings. A limited amount of the work described in the different chapters was originally presented at one or other of the workshops, but the greater part of the book is fresh material specially written for this publication. Taken together, it presents a reasonably representative picture of both the range and the focus of the thinking and approach which are currently of importance in European research on social development in adolescence.

The publication of this book is the fulfilment of a collaborative project involving people from different countries in Europe. As such, it is a happy occasion and one of considerable satisfaction to all concerned. It is therefore particularly sad that the pleasure of our joint accomplishment is clouded by the sudden death of Maria Tyszkowa in July, 1993. Maria was a delightful colleague who brought enormous enthusiasm, commitment and intellectual rigour to her work. We in the European Association for Research on Adolescence will miss her active involvement, her stimulating contributions and her willingness to engage in intellectual debate. Her loss was felt particularly deeply among her colleagues in Poznan where she was an inspirational and supportive leader. We wish them well during the difficult days of re-adjustment which lie ahead. Maria's grandchild may well have served to stimulate her interest in studying the significance of the grandparent/grandchild relation. Certainly he was a constant source of delight to her, and to him and her husband and son, we express our deepest sympathy. She will be greatly missed and we join in their sense of loss.

We wish to express our appreciation to the authors of the different chapters for their active co-operation in the different phases of the preparation of the book. Editors are not always to easy people to live with. Long periods of silence are suddenly followed by demands for instant action in re-phrasing text, modifying tables or substantially reducing the number of pages already written. Such excesses on our part were accepted with patience and good humour. We wish to thank them for this, as well as for their direct contribution to the book as a whole. We also wish to thank Willy Landeweerd and Wolly ten Berge for the secretarial help which they provided at crucial moments and Lammert Leertouwer for assistance in drawing or re-drawing some of the figures. Having overcome his initial hesitancy about an edited book, Michael Forster provided consistent encouragement and support and he, together with others from Lawrence Erlbaum Associates was always ready to provide technical assistance and advice. Finally, we wish to express our appreciation to colleagues in our respective departments and in the European Association for Research on Adolescence for the interest, encouragement and stimulation they offered during the past two years. They offered a supportive social world which, in itself, was an important contribution to the final completion of this book.

Sandy Jackson
Hector Rodriguez-Tomé
September, 1993.

CHAPTER ONE

Adolescence: Expanding Social Worlds

Sandy Jackson and Hector Rodriguez-Tomé

THE SOCIAL WORLDS OF ADOLESCENCE

For the majority of young people, movement into the adolescent years involves a major expansion in the range and complexity of their social life. The nature of relationships with parents changes as the adolescent moves towards greater independence (Smetana, 1988; Steinberg & Silverberg, 1986; Noller & Callan, 1991). Peers begin to occupy a more central role in many areas of the young person's life (Berndt, 1989; Hartup, 1983) and new possibilities for contacts with peers are explored (Silbereisen & Noack, 1988). The amount of time spent with the family diminishes and time spent with peers or alone increases (Csikszentmihalyi & Larson, 1984; Larson & Richards, 1991). Interest and participation in sexual relationships emerges and increasingly influences social activities (Miller & Simon, 1980; Zani, 1991). The nature and demands of the school environment change and this leads to a widening of the social context from one which is primarily based on the classroom, to one which is school-based (Minuchin & Shapiro, 1983). The young person becomes more aware of and occupied by the wider social environment, its possibilities and constraints (Furnham & Stacey, 1991). First experience of employment may occur (Czikszentmihalyi & Larsen, 1984) and career choice and future employment become matters of concern (Santili & Furth, 1987; Banks et al, 1991).

This sketch illustrates the diversity of the social worlds with which the young adolescent begins to become involved. Some of these will not feature prominently until later in adolescence, but even so, the contrast with the situation of the pre-adolescent is vivid. Only a year or two earlier, in later childhood, social activities were likely to be focused primarily on the home and its environs, or on the class-room, and to take place in circumstances where adult supervision and control were more clearly present. Entry into adolescence leads to less direct supervision and control by adults, more involvement with peers, participation in a wider and generally less nurturing school situation and movement within a wider geographical and social environment.

The diverse areas of social activity can be thought of as representing some of the different social worlds within which the young person is likely to be involved. The word "worlds" in this context expresses the relative distinctness of each from the other within the experience of the young person. One such world may differ from the others with regard to participants, demands made, attributed worth and level of personal investment.

This is not intended to imply that social development in adolescence should be thought of in a compartmentalised fashion. Rather, it expresses the diversity of the social contexts in which the young person may find himself and the fact that each of these may involve a variety of new demands. It also expresses the fact that some of these contexts may be relatively isolated from the others, so that participants in one, may have very little awareness of the nature of other social worlds in which an individual is engaged. Peers may be ignorant of the family context from which an adolescent comes. A young person may be involved with different groups of peers which do not overlap with each other; a group at school and another at a sports club, for example. Similarly, parents may not be acquainted with many of their son's or daughter's friends and may know little of the patterns of interaction in which a son or daughter engages at school or when with friends.

The range and influence of these social worlds varies from adolescent to adolescent. One young person may maintain a pattern which differs but slightly from that of the later childhood years, another may rapidly become engaged in a wide variety of new social contexts. Such individual differences are likely to arise from factors such as parental example and encouragement, home conditions, the presence or absence of geographical constraints, personality characteristics, etc.

Social worlds may also vary in complementarity. Parents may express ideas about the significance of school and schooling which tie in with their child's interests, with those of close peers and with the experience and opportunities actually offered by the school. Alternatively, conflicting demands and/or expectations may occur. The young person experiences a mismatch among parental ideas, personal interests, peer attitudes and the reality of the school environment. In circumstances such as these, the adolescent may be more inclined to make sharp distinctions between one world and the other and to communicate little of experiences gained in one, to people who are involved in another.

Variation also occurs in the worth which the young person attaches to different social worlds. Such variation can be thought of in terms of distinctions made at a particular time or period of development, or of change occurring during the process of time. The adolescent may value involvement in a sports club much more highly than the world of school. This may have important implications for the level of personal investment in each. Preparations for a Saturday-night Disco, for example, may be approached with greater seriousness and commitment than revision for end-of-year examinations. Differences of this sort can give rise to considerable tension between the young person concerned and those involved in other social worlds such as the home or the school. Current understanding of why particular worlds, such as those of sport or "pop culture", are so highly valued by some young people that they adversely effect development in others, remains very restricted.

More evidence is available concerning changes over time in the value attached to different social worlds. While adolescence sees a sort of de-idealisation of parents (Steinberg & Silverberg, 1986), most young people continue to turn to parents for advice and support. The extent to which they do so, however, declines over time, and the young person makes increasing use of, first, same-sex friends and then opposite-sex friends for such purposes (Fend, 1990). Similarly, the development of a steady dating relationship leads to changes in the amount of time spent with the same-sex peers and in the value attached to such relationships.

Presumably differences and changes in how different social worlds are evaluated are related to a complex of cognitive processes. Emmerich, Goldman & Shore (1971), for example, found that adolescents distinguish between conduct rules presented by adults and those arising in the peer group and see both sets of rules as demanding high standards. Self-related ideas are also of importance. Fend (1990) has shown that the age at which young people turn more to peers as opposed to parents for support, etc., is related to level of ego-strength. Silbereisen & Noack (1990) report that disparities between the young person's perception of personal state of development and future-time perspective are associated with changes in self-esteem, friendship conceptions and choice of preferred place of leisure. Similarly, Rodriguez-Tomé et al (in press) show that maturational status has different effects on boys and girls where both body-image and relationships with opposite-sex peers are concerned. In short, the evidence suggests that the nature of the adolescent's involvement with different social worlds affects ideas about self, others and social institutions. As adolescence progresses, this process shapes further interactions and engagements into patterns which are specific to the individual.

Another aspect of being involved in different social worlds merits attention. Any one of these worlds may be subject to transition arising from disruption. Relationships with parents may reach a crisis point, a close friendship may be broken, injury may inhibit athletic progress, an examination may be failed, a romantic initiative may be spurned. Where a disruption such as one of these occurs, resources available in another social word may facilitate the process of coping. However, Simmons, Burgeson & Reef (1988) have shown that where disruptions such as change of school, pubertal change, early dating, geographic mobility or family crisis occur in multiple combination, the consequences are likely to be problematic. Simmons et al speculate that their findings might be interpreted in terms of a "developmental readiness" (Simmons & Blyth, 1987) and/or "focal theory" (Coleman, 1974). Taken together, these theories suggest that if change comes too suddenly, too early (in developmental terms) and in too many areas of life at once, the young person is likely to experience personal difficulty and to evince problems in one or more social environments.

The situation may be even more complex, however. In some cases, disruption in one specific social world may have greater effect on other social worlds than might normally be anticipated. In other cases, however, young people who suffer severe disruption in a variety of spheres continue apparently without negative effect, while others in similar circumstances, including siblings, evince a variety of problem behaviours. For such young people, involvement in one or more particular social worlds appears to fulfil a protective function (Rutter, 1989). Such phenomena suggest that more detailed attention needs to be given to the value which individuals attribute to particular disruptive events within specific social worlds and to the way in which social worlds are perceived relative to each other.

The following chapters aim to present a variety of different approaches to the study of the varied social worlds of adolescence. Before describing the broad focus of each of these chapters, let us state clearly that we make no pretence to cover all of the potential social worlds in which adolescents may be engaged. Given the range and richness of work in this area, comprehensive coverage would require a much more substantial volume than the present one. The topics covered by the different chapters, however, do represent areas which are of central importance to the understanding of social development in adolescence. Taken together, they add considerable substance and fresh perspectives to the outline of social development presented in the introductory paragraph of this chapter.

SOCIAL WORLDS CONSIDERED:
PLAN OF THE BOOK

Many of the issues picked up in the preceding section feature prominently in the various chapters of this book. Jackson (Chapt. 2) argues that research on social development in adolescence has given insufficient attention to the cognitive processes underlying the young person's behaviour in different social contexts. He proposes a model for the analysis of social interaction sequences in adolescence which takes account of the cognitive, affective, situational and developmental factors which are involved in social behaviour.

The model emphasises the role played by the information processing systems of both parties who take part in an interaction and points to the greater possibilities for mismatch and misunderstanding which may arise as a result of maturational disparities in cognitive development. Developmental factors may also influence the skill with which a particular social action is carried out and this, in turn, may have important consequences for how it is interpreted. In distinguishing clearly between processing and action, the model emphasises a distinction which is basic to understanding and ameliorating social difficulties in adolescence.

Jackson acknowledges the important inroads in the understanding of social development in adolescence which have resulted from large group investigations. He argues that such approaches require to be complemented by finer grain studies which focus more directly on longitudinal study of the processes involved in individual social cognitive development in adolescence. The social interaction sequence model provides a theoretical framework for initiating such work.

Honess and Robinson (Chapt. 3) also provide a framework for further research. The purpose of the framework, however, is analytical rather than theoretical, though the authors do suggest that it could ultimately contribute to the further methodological and theoretical refinement of studies of adolescent development within a relational context.

The framework is presented by first providing a brief review of the work of each of three prominent groups of researchers in the field of parent-adolescent relationships. In each case, attention is focused upon the methods used, the conceptual model employed and the empirical findings. The authors then assess the degree of consensus between the research groups and the extent to which this is limited by theory and/or methods. This leads to the description of a framework which is used to compare the research approaches. The basic features of the framework consist of four levels: theoretical origins, content focus, subject population and method format. The application of the framework is illustrated by examining research procedures characteristically employed by the different research groups.

The analytical approach provided by Honess and Robinson is particularly timely in a situation where research on various aspects of relationships in adolescence is burgeoning. In such circumstances, a wide variety of research measures are introduced and the full implications of the findings which they produce are often difficult to identify. The framework offers a means of comparing different theoretical approaches and their related measurement techniques and of identifying areas of convergence and divergence between them.

Silbereisen and Kracke (Chapt. 4) first discuss the measurement of maturational timing in adolescence and then proceed to consider the consequents and antecedents of individual variation in this area of development. The consequences of variation in the timing of physical maturation are discussed with regard to self-evaluation, adaptive and maladaptive contacts with peers and substance use. The authors also discuss recent research, including their own, on some of the antecedents of intra-individual timing. The data from such work has been interpreted as reflecting different reproductive strategies. A childhood history of family conflict or father-absence seemed to be related to (early) age at menarche. Silbereisen and Kracke also refer to recent findings which suggest that immigration and problems of inter-cultural contact may also influence maturational timing.

Discussion of physical maturation and its social implication is particularly appropriate at a time when considerable debate is taking place concerning the relationship between physical maturation and intra-familial relations (Belsky, Steinberg & Draper, 1991a, 1991b; Hinde, 1991; Maccoby, 1991). Silbereisen and Kracke provide a useful review of a research area which has important implications for understanding of a variety of aspects of social behaviour in adolescence (cf. Stattin & Magnusson, 1990).

While achievement of sexual maturity has an extended research history, empirical work on dating behaviour has been less prevalent and more fragmentary in nature. At some levels this is not surprising; the very intimacy of the relationship creates problems where detailed research is concerned. Despite this, there is a need to extend knowledge of this area of adolescent behaviour. Problems such as teenage pregnancy, abortion, AIDS and unsafe sex highlight this need, but there is also a range of less dramatic reasons for further research. Zani (Chapt. 5) refers to some of the more important ones. She points out that little is known of the consequences for adult life of different patterns of teenage sexual behaviour, or of the prevalence and nature of sexual difficulties in adolescence, or of the sexual problems of handicapped adolescents, or of the psychological consequences of adolescent parenthood or abortion. There is little doubt that more detailed information concerning these issues is necessary if an effective basis for educational, preventive and remedial work is to be established.

Zani's chapter concentrates on three areas which have been the subject of research attention: the effects of a partner relationship on the young person's wider relational system, the functions and meanings of dating relationships and the relationship between intimacy and identity development. While each of these areas has received considerable question, Zani's review emphasises the many issues which remain unclear and the questions which remain unanswered. She urges the need for more longitudinal research, for more attention to cross-cultural and intra-cultural differences in sex-related expectations and behaviour, and for clearer definition of the age-boundaries being used when carrying out research with adolescents.

Physical maturation and dating behaviour are two characteristics of development which readily spring to mind where adolescence is concerned. The same can hardly be said for relationships between grandparents and adolescent grandchildren which is a topic which rarely features in discussion of social development in adolescence. As Tyszkowa (Chapt. 6) points out, this omission is surprising given the level of contact often maintained between grandparents and the families of their offspring. In some cases, this contact may not always be positively regarded. In a recent study of adolescents aged 13-16, Jackson and Elzen (1990) noted that the "required visit" to grandparents was one of the most frequently cited sources of conflict between parents and adolescents. Tyszkowa's work shows that strongly positive elements also exist in such relationships. Her data indicate that grandparent-adolescent relationships move towards greater reciprocity, that they are increasingly likely to be initiated by the grandchild as adolescence progresses and that they move towards inter-actions on a more psychological level involving self-revelation in both directions.

Much research on adolescence presents an implicit picture in which young people live with their parents in a nuclear family in a Western culture in which they are surrounded by competing peer groups and the occasional teacher! Tyszkowa's chapter corrects this picture in a variety of ways. It reminds us that an additional relative may well occupy the family home, that certain relatives are often assigned a special significance (even in adolescence), that in conditions of joint parental employment or single parenthood grandparents may fulfil an important caring and supportive function and that the pattern and nature of the grandparental role may vary greatly from culture to culture. Her work raises further interesting questions. Do relationships with grandparents offer adolescents a "safe" context for self-disclosure and for developing new strategies for understanding and dealing with social difficulties? Is the care-giving role which may be involved in "looking after" a grandparent itself a form of preparation for the wider supportive roles likely to arise in adulthood? How do close relationships with grandparents correspond to and differ from adolescent friendships?

Kirchler, Palmonari and Pombeni (Chapt. 7) focus on the relationship between successful resolution of developmental tasks and adolescents' interpersonal activities within two social contexts, the peer-group and the family. Their chapter combines a review of research in this area, with presentation of their most recent empirical findings. Their work shows that while the peer group becomes increasingly important during adolescence, the family continues to play a very influential role. Distinctions can be drawn between the roles played by the two groups. While parents are used for discussion and guidance concerning school, future work, etc., peers offer opportunities for recreation, for sharing developmental tasks and for trying out adult activities. Interestingly—despite fears commonly expressed by parents—Kirchler and his colleagues find that the type of group joined by the adolescent is relatively unimportant. What is important is the type of relationship which the young person forms with the group. Young people who identify highly with their group also derive the greatest advantages in developmental terms. High identification with the group does not entail identification problems elsewhere. In fact, Kirchler et al find that identification with the group is positively correlated with identification with family, school-mates and best friend. The reverse tends to be true for those whose identification with the group is low.

These findings raise interesting questions about the origins and nature of identification. Is identification rooted in family processes experienced earlier in development? Can identification be thought of as a special sort of social skill—or perhaps as a combination of social skills? Can potential identification problems be recognised at an early stage so that intervention measures can be taken?

Such questions focus on identification at the level of the individual. As Kirchler and his colleagues point out, however, two-way processes are involved. The family and the peer group both need to allow the adolescent enough "space" for the development of his or her individuality. This raises the possibility that instances may arise where either the family or the peer group may demand too much for the good of the individual. This brings us back to the problem of excessive involvement with a specific social world referred to in the first section of this chapter. Kirchler, Palmonari and Pombeni's work raises the possibility that in such cases, the particular world concerned, whether family, sports club or school, should be encouraged to recognise the need to provide the necessary "room" for development in other worlds to occur.

Seiffge-Krenke and Shulman's review of the literature on stress and coping in adolescence (Chapt.8) provides complementary findings to those of Kirchler and his colleagues on the role of the family. They cite a range of studies which show the extent to which parental behaviour can be helpful or detrimental to the development of effective coping behaviour in adolescence. Where parents emphasise the importance of personal growth —Kirchler, Palmonari and Pombeni might talk in terms of providing "space"—young people develop a sense of mastery and make less use of coping strategies involving withdrawal.

While Seiffge-Krenke and Shulman can point to a considerable body of research on the relationship between family variables and adolescent coping behaviour, much work remains to be done on the role played by the peer group with regard to coping. In situations where identification with the peer group is high, but where the peer group provides "space", a tendency towards positive patterns of coping might be anticipated. Where identification with the peer group is high and "space" is not provided, one might anticipate that positive coping might occur with regard to peer-related hassles or events and the reverse for non-peer group situations. Delinquent gangs appear to provide an example of this type of situation.

One might speculate that the same expectations are also likely to hold for the adolescent's relationships with other social worlds. The most critical of these may turn out to be those in which high levels of intimacy are combined with high identification and little "space".

While little is currently known about issues such as these, Seiffge-Krenke and Shulman's chapter provides indications of some of the directions which future work might take. Means have to be developed to assess more accurately the climate of a group or non-familial relationship in which an adolescent is involved. These should encompass measures of the room provided within the relationship for personal growth. Attention should be given to age- and sex-differences. Such steps should provide a basis for developing understanding of the ways in which different types of relationship can lead to the establishment of coping strategies of a functional or dysfunctional nature. This, in turn, may serve to extend our insight into the nature of protective mechanisms in the adolescent period.

Loneliness is commonly regarded as an undesirable and stressful situation with which people find difficulty in coping. Generally speaking, this view of loneliness tends to be based on the assumption that it involves the lack of company. Marcoen and Goossens (Chapt. 9) point out that the loneliness can also be regarded as a subjective experience which may occur in situations where others are present. Attitudes to being alone may vary. Some may see it in negative terms and see it as a situation to be avoided or reversed as quickly as possible. Others may respond in more positive terms and are happy to prolong the experience. Solitude is also an aspect of being alone. Marcoen and Goossens see this as referring to active, constructive use of time spent alone. It can be distinguished from simply having a positive attitude to being alone, in that it implies wanting to be on one's own for constructive reasons, i.e. to engage in some form of specific activity.

These distinctions between different aspects of loneliness provide a basis for research on the topic. The chapter proceeds first to discuss their implications with regard to the measurement of loneliness and then to discuss the relationship between loneliness in adolescence and features of adolescent development such as identity, intimacy and attachment. The authors then describe the development of a multi-dimensional instrument which measures loneliness in relationships with parents and peers and aversion to and affinity for loneliness. Studies with the instrument reveal that each of these different aspects of loneliness shows a normative developmental trend during adolescence and that they are all related to important features of development in adolescence.

Marcoen and Goossens' chapter is of special interest because of the clear illustration it presents of how analysis of a specific theoretical issue can lead to the development of measurement approaches which open the way to clarification of relationships with other areas of development. As this introductory review has already suggested, topics such as specific types of intra-family relationships, dating behaviour and peer-group climate all require further fine-grained investigation. This implies not only careful conceptual analysis but the development of focused measurement techniques. Marcoen and Goossen's work provides a useful model of how this might be approached.

Most discussion of relationships in adolescence focus on interpersonal activities associated with the family, peers, dating, etc. Emler's chapter (10) focuses on a different type of relationship which becomes increasingly prominent during the course of adolescence, the relationship with the institutional order. Emler argues that the young person's orientation to formal authority is central to their relation to the institutional order. For the great majority of young people, the education system is the most important context for the development of this relationship. The nature of the accommodation made to formal authority is reflected in the level of their involvement in delinquency.

According to Emler, the institutional order can be seen as a system for ordering social relations. Where young people reject this system, they are choosing instead a more informal and personal system of social regulation. Emler considers why an individual leans towards one choice pattern as opposed to the other. He suggests that reasons for a particular choice could be related to factors such as: perceived imperfections of the formal system, personality characteristics, availability of personal resources and social support. Particular combinations of such factors may increase the likelihood of a delinquent solution. But why are adolescents less positive about authority than other age-groups? Emler advances two possible explanations: a developmental progression from childhood idealisation of authority, through adolescent disillusion and cynicism, to adult realism; changes in relationship patterns whereby the peer-dominated pattern typical of adolescence is exchanged for a situation involving a greater generational mix.

The institutional order can be seen as a world which impinges upon adolescents in whatever social worlds they may be involved. Here, as with the other worlds, one might question the extent to which space is allowed for individual development. Emler's review indicates that for certain groups the space allowed, or perceived to be allowed, may be very restricted.

The final chapter (11) fulfils a different function from the rest. The author, John Coleman, was asked to draw the book together by reflecting on the variety of topics introduced in the preceding chapters. Coleman concludes his review by returning to the importance of theory. He considers two theoretical approaches, Lifespan Developmental Theory and his own Focal Theory. He concludes that both have contributions to make in working towards a more realistic conceptual structure. This can serve to provide an "organising framework" which is relevant to the real-life experiences of young people growing up in the many uncertainties of today's world.

While endorsing the call for a coherent theory of adolescence, we wish to make two further observations. In the first place, research on the varied questions relating to adolescent development cannot simply wait until an appropriate theory emerges. There are areas of adolescent experience which remain unsatisfactorily explored and further investigation can both advance further knowledge and enhance the process of adolescent development. Secondly, such further empirical research may itself suggest new possibilities for opening the way to the achievement of a coherent theory.

ADDITIONAL SOCIAL WORLDS

The chapters in this book focus on a number of the different social worlds of adolescence. Taken together they present a relatively detailed picture of current research findings on social development in adolescence.

There are, however, important areas of research on adolescent social development which only feature incidentally and are not treated as topics in their own right. No detailed attention is given to sex differences even though there is considerable evidence that girls and boys approach and think about social behaviour in adolescence in different ways. Similarly, while various authors refer to age-related differences in social behaviour, it is not discussed in any consistent and systematic fashion.

Family relationships in adolescence is an area which might have been expected to occupy a more prominent place. Only Tyszkowa focuses directly on an area of family relationships, but the area concerned is of a very specific type. Honess and Robinson's chapter makes heavy use of selected research on parent–adolescent relationships, but their goal in doing so is to illustrate the analytic framework they have developed. Other chapters deal in some measure with family relationships but not as a topic in its own right. Specific aspects of family relationships or types of family constellation receive no real attention at all. Important examples include: sibling relationships, one-parent families, families under stress such as unemployment or handicap, and relationships following parental divorce. It is clear that these are all topics which are of major relevance to a considerable proportion of the adolescent population. Their omission is not intended to imply the reverse. Recent publications (e.g. Noller & Callan, 1991; Hetherington & Clingempeel, 1992) have focused directly on some of these areas and we refer the interested reader to them.

Let us also briefly refer to four other topics which are pertinent to the social worlds of adolescence but which receive scant attention, if any. Reference is made at various points in the book to problems of social relationships which may arise in adolescence. For some adolescents, such problems are so substantial that professional help is required. While attention might well have been directed to young people in troubled social worlds, the topic was seen as being more suited to a more clinically oriented book.

A related topic, that of intervention, might well have featured. As Seiffge-Krenke and Shulman make clear, not all adolescents develop effective coping strategies and there is also evidence that adolescence can be a period involving considerable anxiety (Rodriguez-Tomé & Bariaud, 1990) and different types of social difficulty (Tyszkowa, 1990a). Recent years have seen increased interest in the application of social skills training approaches (e.g. Hollin & Trower, 1986). To date, however, the long-term effectiveness of such approaches has not been clearly demonstrated and there are uncertainties about the extent to which learning generalises to new situations. Where adolescence is concerned, much more needs to be learned about age, sex and class differences in social skills (Furnham, 1986). There is certainly evidence that a percentage of young people who do not require clinical help may still benefit from the sort of support which social skills training can offer (Bijstra, Bosma & Jackson, in press). We need to build upon such research in order to develop better means of identifying those who could benefit from social skills training, what specific forms of help are needed and which training techniques are most effective. This is more likely to be successful if carried out within a perspective which takes account of the varied developmental processes and tasks with which the young person is engaged during the period of adolescence (Jackson, in press).

Delinquent groups or gangs present another type of problem. Emler touches in his chapter on the potential influences of such groups with regard to the institutional order, but the influence of such groups on their members extends much more widely. Such groups might be seen as representing a classic area of study, which has already received considerable attention elsewhere in the literature.

Finally, little attention is given to the world of work despite the increasingly important role it plays in young people's lives during adolescence. Several different aspects of employment merit consideration: career choice and preparation for employment; the transition from school into employment; the effects of part-time work experience prior to leaving the educational system; and finally, the area of youth unemployment. Again, recent publications have focused welcome attention on this area (e.g. Furnham & Stacey, 1991; Banks et al, 1991).

All of these additional topics might well have featured in the current text. That they have not done so does not diminish their importance. Their omission can be seen as further illustration of the fact that the variety of social worlds in adolescence is considerable indeed. Their exploration and description will continue to be a significant task.

CHAPTER TWO

Social Behaviour in Adolescence: The Analysis of Social Interaction Sequences

Sandy Jackson

Considered superficially, the development of social relationships in adolescence seems to be a very straightforward affair. Much, after all, appears to be known about the social development of adolescents and the area of relationships has long been accepted as one of the significant areas of change in the adolescent years. The change in the pattern of relationships is certainly very evident. During adolescence, the young person moves towards greater responsibility for himself/herself, shifts away from parental control and supervision and becomes more intensely involved with the peer-group. While this does not necessarily mean that parents cease to play a significant role in the context of the young person's social life, subtle changes in the nature and emphasis of parental authority do take place and these are associated with a decrease in the amount of time spent at home or in the company of parents and an increase in time spent with peers.

This description is a drastic condensation of a wide body of research findings concerning adolescent development. Empirical findings discussed in the other chapters in this book add extra substance to this summary. In the present chapter, however, the emphasis is theoretical rather than empirical. It aims to examine the different components which together contribute to social behaviour and social development during adolescence. This approach is necessary because, in recent years, relatively little research attention has been given to the processes underlying social activity and social development in adolescence.

Lack of attention to these underlying processes has led to an inadequate picture of adolescent social cognitive development. Research in this area has tended to remain static and broadly descriptive. This chapter argues that a more analytic approach to social behaviour can provide a framework for further research and that this can lead to the development of new insights into the adolescent's understanding of and participation in the social world. This argument is introduced by considering a series of prototypical social situations involving adolescents and identifying the type of questions which are raised by such situations. Many of these questions have been explored in social cognitive research with adult subjects. However, while such research provides a useful framework for the study of social cognition in adolescence, it has also certain limitations which stem from the characteristics of adolescence itself. With these limitations in mind, a model is proposed for the analysis of social interaction sequences in adolescence. It is argued that this model can provide a clearer picture of the factors which together contribute to young people's responses to different types of social situation. In doing so, it can help clarify the specific areas of social activity in adolescence which require further investigation. Finally, it can be used as a basis for explaining some of the processes which lead to further social cognitive development in adolescence.

Before considering the model in detail, attention will first be given to the type of social situations which can take place in adolescence. This will be done by presenting four scenarios and discussing their implications.

SOCIAL INTERACTIONS IN ADOLESCENCE: FOUR SCENARIOS

During the greater part of adolescence, the majority of adolescents continue to live at home and "negotiate new roles and relationships which are more equal and more mutual" (Noller & Callan, 1991). At the same time, their world beyond the home is expanding, existing relationships may be consolidated or discontinued, new acquaintances are met and new social situations encountered and explored. "Negotiation" at home and facing up to new situations outside the home place new demands on the young person's capacity to respond effectively. At times, the difficulties involved may be considerable. Consider the following scenarios.

Scenario 1. A Parent/adolescent Interaction

John enters the room putting on his anorak. His parents ask where he is going. John answers that he is going out with Harry, a friend who is already known to the parents. One of the parents has just heard from a neighbour that Harry associates with a group of boys who have been in trouble with the police. He/she begins to ask more detailed questions about what John and Harry are planning to do, what they have done in the past, etc. John cannot understand why such questions are suddenly being asked and responds with some irritation. His reaction is interpreted by the parents as indicating evasiveness and guilt, they become more anxious and begin to express reservations about John's friendship with Harry. John reacts angrily, a row erupts and the parents end up by refusing to let him go out.

Scenario 2. Two Adolescents

Helen and Anne are walking along the school corridor. Helen sees an advertisement for a disco. She points it out and suggests that she and Anne should go to it together. Anne has never been to a disco, is unsure about how her parents might react to the idea and answers in a hesitant and unclear fashion. Helen thinks she is being stand-offish and responds sharply, "If you don't want to go with me, I'll get Mary to go instead."

Scenario 3. A Boy and a Girl

Frank sees Katie at a disco and asks her to dance. After a while, they stop for a drink and Frank suggests going out for a breath of fresh air. Katie's friends are still dancing, it's stuffy in the disco, Frank seems nice, in short, there seems no reason not to go out for some air. Once outside, Frank starts to try to kiss her. Katie gets anxious and tries to push him away. Frank thinks she's just teasing and grabs hold of her. Katie screams.

Scenario 4. A Boy and an Adult[1]

David has been skateboarding with a friend and misses the last bus home. As he hesitates at the bus stop, a man drives up and offers him a lift home. David is happy, he'll be home on time after all. The man begins to ask him about his sexual experiences and starts to fondle him. David is terrified, doesn't know what to do. At traffic lights, he wants to try to jump from the car but cannot move. The man takes him to a remote cottage and sexually assaults him. On being released, he doesn't dare tell anyone. His father is "a macho lorry driver" and his parents read the *Sun* (a newspaper) which is "going through a phase of unmasking sick pervert priests". He thinks of himself as "a disgusting pervert".

The first two of these scenarios might be seen as being fairly typical of most adolescents' experience. Tensions, differences of opinion and misunderstandings are common features of most relationships. For a variety of reasons, which will be discussed later in this chapter, adolescent relationships may be particularly prone to such difficulties. The other two scenarios may be thought of as less prevalent, but they can hardly be described as totally outside the knowledge, fantasy or experience of many young people. All, indeed, might be regarded as sharing a number of features in common. In each case, an interpersonal situation takes place to which each of the participants brings their own level of experience, ideas and assumptions. As each situation develops, deficits in experience, insight, understanding of the other, or interpersonal skills lead to difficulties which may lie beyond the coping capacities of one or both of the individuals concerned.

Considered from another perspective, distinctions might be drawn between the first two and the final scenarios. The typicality of the former might lead one to expect few lasting negative effects. The trauma of the fourth, on the other hand, might lead one to anticipate long-term damage which might be particularly likely to affect future relationship patterns and self-related ideas. The third scenario might lead ultimately in one direction or the other. In some circumstances the situation might end in laughter and return to the disco, in others, it might escalate further with the real possibility of serious consequences for one or other of the two young people.

Such distinctions between the scenarios are possible if they are considered as discrete events. Let us suppose that the first or second are seen as being highly typical of John's experience of his parents, or Anne's with her girl friends. In these circumstances, wider and possibly long-term implications for relationships as well as for other aspects of the young person's development begin to become apparent.

Not only the scenarios, but also their potential implications are readily recognised. Despite this, little research attention has been given to the processes actually involved and the ways in which they together contribute to a particular behaviour pattern or developmental pathway. It is clear that some young people leave home early, or experience difficulty at school, or have problems in relationships with peers, or fall victim to delinquency or drug abuse, or cannot relate to the opposite sex, or are more subject than others to aggressive or bullying behaviour. Young people may also develop self-perceptions which inhibit or enhance their ability to respond to new challenges, or styles of interaction which seem designed to work against their best interests.

Some of the circumstances contributing to such negative patterns of development have already been elaborated (e.g. Bandura, 1981; Rutter, 1989) and attempts have been made to map the different types of difficult psycho-social situations which young people may encounter (Goor-Lambo, Orley, Poustka & Rutter, 1990). Evidence has been produced illustrating links between experiences in the childhood years and adolescent patterns of social behaviour (e.g. Holmes & Robins, 1987; Goodyer, 1990b; Feehan, McGee, Stanton & Silva, 1991). In general, however, such work has failed to attend to, or adequately to account for the processes which lead to and serve to maintain these patterns. Research aimed at clarifying these processes remains an urgent need. A possible framework for such research will be described in subsequent sections of this chapter. Before introducing this framework, let us briefly consider the characteristics of current social cognitive research involving adolescent or adult subjects.

RESEARCH APPROACHES TO SOCIAL DEVELOPMENT IN ADOLESCENCE

With few exceptions, current research on adolescent social behaviour is dominated by what might be referred to as an empirical/descriptive approach. A specific area of social activity is studied and descriptions of characteristic patterns of attitudes, traits or behaviour are obtained. Typical recent examples include: external influences on intra-familial processes (review by Bronfenbrenner, 1986); adolescents' understanding of aspects of society such as politics, employment, race (review by Furnham & Stacey, 1991); family relationships, life events and psycho-pathological development (review by Goodyer, 1990a). While the importance of longitudinal approaches is increasingly emphasised, the majority of studies remain cross-sectional in design. Many studies—cross-sectional and longitudinal—adopt a correlational approach and focus upon the relationship between two or more variables, e.g. ego-strength development and social relationships (Fend, 1990), or early maturation and school career, later use of alcohol, relations with peers, etc. (Stattin & Magnusson, 1990).

The range and detail of this work is striking and, taken together, it represents a major development of knowledge concerning social development in adolescence. In general, however, its emphasis tends to be on content rather than on process. Little attention is given to how particular ideas about parents or peers come to develop, even though the fact that development over time has taken place may be highlighted. It is true that reference to social-cognitive development is frequently made. In general, however, this appears to be regarded in stage-theoretical terms, i.e. as a level of understanding which adolescents have (or can be assumed to have) reached.

Even research which focuses specifically on social cognitive development in childhood and adolescence has tended to concentrate on content rather than process. The early studies of person perception (Peevers & Secord, 1973; Livesley & Bromley, 1973) described a tendency to make increasing use of psychological constructs between childhood and adolescence. This work stimulated many similar studies (Barratt, 1977; Honess, 1981;

Barenboim, 1981; O'Mahony, 1986) but the main thrust of such research was concerned with the person-related ideas available to young people as revealed by content-analysis of free descriptions. With few exceptions (Barratt, 1977; Honess, 1979; Jackson, 1987), little attempt was made to examine how such ideas linked together or were applied. Similar observations can be made concerning work on relationships in adolescence (Coleman, 1974) and social perspective taking (Selman, 1980). The former used interview and projective material to identify focal areas of concern at different stages in adolescence, the latter developed a stage model of social perspective taking in childhood and adolescence.

The lack of a more focused and analytic approach means that research on social cognitive development in adolescence remains one-sided and limited. There is a need to progress towards a more comprehensive view in which knowledge of what adolescents say or do is complemented by understanding of the processes which lead to a particular response or action. Conceptions need to be based not only on answers to 'what' questions, but also to 'why' and 'how' questions. At present, much is known about what adolescents think, much less about why the individual adolescent thinks in a particular way and how thinking leads on to action. In sum, more attention needs to be given to the cognitive aspects of adolescent social development.

Research on social cognition has not been confined to developmental issues. In recent years, a confluence of cognitive and social psychological approaches has led to the emergence of a distinctive range of social cognitive research (e.g. Cantor & Kihlstrom, 1981; Fiske & Taylor, 1984; Wyer & Srull, 1984). This work contrasts sharply with the bulk of the developmental literature in that it focuses much more directly on the attentional, attributional, inferential and memory processes involved in social cognition. An important aspect of such work is the attention it has given to the application of models derived from cognitive psychology to social events.

The field of social cognitive research and developmentally oriented work on social cognition (particularly that concerned with adolescence) have remained remarkably distinct from each other. Considered from the standpoint of adolescent research, this division has been unfortunate since it is the cognitive emphasis which is lacking in current work on social behaviour during this period of development. Given this situation, it might appear that one should proceed by simply applying findings from one field to the other. There are important reasons why such an approach is not suitable. Most important of these is the lack of a developmental perspective that takes account of the maturational processes which take place during adolescence: processes which influence patterns of reactions to social stimuli, the responses which are made to social situations and how others in the social environment perceive and respond to the young person.

Social cognitive research, for example, deals almost exclusively with adult subjects. Subjects' previous social experience is assumed to be similar. Subjects are expected to function at much the same cognitive level, unless some form of experimental manipulation has been introduced. In contrast, adolescence sees the emergence of more abstract intellectual capacities which allow social experience to be considered at a progressively more elaborated level. During adolescence and particularly in the early stages social experience is limited relative to that of the average adult. For most adolescents, much of this period of development is also characterised by some level of dependence on their parents. An implication of this is that parental influences often continue to play an important part in a wide range of areas of social behaviour. Nor is this necessarily a one-way situation. Adolescents may continue to seek and value parental guidance, advice and support in connection with social experiences which they have encountered, or are about to encounter (Fend, 1990; Kirchler et al, Chapt. 7).

These characteristics mean that a satisfactory model of social cognition in adolescence has to take account of maturational variations in developmental status. It also has to allow for differences between participants in social situations in terms of developmental level, social experience and awareness of situational influences. Similarly, attention has to be given to the implications of possible variations between individuals in the competence with which social actions are carried out. Finally, it should provide some explanation for the process of social cognitive development itself.

A way of proceeding towards the development of such a model is to focus upon the units which go together to form social behaviour (cf. Newtson, 1973) while trying to take account of the effect of developmental differences among those engaged in the behaviour. Such units might be thought of as comprising social interaction sequences involving characteristic basic features. The following section describes a model of a social interaction sequence involving two individuals. The initial development of the model stemmed from social cognitive research which, in general, was not developmental in orientation (e.g. Cantor, 1981; Higgins & King, 1981; Wyer & Srull, 1984). The elaboration of the model in subsequent sections aims to take specific account of the process of development in which the adolescent is engaged.

A SOCIAL INTERACTION SEQUENCE

Social behaviour might be considered as being made up of a series of interaction sequences, each of which involves certain basic components. Figure 2.1 illustrates the relationship among these components in an interaction sequence involving two actors (A1 and A2).

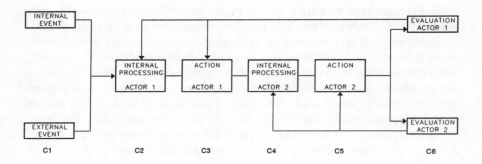

FIG. 2.1. Model illustrating the different components of a social interaction sequence.

An interaction sequence begins with an event (C1) which may be internal or external and which may occur at any point in an ongoing episode of social behaviour. An internal event is a decision or thought such as "I must tell Anne" or "John will be interested in this". An external event is an occurrence in space and time as when Harry opens the front door or Betty trips over the door step. The importance of the event is that it marks the beginning of an interaction sequence involving two people. Since the interaction sequence may occur anywhere within an ongoing episode, the opening event may be preceded by a number of other interaction sequences involving the same participants.

The second component (C2) consists of the inner thought processes which arise in A1 as a result of the event. Inner processes here include thoughts, scripts, value judgements, affects, decisions and similar activities. The range and nature of the inner processes which actually occur in any one interaction sequence can vary widely. Taken together, they dictate the form of the specific action (C3) which A1 takes and which is directed towards A2. C3 may involve spoken language or may be non-verbal and consist of a gesture, glance or a more elaborate form of non-verbal behaviour. How it is executed will depend on A1's personality characteristics and the availability of specific skills or competence to A1 and the extent to which these skills are applied.

The following component (C4) comprises the inner processes arising in A2 as a result the action at C3. These processes will be of a similar nature to those involved at C2 and their nature and the extent to which they feature in this component can again vary considerably from one interaction sequence to another. They lead to a responsive action (C5) on the part of A2. The content of the action will depend on the processes which have occurred at C4, but, as with C3, how it is executed will depend on A2's behavioural repertoire, on the availability of particular skills and personality characteristics.

Component 6 is an evaluative stage. It is dichotomous in that evaluation occurs in both actors (A1 and A2). For each of them, the nature of evaluation is dependent not only on the actions in the sequence (C3 and C5) but also on the thought processes preceding each action (C2 and C4). Since the actors' perceptions of C3 and C5 may differ and the thought processes involved at C2 and C4 are not accessible to both parties, considerable differences may exist between the two evaluations. Participation of each of the parties in a further interaction sequence is influenced by feedback from their own individual evaluation. Thus, feedback may influence thought processes and actions in further interaction sequences and may lead, in time, to psychological development in either or both of the actors.

ELABORATION OF THE MODEL

Figure 2.1 provides a highly simplified picture of an interaction sequence. As the account given earlier makes clear, each of the components is influenced by different schemas and factors or by the employment or presence of particular behavioural patterns, skills or personal characteristics. For the purposes of this chapter, the interaction sequence is always concerned with an adolescent (A2), but the initiator (A1) may not necessarily be an adolescent. The schemas employed by A1 will vary depending on his/her relationship to A2 and the reverse is also true. Before examining such variability, let us consider the type of schemas (etc.) which could be involved in an interaction sequence involving an adolescent child (A2) and a parent (A1).

Suppose that the initial event (C.1) involves an adolescent entering the room while putting on an anorak. The parent responds to the event by saying: "Be in by 11 o'clock tonight." An instruction of this sort is not unusual in the context of parent/adolescent relations and neither party may give it much conscious thought. It can be seen, however, as deriving from an information-processing and decision-making framework (C2), which leads to the action (C3) being taken (in this case, the instruction being given) and which influences the manner in which the action takes place. This is so, even though the parent may not be fully conscious of the various parts which together comprise the framework. The adolescent to whom the instruction is addressed, may be even more dimly aware of the existence of such a framework and its constituent parts. As we shall see, this lack of awareness may have important implications for the further development of the interaction sequence.

Figure 2.2 illustrates the main characteristics of the framework. Each of the constituent parts may be employed in giving the instruction, but this need not necessarily be the case. For example, if only the parent and the adolescent are present and the instruction is given in the usual context, e.g. at home, situational factors may play little, if any role. Similarly, if the instruction is one which has frequently been given and in the same way, values, cognitions and affect are less likely to feature prominently. The very normality of the instruction has important consequences for the further development of the interaction.

The central feature of the framework comprises a nucleus made up of three parts, cognitions, values and affects, each of which influences the others. Cognitions consist of a variety of schemas which relate to the adolescent and which may be either explicit or implicit. Some of these schemas may have a script-like character, e.g. "Young people who stay out late will go to undesirable places. They will encounter demands which lie outside their experience and this will lead them into trouble."

Certain cognitions can be identified which are likely to contribute to this (initial) component of a parent–adolescent interaction. How, for example, does the parent think about parenthood and, specifically, parenthood with regard to the adolescent? Cognitions involved here are likely to include: memories of experiences with own parents; awareness of partner's ideas and approach; perceptions of behaviour of other parents with adolescents of the same age; reflection on previous personal experience of parenting-type situations with an adolescent. Cognitions such as these do not necessarily feature in all interactions. Memories of one's own parents' behaviour, for example, may have little relevance to certain situations, but may be highly relevant—in a positive or negative sense—to another. In addition, cognitions may be contradictory and particular cognitions may be given a higher value than others. For example, the fact that one's partner is a renowned adolescent psychologist may mean that his/her ideas play a more influential role than the unanimous views of friends, neighbours, etc!

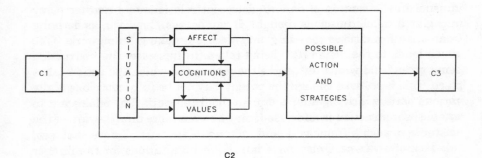

FIG. 2.2. The main features of a social information processing and decision-making framework.

This pattern may not be wholly consistent however. In certain circumstances—for example, when under stress, or in a public situation—the parent might fall back upon cognitions derived from other sources and this might lead to inconsistencies between different interaction sequences.

Other cognitions may be more directly concerned with the adolescent and adolescence. Some of these might be of a general nature and concern what is typical of or appropriate to young people at a particular age-level. Ideas about what is normal behaviour for 15-year-olds may be largely accurate or completely askew. One parent's perception of adolescent independence may be quite different from that of a neighbour. Certain cognitions may be specific to the adolescent child: "He is less mature than others" or "She is too easily led" or "He should only be thinking about his future at this stage." Such considerations may lead to clear contrasts between the approaches adopted towards two different adolescents in the same household. Still other cognitions may be concerned with the characteristics of the young person's companions or the characteristics of the venue for the evening. Knowledge here may be limited or may consist mainly of stereotypes. A parent's ideas about their adolescent's companion may be more strongly influenced by his/her choice of clothing than by other characteristics. Ideas about what actually happens at a modern disco may be primarily based on experience obtained some twenty years earlier, or on what is portrayed on television.

As Figure 2.2 shows, values and affects may be closely involved with cognitions. Religious belief, moral conceptions, political priorities or racially or culturally based ideas may colour these cognitions. Certain behaviour patterns may be regarded as inappropriate for one's own son or daughter, even though they may be recognised as normal within the wider adolescent culture. The idea that it is better if different racial groups do not intermingle may find expression in the instruction "Be in by 11 o'clock tonight" in a situation involving a friend from another racial group, while the same instruction would not be given if the friend was from one's own racial group. The influence of particular values may be still stronger, of course. In some cases they may be potent enough to over-ride all other cognitions. Refusal to permit association with those who do not belong to a particular religious group is one such example.

Affects can have a similar role. Anxiety about the welfare of the young person, dislike of one or more adolescent associates, anger arising from an earlier, unrelated interaction sequence, personal loneliness or insecurity may influence cognitions in a particular way. "Be in by 11 o'clock tonight" might be substituted for the more normal "Try not to be late", for example. As with values, the influence of affects may be so strong that they swamp other cognitions. Where this occurs, everything may be directed to attempting to stop a planned event from occurring.

In certain circumstances these aspects of the central nucleus may be influenced by one or other of two additional factors. Situational factors refer to additional influences which happen to be present when an interaction is initiated. For example, the fact that a neighbour happens to be present may lead to the instruction "Be in ... ", where under other circumstances the question "When will you be in tonight?" would normally be used. In such cases, the cognitions which are normally employed are supplemented by cognitions concerning the ideas, expectations, values, etc. of the other person. Situational factors may link initially with any one of the three parts of the central nucleus. In this example, the influence of the presence of a neighbour is primarily on cognitions. If the neighbour happens to have strong religious beliefs, the influence might be more closely linked to values. Similarly, if the interaction is being initiated in a different setting from normal—while on holiday in another country, for example—heightened uncertainty or anxiety may mean that the main influence is on affects.

Situational factors occur within a broader social and ideational context. A particular sub-cultural group may have particular ideas about adolescence, parental responsibility, appropriateness of certain activities, etc. In a particular historical period, the prevailing culture may be more open or more opposed to a specific view of adolescence. Such broader viewpoints are likely to influence the direction of parental thinking and decision-making. Where they are generally held within a culture, little problem is likely to arise since their generality is likely to encourage consistency. Where differences exist—for example, in situations where parental thinking refers back to a sub-culture which espouses views which differ widely from the prevailing culture—problems may arise. The same is likely to be true in situations where there are wide divergencies between the wider culture, which serves as the parental source of reference and a specific adolescent sub-culture to which sons or daughters refer.

Additional parental pre-occupations may have somewhat similar consequences, though generally, they are less likely to influence values. On the other hand their effect may be dramatically different. If the parent is already strongly pre-occupied with other activities, an event may be initiated unthinkingly and further development of the interaction sequence may be largely ignored. Situations where this might occur include: where another child is demanding attention, where a close relative is seriously ill or where the marriage relationship is in jeopardy. Sometimes, of course, pre-occupation may be at a much more trivial level as when the parent is simultaneously involved with the dramatic dénouement of a television programme.

The final part of the framework lies between the processing phase and Action 1. It is a decision-making phase in which A1 decides what action is necessary and selects a specific response from the interaction repertoire available to him/her. On many occasions, selection is likely to be a routine affair in that an habitual interaction style will be adopted. This is particularly likely to occur in circumstances where the two participants in the interaction sequence are related or very well known to each other. Sometimes, however, other types of interaction style may be necessary. This is probably most likely where values or affect are involved, or where situational factors are involved. Depending on the circumstances, an interaction style may be employed which is authoritarian, or placatory, or wheedling, etc. As illustrated by the various forms of the "time to come home" theme which were employed earlier, these different styles are likely to involve the use of quite different forms of utterance.

The cognitive processes in C2 lead A1 to carry out a specific action (C3). Note that this action can be carried out in a variety of different ways. An utterance may be made confidently or hesitantly. A movement may be executed smoothly and purposively, or it may be clumsy and ineffective. A statement may be phrased and expressed with great clarity or so loosely strung together and mumbled out that meaning is lost in ambiguity. Variation in the manner in which C3 is carried out may be related to the processes carried out at C2. A1 may be aware of inconsistencies or contradictions at C2, or anxious because of particular situational factors. As a result, C3 may be adversely affected. On other occasions, however, variations are likely to be related to the extent to which communication skills have been developed or to A1's individual personality characteristics.

The next component in Figure 2.1 (C4) is again concerned with cognitive processes, those arising in A2 as a result of Action 1. As with C2, the processes involved are potentially very complex. This is so whatever the characteristics of A2, but in the present case, where A2 is an adolescent, the situation is further complicated by developmental factors and specifically, those which relate to level of social cognitive development.

The framework presented in Figure 2.3 illustrates the different cognitive processes involved in C4. As was the case with Figure 2.2, each of the constituent parts may be involved in considering C3, but this need not necessarily be the case. For example, the event may be so routine that it is barely considered at all. There is still another possibility. If the adolescent concerned is quite young and social cognitive development is comparatively undeveloped, certain parts of the framework may not be employed. The development of processing power which is likely to arise as the adolescent grows older is illustrated by the concertina-like extensions of the framework as a whole.

C4 resembles C2 in that two basic phases are involved, processing and decision making. It differs in that in adolescence, the amount of activity

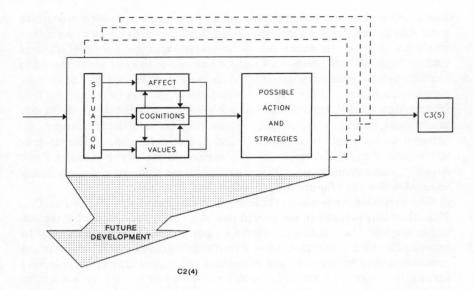

FIG. 2.3. A social information processing and decision-making framework within a developmental context. The stippled lines and arrow illustrate the variability in the elaboration of the framework associated with developmental processes.

involved in each of these two phases is dependent on a variety of factors relating to the young person's developmental level. Examples include: the nature and range of prior experience, the extent to which capacities for abstract, reflective thought have developed and the range of social strategies available to the young person.

The main constituents of the processing phase are the same as those at C2. Perception of the action (C3), whether it is initially directed at A2 or not, leads to internal processing which may involve cognitions, affects and values. In view of the similarity between the processes occurring here and those at C2, it is not necessary to describe all of them in detail again. However, certain differences are worth noting.

The first concerns the action which triggers processing on the part of A2. Whereas the beginning of the interaction sequence (C1) was either an internal or an external event, C3 is always an external event—in the present sequence, a parental action. Whether the action is directed explicitly at the young person or not, it has the effect of triggering internal processing. How the action is perceived is part of that processing. Which parent is involved; the action's consistency with previous parental behaviour in similar contexts; the manner in which it is carried out; its affective tone; its appropriateness: issues such as these can influence the direction and quality of the processing phase. Suppose, for example, that the parental instruction to be in by 11 o'clock has not been used for many months. In such circumstances, it is likely to cause surprise and irritation and may invoke previously held ideas about parents, together with ideas relative to self and adolescence. It is important to note that the young person's perception of C3 may not be accurate. A tone or a look may be misinterpreted. Perception may be biased by other factors such as the adolescent's anxiety about being too late to meet up with friends, or the emotional carry-over from an earlier argument with the parent concerned, or irritation about a favourite shirt not having been washed. On the other hand, it might be biased by the fact that the young person's social interpretative skills are inadequately tuned to take account of all of the factors which may have influenced the parental action.

A second difference concerns the role of values. We have seen how values, together with cognitions and affects, may be involved in the parental processing which occurs at C2. While all three may potentially be involved with the adolescent, values are less likely to feature in a distinctive way unless the parental action appears in some way to be inconsistent with his/her normal pattern. This is so because of the generally close similarity between the political, religious and moral values of parents and their adolescent children (e.g. Youniss & Smollar, 1985).

These differences apart, the main features of the processing occurring at C4 correspond with those at C2. The nature of the internal processes will be different, however. This is so because another person is involved (A2) and because he/she is an adolescent. The fact that another person is involved raises the possibility that cognitions, affects and values at C4 will be discongruent with those at C2—individuals vary in their thought processes, their values and in their affective reactions. That A2 is an adolescent brings in a developmental dimension and this may increase the likelihood of discongruency. This is especially the case where A1 assumes a level of functioning which is too advanced for A2, or where A2 cannot comprehend the various dimensions of the parental situation, or where either A1 or A2 is insufficiently sensitive to the difference between parental priorities and adolescent priorities.

For example, the parent might attempt to give a coded message to the young person. "Be in at 11 o'clock tonight" refers back to an earlier discussion in which the adolescent has talked about his/her difficulties in resisting a companion's pressure to go, after the cinema, to a particular café with a bad reputation for trouble late at night. The instruction may be seen by the parent as something which can be invoked in order to get out of a difficult situation. The young person may interpret it in a much more immediate way as a statement about personal independence or about the companion for that particular evening.

Alternatively, the adolescent may be unaware of the difference that the presence of a certain neighbour makes to the parent's behaviour. The parental instruction is heard and responded to solely within the context of the dyadic relationship between parent and child. No account is taken of the possibility that the neighbour has a particular position, or holds certain opinions and that this has bearing on parental behaviour.

Insensitivity to the priorities of the other means that one of the two people concerned takes insufficient account of the other person's situation. The adolescent may fail to recognise legitimate responsibilities, anxieties or needs on the part of the parent. This may lead to resentment being expressed because the parent wishes to have some indication of the plans for the evening, or to hostility when anxiety is expressed about companionship with drug-users, or prevarication when assistance is sought with a household task. Thrusting for independence in the context of the attractions and competing demands of the new world outside may encourage the young person to dismiss parental concerns as little more than attempts to deny the reality of the movement away from child-hood.

The parent, on the other hand, may be unwilling to recognise the pressures which the young person is experiencing. Uncertainty about personal competence, fear of being unpopular—the odd man out—worries about physical appearance and anxiety about being at the centre of everybody's attention (Elkind, 1974) are characteristic features of many young people's experience of adolescence. Parents may ignore or decry such feelings, or even strengthen them through inopportune comments in the presence of others. Such failures to take account of the other's position are not confined to parent/adolescent relationships of course. The presence of a developmental dimension, however, may increase the risk of discongruency in the relationship. The parent needs to take account of the shifts in the young person's position which development brings. This entails not only recognition of physical change, but also awareness of the need to give more room to achieve greater independence, to face up to new experiences and to make one's own mistakes. Sensitive tuning-in of this sort is not necessarily easy and this is especially so when the young person's behaviour may appear to be more indicative of regression, than of capability of looking after him/herself.

The restricted nature of current knowledge of how social cognitive development proceeds means that currently it is not possible to provide a detailed description of the effects of developmental change on the pattern of parent/adolescent relationships. It seems reasonable to assume that the less advanced the individual's understanding, the greater the chance of unawareness of the complex factors which may lie behind a parental action, the greater the ignorance of the contribution of his/her own behaviour to the event and the more restricted the ability to express personal thoughts or emotions in an effective way. When such deficiencies are present with the adolescent involved at C4 in an interaction sequence, the most likely outcome is rapid movement to the decision-making phase with limited and superficial processing. In the context of an adult/adult interaction sequence, one might refer to an ill-considered or precipitate decision. With the adolescent this description is hardly appropriate. Consideration remains restricted, but it does so because the appropriate abilities remain undeveloped or are inadequately developed.

The decision-making phase is similar to that which occurred at C2 and which led directly to the choice of a specific action (C3). In the light of the processing which has occurred, A2 decides what sort of action is necessary and selects a specific response from his/her action repertoire. As with the processing phase of C4, however, its range of operation is dependent on the young person's level of social cognitive development. More specifically, it depends on: the nature and extent of the young person's previous social experience; the perceived relevance of that experience to C3; the range of the potential responsive actions which are available; and finally, the level of awareness of the possible impact of particular responsive actions on the parent.

Generally speaking, the younger the adolescent the greater the likelihood that each of these aspects will be restricted, with the result that the choice options available to him/her will also be limited. Increasing age, experience and social understanding bring not only new insights, but also a wider range of action possibilities. Seen in these terms, the quality of the decision-making phase is ultimately a product of the complexity of C3, the range and depth of the processing phase and the number of action choices available to the young person.

The next component of the interaction sequence, C5, is the execution of the decision reached at C4. Here, as with C3, the manner in which C5 is carried out varies according to the nature of the young person's internal processing (C4), the level of acquired social skills and personality characteristics. The young person may feel that there was more to C3 than met the eye, feels uncertain, acts in terms of limited understanding and does so at a very tentative level. On the other hand, what has happened and what should be done may be very clear, but the adolescent may lack the skills necessary in order to put it into effect. Alternatively, personal characteristics of a more ongoing nature may intrude and may influence what the young person does. In adolescence, uncertainties relating to self, for example, might adversely effect the way C5 is approached and carried out.

The final part of the sequence, C6, is an evaluative phase and involves both parties, A1 and A2. Each considers what has occurred at C5 from their own individual perspective. For A1, this evaluation is likely to be at two different levels: what happened at C5 and how it relates to C2. The former refers to what A2 actually did and how and why it was done. The latter is concerned with the level of congruence between the thoughts, emotions, expectations, etc., which occurred at C2 and what A2 did, or apparently did.

For A1, this evaluative procedure feeds back and contributes to new interaction sequences involving A2. This may occur immediately or may occur after an interval of time. In the latter case, it may either form the initiating (internal) event of a new interaction sequence, or it may inform the processing which occurs at C2 (or C4, if the sequence is initiated by A2). Suppose, for example, that A2's reaction to "Be in at 11 o'clock" is an angry "That's far too early" followed by a slammed front door. In this case the interaction sequence has been abruptly terminated. A1 may be angered by the tone of the reaction, but may realise that the instruction was given at an inappropriate moment and without adequate explanation. A1 decides not to say anything more if A2 arrives back on time. Even if A2 is on time, future interactions may continue to be influenced. For instance, later processing may include memories of the angry response and a determination not to stand any nonsense. Alternatively, more attention may be given to the provision of fuller explanation of why a particular instruction or request is being made.

Evaluation on the part of A1 may have still wider implications. One or more features of the interaction sequence may be seen as relevant to parenting, to adolescence, or possibly even to values. As a result, the processing which occurs in other types of interaction sequence involving A2, or in sequences with other adolescents or children may be modified by the outcomes of this evaluation phase. Put differently, the evaluation and feedback which arises from it serve as the basis for inner change and hence for alterations of approach to new interactions.

The evaluation in which A2 engages is potentially of a similar nature but its range and quality are defined by the social developmental level which has been attained. Younger adolescents are generally less likely to reflect in any detail on the various components of the interaction, including the appropriateness of their own processing and decision making or the effectiveness with which they acted. This may explain why early adolescence is the period when most arguments between parents and young people take place (e.g. Steinberg, 1987). With increasing age, the pattern changes and the adolescent begins to reflect on personal actions, etc., in the same way as the parent. How this change comes about is not clear. It may be stimulated, in part, by reference back on the part of the parents to previous interaction sequences. In doing this, the parent may describe something of his/her own reasoning processes, or allude to aspects of a sequence which the adolescent should have taken into account. Such referral to the potential elements of an interaction may stimulate the adolescent to engage in more extensive reflection on his/her part in a new sequence. Once such reflection has begun to take place, however, it seems likely that this, as with A1, forms the basis for change in how future events are processed and acted upon and that this process does not remain restricted to interactions involving one person.

In this section attention has focused on a single interaction sequence involving two people—a parent and an adolescent. It is evident that the vast majority of such sequences occur within a much more extended pattern of interaction than has been examined here. Such a pattern might be described as consisting of a series of linked interaction sequences in which the action C5 can be regarded as the starting point for a new sequence and in which the evaluation (C6) contributes to the further processing at C3. Such sequences and the internal processing, responses and evaluations they entail lead gradually to new forms of accommodation to each other which involve changed conceptions and expectations.

RELATIONSHIPS WITH PEERS—SAME SEX

The parent/adolescent relationship is of great importance in adolescence, but it is also a relationship of a highly specific nature. The two parties differ in age, knowledge, experience and in the nature of their responsibility for each other. In most cases, the relationship has a history which extends back into the childhood years. This offers both parties the advantage of having experience of each other's varied characteristics in a wide range of different interactional contexts. What the other thinks and expects is forecastable and most expectations probably tend to be confirmed. On the other hand, the one's ideas about the other may be somewhat inflexible, so that adoption of a new perspective (concerning the other) may be difficult. This may be particularly true of the early adolescent period, when various pressures towards change occur, but concurrence about the extent and speed with which change should be embraced might be difficult to achieve.

The asynchronous nature of the relationship (Damon, 1983) may mean that change during this period is more difficult for the parent, since he/she is put under pressure to modify ideas concerning a son or daughter, while the reverse is less true. The adolescent is also under pressure to change, of course, but the pressure to do so comes from his/her increasing awareness of personal resources, the example of age-mates and the attractions of the world outside the home. While the parent's experience of the wider world is juxtaposed with perceptions of a young person who remains something of a child, the relatively restricted nature of the adolescent's view and experience may encourage over-simplification of the potential problems and excessive optimism about personal capacities to work everything out. In this context, the parent may be perceived as a source of constraint, but for most adolescents, this perception is likely to represent little more than a continuation of earlier perceptions.

Relationships with peers present a very different situation. Age-levels are similar and each member of a dyad is on a roughly equal footing with the other. Even where the relationship extends back into childhood, areas of common experience are more restricted and features such as authority and responsibility are largely absent. As a result, knowledge of the other is more limited and this means that expectations are less likely consistently to be confirmed. In early adolescence, in particular, young people's levels of both social insight and understanding are likely to be limited and also their capacity to deal effectively with awkward social situations. This increases the likelihood of communication difficulties and misunderstanding so that "falling in and out of relationships" (Erikson, 1968) is more likely to occur. The more short term the relationship, the greater the lack of knowledge of the other and the greater the uncertainty as to how he/she will act in new circumstances. As a result, it might be anticipated that relatively new relationships in early adolescence will be less durable than relationships which extend back into the childhood years.

Let us consider these broad differences in the context of an interaction sequence. The basic components of a sequence with two same-sex peers are the same as those in a parent/adolescent interaction (Figure 2.1). As indicated earlier, however, potential limitations in social cognitive development, in shared social experiences and in social skills, create more room for misunderstanding and inappropriate response within the sequence.

Since these limitations hold for both parties in the interaction, almost all of the components (C2–C6) may, in some measure, be adversely affected. Note that this is less true of parent/adolescent interaction, where the parent's more developed social cognitive functioning and social skills and more extensive shared experience mean that misunderstandings, misperceptions, etc., are more likely to be confined to C4 and C5.

The basic similarity in the underlying processes means that it is unnecessary to work through the different components of an interaction sequence involving two adolescents in the same detail as in the previous section. Instead, attention will be confined to specific parts of the information processing activities involved.

Suppose that the initial event (C1) consists of A1 noticing an advertisement for a disco. As with the parent/adolescent interaction, the following component (C2) in the sequence involves processes in which cognitions, affects, values and situational factors may all feature in some measure. Figure 2.4 illustrates how part of this processing may proceed.

Let us assume that the start of the flow-chart in Figure 2.4 is A1's idea that a disco is something for young people. This thought leads on to a reference to personal experience. Where social cognitive development is not far advanced, processing is likely to be at a shallow level. In the absence of previous experience, this might take the form of a statement such as, "I wouldn't go to that." It might lead to a straightforward information-seeking question "Do you know what they're like?". Alternatively, an utterance such as "Fancy going to that!" might be used.

Where A1 has already attended a disco, reference back may lead to a positive or negative reaction. In the case of the former, it might take the form of "That's great, let's go!"; with the latter, "I wouldn't go to that" or "Who'd want to go to that!".

Responses such as these can be seen as shallow in that they take little account of the possible position of the other participant in the interaction. The negative reactions expressed by A1 indicate either no interest in what A2 thinks, or an assumption that A2's thinking on the matter will be the same. No attempt is made to consider A2's position and whether it might be different from that of A1. The same is true of the positive reaction. A1 is caught up by his positive feelings and A2 is simply expected to tag along.

The question, "Do you know what they're like?" can be regarded slightly differently. On the one hand, it might stem from idle curiosity. A1 has never been to a disco, wonders if A2 has and, if so, what he thought of it. On the other hand, it may have a different purpose. It may be a means of opening

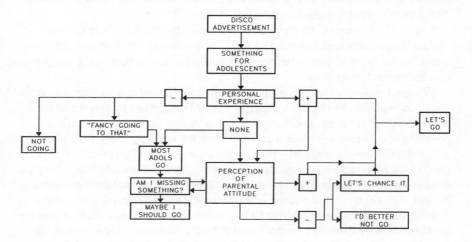

FIG. 2.4. Flow-chart illustrating the information processing in which a young person might engage in response to a disco advertisement.

up a topic which A1 would like to explore in more detail. No personal position is expressed, but depending on how A2 responds, it may be possible to introduce questions concerning issues such as the possibility of attending. The presence of such motives can be taken to indicate that A1's level of social functioning goes deeper than in the other examples. Identifying their presence can only occur as succeeding interaction sequences take place.

The exclamation "Fancy going to that!" raises another type of issue. With only slight changes of tone and stress it might be taken to be a question rather than an exclamation. The difference in interpretation could make a crucial difference to the further development of the sequence and to the part it plays in a broader social episode. Factors such as the quality of A1's communication, A2's knowledge of A1's probable position on discos and A2's enthusiasm, or otherwise, for discos could play a significant part in deciding whether misinterpretation occurs or not.

Figure 2.4 shows that processing may move beyond the shallow level associated with inadequate social cognitive development (or with insufficient interest or attention). Progress through the flow-chart leads into issues and questions associated with processes which are not qualitatively different from those involved at C2 in Figure 2.2. Here, as previously, A1 is engaged in trying to assess or anticipate other people's ideas and feelings, to weigh these against personal goals and assumptions, to take account of the immediate situation or the wider social context. The extent to which this occurs and how effective it is will depend on A1's level of development, as well as attentional, motivational and similar factors. The figure provides some illustration of this.

Take, for example, the positive response to previous experience. In Figure 2.4, movement beyond the shallow level may involve two separate considerations: deciding whether A2 should be asked to go and weighing up the parental position.

Where the former is concerned, issues considered might include: A2's possible reaction to the idea; his/her possible reaction to the disco itself; his/her suitability as a companion to a disco; comparison with other possible companions; consideration of how A2 might get on with some or all of these others; etc. Note that some of these considerations might be guided by relatively inadequate or inappropriate information. A2 may be a class-mate with whom contact is restricted to school situations. Knowledge that A2 has a keen interest in sport may lead A1 to assume a similar attitude towards discos. Other possible companions may be known within a totally different context and A1 may have no experience of them in a disco-like situation. Considerations more closely related to adolescence may also play a role. In the context of going to a disco, level of physical maturity may be an important plus point, or the opposite. Liking for a particular style of clothing may have similar positive or negative effects. The same may be true for A2's membership of a particular religious or racial group.

With all such issues, A1's actual knowledge or experience of A2's actual position may be extremely limited. In general the shorter the duration of the relationship, or the more limited the context in which it has developed, the greater the likelihood that perceptions will be mistaken. The possibility of misperception is still greater in circumstances where A1's level of social cognitive development is comparatively low. Perhaps it is for this reason that many of the relationships of early adolescence tend to be based on cliques (Dunphy, 1963). Associating with the clique may help to avoid many of the situations in which potentially damaging social errors can occur. At the same time, it provides the opportunity for acquiring better knowledge of other members through joint association and mutual observation. Such knowledge may lead to more informed choices with regard to specific activities and may ultimately serve as the basis for the development of more long-lasting friendship choices.

Weighing up the parental position about going to a disco raises quite different ideas. These may include: what the parents think about discos; what they think about A1 going to one; what they think of A1 as an adolescent; what are the risks involved in going without telling them; what would be their likely reactions if they should find out. Questions such as these relate in turn to personal wishes, to ideas about self and how self should be presented, or is perceived and to ideas about personal (adolescent) rights as opposed to parental rights. The latter might also be strongly influenced by how A2 is perceived, A2's importance as a friend, what is known about A2's relationship with his/her parents and the implications of revealing personal anxieties about the parental position.

These two examples illustrate the complexity of the inner processing which may be involved as an interaction sequence, based on a situation which is fairly typical of adolescence, starts to unfold. As with the equivalent component of the parent/adolescent sequence, cognitions, affects, values and situational factors are all potentially involved. The nature of these is influenced by features which spring directly from the characteristics of adolescence and the level of adolescent development the individual has attained.

The remaining components of the adolescent/adolescent interaction sequence do not need further detailed discussion. The developmental correspondence between the two participants means that the previous remarks apply to the way in which A2 processes the action (C3) carried out by A1. Similarly, the characteristics of the two action components (C3 and C5) and the evaluation component (C6) are the same as those which feature in the equivalent components of the parent/adolescent sequence except, of course, that both participants are adolescents.

RELATIONSHIPS WITH PEERS—
OPPOSITE SEX

In the preceding two sections, attention has focused on the various factors which are involved in two different types of interaction sequence. One factor, sex, was not considered with regard to either, though clearly it is potentially of great importance. The sex of both the parent and the adolescent is likely to influence the part which each plays in an interaction sequence. Both parents may respond to the entry of a daughter putting on an anorak with the "Be in at ..." instruction, for example, while only mother may react in this way with a son. Similarly, in a peer/peer interaction, it can be anticipated that the sex of the two participants will play an important part in defining what takes place. In the case of the advertisement for the disco, for example, the processes involved in the interaction as well as the final outcome might vary considerably depending on whether two boys or two girls were involved. Such variation could stem from a variety of factors including: different socialisation experiences; different levels of parental control over social activities; maturity level; perceptions of opposite-sex peers; ideas about discos; etc.

Factors such as these are of particular significance in an interaction sequence involving a boy and a girl. The basic components remain the same (see Figure 2.1) and, as was the case with the other two types of interaction sequence, variations in adolescent social cognitive development may influence the nature of the information processing components (C2 and/or C4). However, the fact that there is a sex difference introduces an additional dimension which is likely to play a part in all of the component parts of the sequence. Figure 2.5 illustrates the role of sex-related cognitions at C2 and C4. It also illustrates possible variation in the salience of these cognitions. As previously pointed out, the special place given to sex-related cognitions is not intended to imply that such cognitions do not occur in other types of interaction sequence. They may feature—even very prominently—in parent/adolescent or peer/peer interactions. Consider, for example, a situation where a parent interprets an adolescent's behaviour as sexually inappropriate, or more extremely, where an action, by parent or adolescent, is sexually provocative. The prominence given to sex-related cognitions in Figure 2.5 emphasises the fact that within a cross-sex sequence, cognitions relating to sex are always likely to have some influence.

A boy/girl interaction sequence resembles the parent/adolescent sequence, in that there is always a basic difference between the two participants. This difference is rooted in the contrasting socialisation histories which the two have experienced throughout their childhood years and into adolescence. Each young person enters adolescence with an

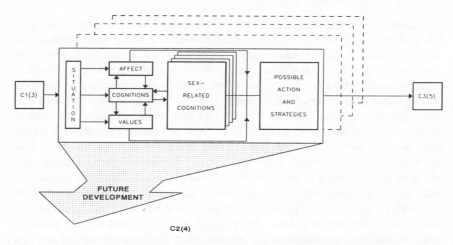

FIG. 2.5. Sex-related cognitions in the context of a social interaction sequence.

individual socialisation history, of course, so that even in a same-sex relationship, socialisation differences will have some effect. Where opposite sexes are concerned, this effect will generally be more significant and probably also more marked. The young person will have grown up learning to think of himself/herself in a particular way and to think of the opposite sex differently. Part of this difference will go back to parental ideas about maleness or femaleness and how these have influenced the child-rearing process. Part will stem from the pressures, expectations and examples offered by the wider environment. The physical changes associated with early adolescence serve further to consolidate perception of self in terms of having a particular sexual identity. This identity is associated, in turn, with a network of ideas, assumptions and stereotypes concerning characteristics of members of the same sex and those of the other.

Each of the participants in a cross-sex interaction sequence brings at least some elements of this socialisation background, sexual identity and network of ideas into the interaction. However, the salience of these sex-related aspects varies greatly from sequence to sequence. Take a classroom context where two young people are regularly engaged together in class tasks, for instance. Here the difference in sex between them may play a relatively insignificant role. The situation is familiar and highly structured. Each may see the other primarily as the possessor of specific skills or knowledge which is relevant to the task in hand. Sex-related aspects in this case may be restricted to the way the task is approached, to how one talks or responds to the other, or to the extent to which physical contact occurs.

Imagine a slight change of situation. The task in which they are engaged requires them to visit another part of the school. They walk along the corridor and A1 notices the advertisement for the disco. Whatever the processes which occur at C2, we can assume that the fact that A2 is of a different sex is likely to be more salient than in the familiar, structured setting of the class-room. The dismissive "I wouldn't go to that" or even the interrogative "Do you know what they're like?" seem less likely in such a situation. Perhaps a more neutral form "Are you going to that?" might be used, or even the more direct "Do you like discos?". The essential point is not what is actually said, but the likelihood that certain formulations will be replaced by others of a different content and tone. The change can be attributed to a complex of ideas associated with the nature of discos, knowledge that boys and girls may see them in different ways, uncertainty about A2's perspective, anxiety to avoid revealing too much of one's personal feelings, attitudes or experience, etc. Whatever the sex of A1, the nature of these ideas will be rooted in the nature and range of his/her experience of peers of the opposite sex. As with adolescent processing in other types of interaction sequence, the complexity of the ideas will be dependent on A1's level of social cognitive development.

Where sex-related cognitions are highly salient, affects, values and situational factors may all be strongly involved in a sequence. Strong attraction to A2 may lead to a considerable increase in affect, thereby limiting the range of action strategies available and influencing the content of what occurs at C3 and the manner in which it is presented. Values may also be involved and at a variety of levels. Particular ideas about appropriate or inappropriate sexual behaviour may be taken over from parents. The young person may become aware of considerable variance between peer group norms and parental ideas. Knowledge, however accurate, of diseases such as AIDS may influence the perception of and response to certain types of situation. Attributions about the (sexual) values of another may be made on the basis of his/her friendships or participation in activities such as attending discos or drinking alcohol. As with affect, reference to value systems and to the implicit or explicit ideas sustaining them, may serve to channel the processing and decision-making component and modify the behaviour response in a particular way.

As with other types of interaction sequence, situational factors may also influence the nature of the cognitive processes in a cross-sex interaction sequence. The presence of others or the physical situation itself may inhibit or encourage particular ideas. The presence of a friend, for example, might lead to inaction on the part of A1, or to a rather vague, indecisive overture to A2, or to even to ribald types of behaviour. In such situations, the patterns of discussion and behaviour relative to the opposite sex within one's same-sex peer group might place the individual under pressure to act in a certain way. This broader context may also be important at another level. For many young people, particularly those in early adolescence, personal sexual proprieties are ill-defined. Little parental guidance on such matters may be given, so that what is culled from the wider youth context may serve as the main guide for the young person's initial explorations.

Variation in the salience of sex-related cognitions between A1 and A2 appears likely to increase the possibility of misunderstanding between the two. On occasions this may lead to serious misunderstanding or even to a dangerous situation. The young girl at the disco may respond positively to the young lad's suggestion that he see her home, because it offers safety, companionship and perhaps a goodnight kiss or two. The lad may make specific assumptions about young girls who go to discos, see her agreement as indicating a willingness to go out with him on other occasions, or as being prepared to have sex with him. Each individual's reaction as the divergent assumptions become evident may lead to situations in which bitterness, anger or even aggression emerge.

The varied cognitive processes (at C2 and C4) lead to a decision concerning what should be done at C3 (C5). The nature of this decision will depend on the range of possible actions and action strategies available to the participant concerned. As indicated earlier, affects, values or situational factors may reduce of possibilities open to the individual in a specific interaction sequence.

The following component (C3 or C5) might also be influenced by the fact that the interaction is between the sexes. This may be true not only of the form of utterance used, but also the way in which it is said. A1 may find it difficult to talk freely to A2 outside the well-known, structured context of the classroom. The resulting hesitancy or awkwardness might contrast starkly with the freedom and spontaneity of speech with which a same-sex friend would be addressed in similar circumstances. On the other hand, considerable experience of members of the opposite sex in a variety of situations—e.g. the presence of brothers/sisters at home—might lead to an easy, bantering approach.

As with the other types of interaction, the manner in which C3 is carried out, together with its content informs the processing activities which result at C4. Here too, sexual factors may vary in salience. In the classroom context, what A1 intends as a deprecatory remark about the task, might be interpreted by A2 as a statement about him/her. A disco remark might be seen as emphasising A1's ignorance, or maturity, or flirtatiousness relative to others of the opposite sex. Such reactions might serve to trigger a range of thoughts, emotions and value judgements concerning issues such as, why A1 had made the utterance, what lay behind it and what it suggests about how A2 is perceived.

SOCIAL INTERACTION SEQUENCES:
A RESEARCH PERSPECTIVE

The interaction sequences discussed earlier refer to three situations which are fairly typical of adolescence. It is clear that a variety of other types of interaction can also feature prominently during the adolescent period: examples include, interactions with siblings, with a step-parent, with members of other cultural groups or with authority figures. Interactions may also be bedded in group situations involving more than two people. In all such additional interaction sequences, certain cognitions may occupy a more salient position than in the examples given here. In general, however, it is safe to assume that the basic characteristics of the sequence will remain the same.

Analysing social interactions in adolescence in this way has important implications for research and applied work with adolescents. The basic framework of the interaction sequence emphasises the role played by the information processing systems of both of the parties involved. It indicates that even though the two parties are interacting with each other, individual differences at the processing level may lead to quite different interpretations of what is taking place (cf. Belsky, Lerner & Spanier, 1984). The more this is so, the greater the likelihood that each participant will evaluate the sequence in a different way from the other and this, in turn, may influence the way in which subsequent interaction sequences are approached and interpreted. The tendency for most conflict between parents and adolescents to occur between early and mid-adolescence (e.g. Hill et al, 1985; Steinberg, 1981) may be partially explained by such misinterpretation. The ideas about the young adolescent which are most readily accessible to the parent are dominated by notions developed in the childhood years. The adolescent, on the other hand, is entering an expanding world of experience in which ideas may vary greatly in their availability and salience. Such circumstances seem likely to increase the chances of misunderstanding and misinterpretation. As progress through adolescence takes place, parents accommodate to the changed circumstances of son or daughter and the latter become more focused and settled in their interests and ideas. This leads to a reduction in the number of conflicts from mid-adolescence onwards.

While this may be a plausible explanation for conflict in early adolescence, it requires empirical verification. Attempts to do this need to be able to explain other findings which indicate that relationships between adolescent girls and their mothers involve considerable conflict up to and even slightly beyond the point at which the daughter leaves home (Honess & Lintern, 1990). The apparent contradiction between the two sets of findings emphasises the need to adopt a research approach which takes account of possible differences between cultures, between social groups and between the sexes in the way in which adolescence is experienced.

One of the important aspects of the processing component is the reference back to previous experience and to previous socialisation history. A feature of the adolescent phase is that the young person is liable to encounter situations which fall outside his/her personal experience, i.e. situations where it is not possible to refer back. The result is that capacity to respond or to cope effectively is diminished. In such circumstances, ideas advanced by another adolescent, assumptions about what most adolescents do, or particular situational factors may exert a disproportionate influence on behaviour. For some young people, this may lead to early involvement in risk-taking behaviours involving alcohol, drugs, sexual behaviour, or delinquent acts. It may be that young people who mature early are at greater risk in this respect since the extent of their experience may not match their level of physical development (Stattin & Magnusson, 1990; Silbereisen & Kracke, Chapt. 4). This is not to argue that lack of experience is the sole explanation for such patterns of behaviour. Factors such as modelling processes, the shaping effects of the wider environment or specific stressors may also play a role. All of these, however, are likely to involve some degree of reference back to individual socialisation experience.

A further important feature of the processing system is that certain cognitions may be more salient in one type of interaction sequence than in another. In the previous section, for example, sex-related cognitions played a salient part in cross-sex sequences in that they influenced other aspects of the information processing and decision-making system. As a result, thinking and action emerged as showing a different pattern from that typical of same-sex relations. Salience refers to a situation where a particular idea or construct has special prominence in an individual's thinking (Higgins & King, 1981; Markus & Sentis, 1982). This does not mean that it necessarily features in all interactions. Whether it is triggered or not depends on the nature of the situation itself or the actions of the other participant or on additional (chance) factors. The more salient a construct, the more accessible it is likely to be and therefore, the more likely to be frequently employed. A self-related construct such as being overweight, for example, may mean that in interactions with others particular attention is focused upon their slimness or fatness. Similarly, anothers' behaviour towards oneself may be interpreted as a response to one's physical characteristics. To date, little attention has been directed towards the implications of highly salient stored constructs. During a period such as adolescence, when new and significant experiences follow each other in rapid succession, one might anticipate that the study of the influence of prominent and accessible constructs on social behaviour could prove to be a particularly fruitful area of study.

The framework makes a clear distinction between processing and action. This distinction seems to be of particular importance in adolescence since each of these activities may be influenced by developmental factors. Level of social cognitive development may mean that processing occurs at a superficial level, though the action which follows may be carried out in a socially skilful manner. Similarly, deficient social skills need not indicate inadequate processing.

Research and applied programmes have tended to focus primarily on action and little attention has been given to the processing component. Where social skills are deficient, intervention has generally been approached within a social learning paradigm in which emphasis is placed on describing what (or what not) to do in specific social situations and using modelling and role-play techniques to develop the necessary skills (e.g. Goldstein, 1981). Reference to the different components of the social interaction sequence suggests that this approach is too limited and that account needs to be taken of the processing as well as the action components of social behaviour.

In contrast, research on coping behaviour and social competence has emphasised the relationship between the two components. Primary and secondary appraisal (Lazarus & Folkman, 1984; Seiffge-Krenke & Shulman, Chapt. 8) are seen as important aspects of the coping process and various authors have described social competence in terms of a combination of cognitive, affective and behavioural activities (e.g. Dodge, 1986; Ford, 1985; Waters & Sroufe, 1983). Despite their acknowledgement of the role played by such processing, both approaches could benefit from clearer articulation of the development of information processing capacities as adolescence proceeds. Currently, we know little of the establishment and functioning of information processing in circumstances where rapid changes in knowledge, experience and exploration are taking place. In situations where experience is limited, for example, the adolescent may fall back on scripts which are inappropriate or inadequate. Behaviour which is apparently regressive may be thought of in these terms. Similarly, a phenomenon such as foreclosure (Marcia, 1980) may occur in circumstances where self-related constructs are well established and constructs relating to the broader social environment remain restricted to a limited number of global and ill-developed ideas.

Possibilities such as these will be clarified by a research approach which focuses upon how information relating to self and other is acquired and processed during the adolescent years. Consideration of the social interaction sequence described in this chapter suggests that this approach needs to take account of the role played by other important participants in this process. In the context of parent/adolescent relationships, attention might be directed, for example, to the ways in which parent and adolescent construe adolescence and the parental role relative to an adolescent son or daughter, or to how changes in perceptions of others occur as a significant new relationship establishes itself.

Beyond this, it needs to be approached within a longitudinal perspective which attempts to map ways in which information processing develops and changes as significant new life events take place. We know little of the processes which lead the young person to define him/herself as unable to compete with others in certain activities, or as being incompetent in a particular activity, or as belonging to a particular sub-group, or as being a reject. Such knowledge as we have, needs to be complemented by a more analytical approach which examines the individual within the social context and explores how change and/or consolidation of particular ways of processing ideas relating to self, significant others and the broader environment takes place. The social interaction sequence provides a model of a potential approach to this endeavour.

The approach to social cognition presented in this chapter is not particularly new. In some respects in might be seen as referring back to Mead's "conversation of gestures" (Mead, 1934). Much more elaborate models of social information processing have also been developed which take more satisfactory account of memory processes (Hastie & Carlston, 1980) and information processing (Wyer & Srull, 1980). What is new is the attempt to approach social activity in adolescence from a viewpoint which takes explicit account of the processing activities in which the young person is engaged. Approaching social activity in this way, offers new possibilities for developing knowledge of how social thinking develops over the adolescent years. It suggests the need to combine the broad band approaches which have characterised the bulk of recent research on adolescence with a more detailed, fine-grain research strategy where more attention is given to the way in which individuals process familiar and novel aspects of their experience. It provides a framework which may serve as a basis for further research into some of the contradictory and anomalous features of social development during the adolescent years. In doing so, it offers further possibilities for extending our understanding of how adolescents develop into new social worlds.

NOTE

1. This example is based on an article entitled "Against their will" published in the *Guardian*, 23.7.91.

CHAPTER THREE

Assessing Parent-adolescent Relationships: A Review of Current Research Issues and Methods

Terry Honess and Margaret Robinson

Researchers studying adolescent development within the context of the family share the basic premise that development is influenced by the quality of the parent–adolescent relationship. However, researchers have been influenced by a variety of theoretical perspectives including family systems theory, family therapy, psychoanalytic theory and cognitive developmental theory (Anderson & Fleming, 1986; Cooper, 1987; Sabatelli & Mazor, 1985) and they have used numerous assessment techniques in their research. Together, these factors have led to a degree of conceptual confusion (Cooper, 1987; Galligan, 1989; Grotevant, 1989) and data which is difficult if not impossible to compare and accumulate across studies (Powers, 1989). Moreover, it is increasingly argued that a unified theory is necessary (Cooper, 1987; Galligan, 1989; Grotevant, 1989; Powers, 1989).

In spite of these problems, this decade has seen an emerging consensus in recognising that it is necessary to go beyond "unilateral" concepts such as parental warmth or restrictiveness to more reciprocal "relational" constructs (see Maccoby & Martin, 1983 and the series of research contributions in the work edited by Grotevant & Cooper, 1983). For example, Bell and Bell (1983) talk of a "paradigm shift that conceptualises individual behaviour as constrained by and nested in ongoing systems of relationships of which the family is the primary representative". Indeed some authors (e.g. Oliveri & Reiss, 1981) see adolescent behaviour as an inseparable part of family functioning so they focus on "family paradigms" and see the family as the basic unit of analysis.

A common feature of such work, suggest Grotevant & Cooper (1985), is the analysis of adolescent identity construction through the "renegotiation" of adolescent-parent relationships, rather than the more common concern with parenting styles that would facilitate adolescent "autonomy", i.e. a disengagement from parents. Youniss (1983) takes a similar line in arguing "the notion that there is a developmental course to the parent-adolescent relation is not widespread". Nevertheless, within the emerging body of research that takes such a perspective, different assumptions and practices are clearly evident.

The task of this chapter is to set out similarities and differences in both theoretical assumptions and research methods, and to suggest a framework for helping carry forward the study of parent-adolescent relationships. This will be done by:

1) Providing a review of the work of a representative selection of key researchers, namely: Grotevant and Cooper, Hauser and Powers, and Adams and his associates. These researchers have been selected because their research has consistently and systematically added to the core of empirical findings and has influenced the work of other researchers. Moreover, their work illustrates the range of theoretical, conceptual and methodological influences evident in this area.

2) Developing the review of the three selected research teams by discussing related research techniques and empirical findings to assess the degree of consensus in such research and the limitations which are placed on this by the differing theoretical and methodological approaches used.

3) Providing a framework for comparing the best known or the most promising of the different methods, and identifying possible directions for further methodological and theoretical refinement and development.

SELECTIVE REVIEW OF REPRESENTATIVE RESEARCH WORK
Grotevant and Cooper

Overview of Methods.   Grotevant and Cooper have been influenced by family systems theory and family therapy. They have studied the family system's effect on adolescent psychosocial development—specifically identity development (measured by the Ego Identity Interview, Marcia, 1966) and role taking ability (measured by the Role Taking Task, Feffer, 1959a). The family system is assessed through encoding family communications (Condon, Cooper & Grotevant, 1984; Cooper, Grotevant & Condon, 1982) which are stimulated through family discussion of plans for an imaginary two week family holiday; this is called the Family Interaction Task. When coded, each dyadic relationship (i.e. adolescent and mother, adolescent and father, mother and father) is measured across two relationship dimensions: "individuality" and "connectedness". The authors have proposed that a balance between these dimensions is the optimal context for psychosocial development, and a dyadic relationship which exhibits this balance is called an "individuated" relationship.

Conceptual Model. The conceptual model of "individuality" and "connectedness" has been supported by factor analysis of data on frequency of various interpersonal communication behaviours (Grotevant & Cooper, 1986). Four factors were extracted which corresponded to the four properties of the model namely: self-assertion, separateness, permeability and mutuality. Self-assertion and separateness behaviours are associated with the concept of individuality, and permeability and mutuality with connectedness. Self-assertion involves being aware of one's own point of view and of taking the responsibility for communicating it clearly to others; it is demonstrated through the ability to make direct suggestions. Separateness is related to the ability to express differences between oneself and others; it is demonstrated through statements of personal difference, direct or indirect disagreements, requests for action and making irrelevant comments. Permeability is associated with openness and responsiveness to the views of others and is demonstrated through agreements, requests for information, complying with requests, making relevant comments and acknowledging others. Mutuality consists of behaviours which indicate sensitivity and respect for the views of others. This includes making indirect suggestions, initiating compromise, responding to requests for information and reporting the feelings of others.

From the family systems perspective, individuality is important to adolescent development because it relates to making decisions and commitments (self-assertion) and the demonstration of one's individual personality (separateness); connectedness is important because it fosters openness to others and to novel stimuli (permeability) on which personal development can be modelled in a supportive and encouraging environment (mutuality). Further, the adolescent's experience of individuality and connectedness within the context of family is held to affect their development outside the family and to influence interactions with non-family members including peers (Cooper & Ayers-Lopez, 1985).

Empirical Findings. Empirical evidence has shown the concepts of "individuality" and "connectedness" in family interactions to be adaptive for adolescent development (Cooper, Grotevant & Condon, 1983; Grotevant & Cooper, 1985). In general, adolescents' expressions of both permeability and separateness were found to be positively associated with identity exploration and role taking. Findings have indicated that different interaction patterns in dyadic interactions were associated with these two psychosocial variables.

For example, different adolescent-father interactions were associated with high identity exploration for sons and for daughters: sons with high scores on identity exploration were more likely to express direct suggestions (indicative of self-assertion) and separateness with their fathers; fathers reciprocated with expressions of mutuality and a low frequency of expressions of separateness. In contrast, high identity exploration daughters made indirect suggestions (indicative of mutuality) while fathers showed a high frequency of relevant comments (indicative of permeability) and low frequency of indirect suggestions. In mother-daughter dyads identity exploration was negatively correlated with mothers' expressions of mutuality. High scoring identity exploration daughters expressed high frequencies of indirect and low frequency of direct suggestions (indicative of self-assertion) while their mothers were more likely to make direct than indirect suggestions. In the father-mother dyad fathers' expressions of high separateness and low mutuality to their wives were associated with high levels of identity exploration in daughters; mothers who expressed mutuality to their husbands were associated also with high levels of daughter identity exploration. Such findings indicate that the family interactions and adolescent intra-psychic development are complexly interrelated.

Summary.   The Grotevant and Cooper model, which operationalises various family systems theory concepts, has been empirically supported; empirical evidence has been found too for their proposition that individuality and connectedness in family interactions provide an adaptive context for adolescent development (Grotevant, 1983). Further, since it has been suggested (Grotevant & Cooper, 1985) that connectedness and individuality may also be indicators of adult intra-psychic development, this model must be considered of potential value for both contemporary adolescent and life-span developmental research.

Hauser and Powers

Overview of Methods.   Hauser and Powers have adopted a structural-developmental perspective and have proposed that adolescents require a cognitively stimulating physical and social (family) environment to promote ego development. They assess ego development using the Sentence Completion Test (Loevinger & Wessler, 1970), and the family context through encoding family communications. Family communication is stimulated by a "revealed differences" task (Strodbeck, 1951) where the family discuss issues on which they disagree with the aim of reaching a family consensus. The communication is coded using a technique specifically developed for this research (Hauser, Powers, Jacobson & Noam, 1986) and the stimulus material for discussion uses Kohlberg's moral dilemmas (Colby, Kohlberg, Candee, Gibbs, Hewer, Kaufman, Power & Speicher-Dubin, 1986).

Conceptual Model. Hauser and Powers examine the influence of four types of family behaviour on ego development: cognitively stimulating behaviours, cognitively inhibiting behaviours, affective support and affective conflict. Cognitively stimulating behaviours and affective support are termed enabling behaviours and include explaining, focusing, problem solving, curiosity, acceptance and empathy; it is proposed that enabling behaviours provide an emotionally supportive, challenging and stimulating environment through which adolescents can actively develop their ego. Cognitively inhibiting behaviours and affective conflict are termed constraining behaviours and include distracting, withholding, indifference, being judgmental, emotional excess and devaluing; it is proposed that constraining behaviours are not conducive to ego development.

Empirical Findings. Hauser and Powers (Powers, Hauser, Schwartz, Noam & Jacobson, 1983) found empirical evidence for their proposal that family interaction patterns were valuable predictors of adolescent ego development. For example: parents' cognitively stimulating behaviours and support were both positively associated with adolescent ego development while families which demonstrated a high degree of cognitively inhibiting behaviours and high affective conflict had adolescents with low levels of ego development. Adolescents at higher levels of ego development themselves engage in more cognitively enabling interaction (such as problem solving and curiosity), while those at a lower level of ego development behaved in a more constrained manner (e.g. devaluing, emotional excess and withholding).

It was noted also that mothers with higher levels of ego development contributed more frequently to family discussion and that fathers' contribution to discussion was negatively correlated with mothers' ego level. A study focusing on family verbal interactions (Hauser, Book, Houlihan, Powers, Weiss-Perry, Follansbee, Jacobson & Noam, 1987) showed that girls and boys spoke more to their fathers expressing problem-solving and accepting behaviours, while fathers expressed cognitively enabling behaviours: the observation was made that this may be a reciprocal pattern of interactive behaviour. It was found that mothers expressed more distracting (i.e. constraining) behaviours while both parents were more devaluing (a constraining behaviour) to sons than to daughters. The associations between mothers' ego development, fathers' and mothers' frequency and style of contributions to discussion, adolescent gender and adolescent ego development have not been fully unravelled, but, as Hauser, Powers and colleagues have demonstrated (Hauser et al., 1987; Leaper, Hauser, Kremen, Powers, Jacobson, Noam, Weiss-Perry & Follansbee, 1989), the links between family patterns of interaction, gender and ego development, although not straightforward, are clearly demonstrable.

Summary. Hauser and Powers have focused on enabling and constraining behaviours in family interactions and the influence of these on adolescent ego development. Their research has shown these concepts to be identifiable and to be associated with different level of adolescent ego development. Given this, these concepts should be considered of potential use in investigating adolescent intra-psychic development within the context of the family.

Adams and Associates

Overview of Methods. Adams and associates are engaged in a longitudinal project with threefold aims: the empirical study of adolescent intra-individual ego identity development and the contribution of family to this; the interpretation and empirical testing of Erikson's psychosocial theory from which the research stems; and the development of the Extended Objective Measure of Ego Identity Status (EOMEIS), a self-report technique which operationalises Eriksonian theory and Marcia's (1966) Ego Identity Status Interview. The EOMEIS (Adams, Bennion & Huh, 1987) assesses exploration and commitment to issues pertinent to adolescence (e.g. occupation, friendship) and through it adolescents are assigned to one of four ego identity statuses: achieved, moratorium, foreclosure or diffusion. Of these statuses, achieved is the most mature outcome, followed by moratorium, then by foreclosure and lastly by diffusion as the least mature outcome.

Conceptual Model. Adams, Montemayor, Dyk, & Lee (1991) have further interpreted Erikson's writings; they contend that he implied social equivalents for the psychological differentiation and integration which underpins ego identity development. Social differentiation and social integration are held to influence the adolescent's psychological differentiation and integration and, in this way, social differentiation and social integration are taken to affect ego identity development. This proposition echoes the general working assumptions made by Bell and Bell, Grotevant and Cooper, and Hauser and Powers that social (i.e. family) contexts facilitate or inhibit intra-psychic development.

Adams and colleagues have constructed a model which combines the Hauser and Powers' notion of enabling and constraining behaviours influencing development and the Grotevant and Powers' view that quality of relationship (i.e. degree of connectedness and individuality) influences development. The resulting "Family Interaction Model" can be seen as an attempt to address explicitly how family behaviour influences the family relationship which in turn affects adolescent psychological development. This model is discussed following the review of their empirical work.

Empirical Findings.   In a three year longitudinal study, Adams and Fitch (1982) identified three developmental trajectories: progression which was an advance in ego identity formation; regression which was the opposite of progression; and stability where no change in ego identity status is recorded. Findings indicated that ego identity formation was associated with psychological differentiation defined by Adams et al. (1991, p. 27) as "... self-awareness of distinct and sometimes contradictory selves, recognition of possible selves and identification of multiple personal choice" and integration defined (op. cit.) as "... the selection of preferred distinct parts of self based on personal choice and the organisational self-selection into a meaningful and harmonious whole". Levels of psychological differentiation (assessed through locus of control) and integration (assessed through self-acceptance) were also predictive of different developmental trajectories: high levels of differentiation and integration predicated a progressive trajectory while low levels predicated a regressive trajectory. This empirical evidence was taken as support for the theoretical proposition that ego identity formation was "underpinned by increasing differentiation and integration" (Adams et al., 1991).

Evidence of a family contribution to ego identity development has also been sought: initial studies (Adams, 1985; Adams & Jones, 1983; Campbell, Adams & Dobson, 1984) indicated that parental relationships which exhibited rejection, withdrawal and control were associated with low level adolescent ego identity while high ego identity level was associated with parental warmth, support and the encouragement of the adolescent's move towards independence. A recent study (Adams et al., 1991) extended this line of research: the influence of family interaction patterns on intra-individual developmental trajectories was assessed. Findings indicated that family interaction patterns were strong predictors of development: progressive and stable ego identity trajectories were associated with more open family conflict and less family cohesion than the regressive trajectory. Also adolescents with a progressive trajectory had families who were less controlling than those adolescents with stable and regressive trajectories. (Note: "Conflict" was regarded as functional and not dysfunctional; it can be understood as open disagreement and discussion among family members rather than destructive conflict.)

Together these study findings led Adams and colleagues (1991) to conclude that regressive ego identity development was related to rejection, over-control and emotional withdrawal in the family context while progressive development was related to the open expression of conflict, a moderate level of cohesion and low parental control. Overall, findings lent empirical support to theory in demonstrating that a nurturing family environment was conducive to ego identity development.

The Family Interaction Model

In this model, developed by Adams and colleagues, connectedness is reconstrued as social integration in family interactions and individuality as social differentiation in family interactions. It is proposed that social differentiation and social integration are influenced by enabling or constraining family behaviours; in turn social differentiation and social integration affect the adolescent's psychological differentiation and integration which underpin ego identity formation. Table 3.1 depicts the Family Interaction Model giving definitions for the enabling and constraining behaviours.

Empirical Support. To date, the Family Interaction Model has been used in one three year longitudinal study (N = 49 families; adolescent age 15-16 years) examining family influence on intra-individual ego identity development; an alternative way of expressing this is that the study assessed social differentiation and social integration (through family influence) on psychological differentiation and integration (assessed by ego identity development).

The model's dimensions were assessed using both self-report techniques e.g. Parent-Adolescent Relationship Questionnaire (Sullivan & Sullivan, 1980); Family Adaptability and Cohesion Scale (Olson, Portner & Bell, 1984) and an interactive assessment technique which engaged the family in discussion. Adams and colleagues developed their own system for coding family discussion. Adolescent ego identity development was assessed using the Extended Objective Measure of Ego Identity Status (EOMEIS).

Findings indicated that: lack of social differentiation predicted regressive development while high social differentiation predicted progressive or stable development; families which showed high social integration impeded progressive development but facilitated regressive

TABLE 3.1

The Family Interaction Model

	Social Differentiation (Individuality)	Social Integration (Connectedness)
E N A B L I N G	**SELF-FOCUS** Clarifying uncertainty or confusion about other's point of view.	**PERMEABILITY** Acknowledgement which includes affirmation, openness to and union with speaker and compliance with a request for action.
	ACCEPTANCE Paraphrasing and giving positive feedback reflecting understanding, warmth or encouragement to continue speaking.	**MUTUALITY** Sensitivity and respect for other's view, constructive proposals to address and solve differences and initiation of positive solutions surrounding differences through mutually beneficial compromise.
C O N S T R A I N I N G	**DISTORTION** Inaccurate representation of another's view or incorrectly perceiving communication.	**NEGATIVE SEPARATENESS** Indicating speaker is unpleasant and distinctly separate from others.
	DISAGREEMENT Disagreeing, blocking off, challenging, stating objection.	**JUSTIFICATION** Creating defensiveness by demanding explanation and justification for an action.

development. Adams and associates concluded that the findings indicated that a "balance" between social differentiation and social integration in the family environment best facilitates progressive development.

Summary.   Adams and colleagues study adolescent intra-individual development from an Eriksonian perspective. They have gathered empirical support for this perspective. They have identified three developmental trajectories: progression, stability and regression, establishing that increased psychological differentiation and integration underpin progressive growth. They have found evidence for their proposal that these underpinnings of psychological development are affected, in their turn, by social differentiation and social integration. The Family Interaction Model illustrates how social differentiation and social integration are enabled and constrained by family behaviours. A recent study used this model to study how psychological differentiation and integration (as assessed by ego identity development) were influenced by their social equivalents. Findings indicated that regressive ego identity development was facilitated by a family which provides too little social differentiation and too much social integration while progressive ego identity development was facilitated by a family which gave some social differentiation and moderate amounts of social integration. This study also demonstrated the potential of the Family Interaction Model.

Overall, the Adams and associates' research can be viewed as a significant step forward in the study of adolescent social development. Their longitudinal studies have allowed them to assess the role of family on intra-individual development rather than examining how individual differences in development are associated with different family interaction patterns as was the case for Grotevant and Cooper, and Hauser and Powers.

GENERAL REVIEW AND DISCUSSION OF FINDINGS

In this section, the studies already cited are discussed along with other research in an attempt to identify consensus among researchers and the extent to which the various conceptual interpretations and methodological tools used limit or facilitate cohesion and progress.

Family Context and Adolescent Psychological Development

All of the studies reported give at least tentative support to the proposition that family context influences adolescent psychological development. Grotevant and Cooper, and Hauser and Powers examined individual differences in adolescent development and patterns of family interaction: in general they found consistently that adolescents at advanced levels of development experienced a warm, supportive family environment, but such evidence is insufficient to indicate that family context caused the observed developmental outcome. The studies of Adams and associates go further towards establishing a causal link, for in studying intra-individual development longitudinally they have found that an individual's future level of development can be predicted by style of family interaction. These studies add weight to the supposition that psychological development is influenced by family context, but the causal relationship still has not been established: the family's behaviour may foster the adolescent's development but so might the individual adolescent "cause" the family to behave in a particular manner; the intricacies of this interaction are undoubtedly complex and still await detailed examination.

In general, researchers are agreed that a warm, supportive context in which family members felt comfortable expressing and discussing their individuality, differences of opinion etc. is a facilitating context. It is feasible that this type of family context offers the adolescent the opportunity to observe, discuss and practise being "individual" in the secure knowledge that the family will be accepting and tolerant and not rejecting (Grotevant & Cooper, 1985).

The Role of Family in Wider Social Interactions

Researchers who comment on social interaction outside of the family tend to assume that the family's own interaction pattern affects interaction in other situations; but this is understood in different ways. Grotevant and Cooper (1985) have a "flexible" view of the family's role for they regard the family context as giving the adolescent the confidence and skill to extend the developmental experience beyond the family and into the forum of social relationships. In contrast, Bell and colleagues, and Reiss, Oliveri and Curd (1983) can be seen to have a more deterministic view of the family's role, for they regard the family as providing a model for social interaction.

The more "deterministic" interpretation can be supported by citing the Bell, Cornwell and Bell (1988) study where it was hypothesised that level of "connectedness" in family interactions would be parallelled in peer relationships; and the Reiss, Oliveri and Curd (1983) study hypothesised that adolescent behaviour patterns within the family would be reflected in other social interactions. In both these studies the hypothesis was supported but whether this indicates the strength of influence of the family interaction pattern or its immutability is open to debate and empirical testing. For example, do ongoing non-family interactions remain as mirrors of family interactions or do they come to influence family interaction patterns? While researchers agree on the general point that family interaction patterns influence wider social interactions they are not agreed on the finer details; and since their studies are not directly comparable (conceptually or methodologically) the questions cannot be answered at present.

A Redefinition of the Parent-adolescent Bond

Research clearly indicates that when adolescent intra-psychic development occurred within the parent-offspring bond it seems possible, if not inevitable, that this bond will be "transformed and renegotiated" (Grotevant & Cooper, 1985) to accommodate the adolescent's development: this is yet another matter on which there is general agreement. Moreover, empirical support is readily forthcoming: Honess and Lintern (1990) and Youniss and

Smollar (1985) find that during adolescence, relationships with parents did undergo radical transformation. Sometimes this involved moving to a more mutual and symmetrical relationship, in other cases to a more distanced relationship with a greater psychological distance between adolescents and their parents. Similarly, White, Speisman and Costos (1983) reported that the redefinition of the parent-offspring bond continued into young adulthood and that, in time, it became more "peer-like" in character.

The review presented in this chapter has also clearly demonstrated that the interaction between relationship patterns and intra-psychic variables is a complex one. In particular, there is evidence that changes in the parent-offspring bond are different for the dyadic relationships between mother and adolescent and father and adolescent. For example, Bell and Bell (1983) noted that while maternal support had a positive effect on adolescent daughters' development, paternal support was negatively related. Grotevant and Cooper (1985) found that fathers' expressions of "mutuality" were positively associated with development while mothers' expressions of "mutuality" were negatively associated. Hauser and Powers (Hauser et al., 1984) showed fathers with offspring at high levels of ego development expressed "enabling" behaviours, while the mothers of these adolescents had a tendency to express "constraining" behaviours. And Adams et al., (1991) found that fathers', but not mothers', differentiation behaviour was predictive of the adolescent's developmental outcome. Such findings clearly suggest that "... mother-adolescent and father-adolescent relationships contribute differentially to psychological development ..." Youniss and Ketterlinus (1987, p. 265).

Gender Differences:
Unifying the Theoretical Accounts

Given the importance of the separation-merger polarity in the family systems accounts, and their reports of "sex differences", it is surprising that such authors appear to be relatively "gender blind" in their theoretical accounts. There appear to be fruitful possibilities of integration with aspects of the gender socialisation literature that posits the separation-merger polarity as central, and which, moreover, seeks to encourage a relational perspective for interpreting the psychological development of individual men and women.

The most common set of theories which provide an explicitly gendered account are those derived from Freudian roots which therefore posit a fundamental conflict between daughters and mothers. One reference to Freud will serve to remind the reader: "and the embitterment of so many daughters against their mothers derives, in the last analysis, from the reproach against her for having brought them into the world as women instead of men" (Freud, 1973). Reference to neo-Freudians (e.g. Friday, 1979; Chodorow, 1979) concerned with mother-child relations reveals an emphasis on the pre-Oedipal period for an establishment of mother-child, especially mother-daughter, "connectedness". However, such neo-Freudians sustain the conflict model between mothers and daughters for interpreting later stages of development. Moreover, even for those writers who specifically eschew Freud's position in seeking to describe mother-daughter relations (e.g. Arcana, 1981), and refer to socio-cultural practice, conflict is still the central frame: "Mothers socialise their daughters into the narrow role of wife-mother. In frustration and guilt, daughters reject their mothers ...".

The position for boys is generally argued to be less conflicted, but more distanced. Thus, Chodorow (1979), for example, describes how mothers experience their sons as a "male opposite ... a sexual other". Girls, as indicated earlier, remain involved in issues of "merging and separation", while boys develop a "more defensive firming of ego boundaries". Similar outcomes are posited from more behaviourally oriented theoretical positions (e.g. the modelling approach put forward by, for instance, Maccoby & Jacklin, 1975).

These theoretical formulations find some support in the Youniss and Smollar (1985; 1990) findings. They describe how for both adolescent boys and girls (in what they describe as their "white, middle class sample", the relationship with mother is generally more complex than that with father: an "authority tempered by intimacy and moments of equality". The mother is typically involved in household rules, emotional and interpersonal matters, which allow more co-operative forms of relationship to emerge, allowing mothers to "become people" sooner than fathers. The latter's sphere of involvement tends to be with relatively "objective" concerns such as school performance, wherein they appear to make demands without modifying them in the light of the adolescents' perspective.

Honess and Lintern (1990) provide further details on gendered changes but this time in respect of sons' and daughters' different relationships with their mothers. Although both boys and girls were found to develop interdependent styles of relating to their mothers, the potential for conflict (consistent with the Freudian arguments) may be a significant element in accounting for adolescent girls social development. However, the study did not provide evidence of enduring conflict: on reaching early adulthood, the young women had typically reached a stage of interdependence with their mothers.

Other more recent interpretations of gender socialisation, like those from the family relations literature discussed earlier, also challenge the assumption that adolescent development necessarily involves increasing autonomy and independence from others (e.g. Gilligan, 1982; Hare-Mustin

& Maracek, 1986; Bush, 1987). For example, Bush suggests that the meanings of polarities such as "instrumental focus (typically male) vs. popularity focus (typically female)" are themselves changing. Bush argues that the adolescent girl who eschews the traditional passive dependent role does not necessarily reject a concern with connectedness, instead, she may, in effect, redefine what it means to be independent. Put simply, it can be said that "interdependence", which involves relating with others, can be of a positive kind for both girls and boys, where decision-making is shared in a way that is considered appropriate by both parties. This is consistent with the mutuality orientation of Cooper et al. (1983), and others who adopt the relational paradigm.

FRAMEWORK FOR DESCRIBING DIFFERENT RESEARCH METHODS

The literature review has demonstrated both the potential and the problems facing this contemporary field of research. Consensus has been indicated on a number of basic tenets including that: the parent-offspring bond is maintained during adolescence; the "quality" of the family relationship is associated with different developmental outcomes; the adolescent's experience of family plays some role in social interactions outwith the family unit; mothers and fathers contribute differentially to the adolescent's development.

Despite this agreement on general findings, the way forward in respect of a more sensitive understanding of adolescent development within the family context is problematic. Although the need for a unified theory may be important, it is the lack of demonstrable comparability between measures and procedures which is the most pressing concern. The literature review has demonstrated considerable overlap and convergence in ideas, but investigators typically devise their own measures, with scant regard for issues of convergent and discriminant validity. Guidelines that provide a priori reasons for assuming convergence of measures should encourage such comparisons.

A four-level framework for the description and preliminary evaluation of research methods suited to studying adolescent development within a relational context follows. The four levels are (1) theoretical origins, (2) content focus, (3) subject population, and (4) method format. The framework (see Table 3.2) is illustrated with reference to six procedures that have been reported in the literature, which measure dimensions generally considered relevant, and they illustrate fully the descriptive framework. The six procedures are identified under "method format".

TABLE 3.2
A Framework for Grouping Research Methods

LEVEL 1: Theoretical Paradigms

A.   Directly linked to relational paradigms

B.   Developed from traditions with adolescent focus

C.   Taken from distinctly different theoretical origins

LEVEL 2: Content Focus

A.   Family relationships

B.   Adolescent ego/identity development

C.   Maturity of adolescent interpersonal skills

LEVEL 3: Subject Population

A.   Family group or family dyads

B.   Adolescent only

LEVEL 4: Method Format

A.   Reactive methods/quantitative scoring
     Examples:
        1. Extended objective measure of Ego Identity Development Status
        2. Relationship Questionnaires

B.   Projective methods
     Examples:
        3. Role Taking Task
        4. Sentence Completion Test

C.   Interview methods/qualitative analysis
     Example:
        5. Paired Interviewing

D.   Interactive methods/family discussion
     Example:
        6. Family Interaction Task

Note: Procedures 1–6 are used to illustrate the Framework.

Consider level 1 (theoretical origins): Origins at 1A are the most promising for technique selection, followed by 1B, where a focus on adolescent adjustment, for example, can be interpreted with reference to the broader family system. However, even with such a justification, a focus on the individual *per se* may need considerable theoretical work to bridge the gap to an orientation that gives primacy to relations between people (see Semin, 1986, for a general discussion of the individual/society interface, and Honess & Edwards, 1990, for such a discussion with particular reference to adolescents).

Origins at level 1C are likely to prove the most problematic for interpreting the data derived from a particular technique. For example, a Piagetian framing will inevitably be "individualistic" (see comments on 1B origins) as well as involving potentially redundant theoretical baggage. Only an exceptionally promising technique should be drawn from unrelated theoretical origin.

Similar considerations apply to level 2 (content focus), where a content focus on domains B and C is likely to require the use of additional methods that explicitly focus on domain A.

In respect of level 3 (subject population) there is a prima facie case for selecting 3A. Any interactive methods are ruled out if 3B is chosen, as is any analysis which builds on the different perspectives of family members. Hence, the choice of using the adolescent only requires particular care. Level 4 decisions (method format) are discussed after consideration of the six procedures chosen to illustrate the framework:

Objective Measure of Ego Identity Development
(Adams, Bennion and Huh, 1987 et seq.)

Theoretical Origins: (1B) Erikson's theory of adolescent identity development.

Focus: (2B) Adolescent ego identity status. During adolescence the individual is held to explore and make commitments to ideological (personal) and interpersonal (social) issues. This exploration and commitment influences the normative process of identity development and formation.

Subject Population: (3B) Adolescent only.

Method Format: (4A) The EOMEIS is a self-report technique developed from Marcia's (1966) semi-structured interview. It has 64 items and takes approximately 25 minutes to complete.

Validation and Use: The EOMEIS has been developed in a psycho-metrically rigorous manner and yields high levels of reliability and validity. The manual is comprehensive and gives details of the history, rationale, development, administration, reliability and validity studies of the EOMEIS. As can be seen from the review of Adams' work, the necessary theoretical links have been made to relational ideas, and the use of the procedure has been strengthened by using it in conjunction with family relationship measures. The technique is becoming increasingly widely used.

Relationship Questionnaires
(Youniss, J. and Smollar, J., 1985 et seq.)

Theoretical Origins: (1A) Relational paradigm.

Focus: (2A) The characteristics of different relationship structures, specifically those between adolescents and parents and adolescents and friends.

Subject Population: (3B) Adolescent only.

Format: (4A) A set of seven reactive methodologies, divided into two parts, are administered to adolescent respondents. Total completion time is approximately 80 minutes.

Validation and Use: Valuable descriptive data is reported by the authors, but no clear or validated scoring system has been published, nor has the procedure been strengthened by using it in conjunction with family relationship measures that move beyond the adolescent perspective alone. Published work has to date only emanated from the Youniss team.

Role Taking Task
(Feffer, 1959)

Theoretical Origins: (1C) Piaget's stage theory of cognitive development.

Focus: (2C) Role taking: a measure of ability to decentre from one's own point of view, to consider others' perspectives.

Subject Population: (3B) Adolescent only.

Format: (4B) The Role Taking Task is a projective test. The adolescent is presented with a TAT style stimulus. The subject makes up a story about the stimulus picture and then retells the story from the point of view of self and then of the other characters. The completion time is approximately 25 minutes.

Validation and Use: The Role Taking Task has been administered to a wide variety of subjects and has reported high levels of reliability and validity. However, it was not developed specifically for use in the study of adolescent development. Other researchers have developed more appropriate scoring systems. For example, Cooper and Grotevant (1979) report a scoring procedure with four dimensions: simple refocusing, character elaboration, perspective elaboration and change of perspective. At best, the Role Taking Task provides information on just one component of relationship skills. The conceptual and methodological bridge with the relational paradigm remains to be properly established.

Sentence Completion Test
(Loevinger, J. and Wessler, R., 1970 et seq.)

Theoretical Origins: (1B) A stage theory developed and refined through empirical study.

Focus: (2B) Measures stages of ego functioning. No definition of the ego is provided by Loevinger but it can be understood as being a unitary entity which provides the framework through which one understands and interprets the world.

Subject Population: (3B) Adolescent only.

Format: (4B) The Sentence Completion Test is a 36 item projective test with different versions for men and for women. The items are in the form of sentence stems which the subject completes in a way they feel appropriate. For example, "Rules are ...". Completion time is approximately 20 minutes.

Validation and Use: The manuals are comprehensive. They provide details on reliability and validity, and an intensive training programme for rating the Sentence Completion Test. The focus of the Sentence Completion Test is life-span ego functioning, it is not specifically a measure of adolescent ego functioning. The technique is widely used but conceptual and methodological links with the relational paradigm have not been fully established.

Paired Interviewing
(Honess and Lintern, 1990)

Theoretical Origins: (1A) Relational paradigm

Focus: (2A) Changing parent adolescent relationships with particular reference to particular interaction styles as construed by both members of the dyad.

Subject Population: (3A) Adolescent and parent dyads.

Format: (4C) A technique which exploits independent interviews with dyads, the members of which are asked parallel questions. A coding procedure is described that is based irreducibly on both the parent and the child perspectives.

Validation and Use: A new procedure that allows complementarity, disagreement and accuracy between members of a dyad to be assessed in order to operationalise the concepts of conflict, dependence, independence and interdependence. Data are available on parent-adolescent pairs, and mothers and post-adolescent daughters, but to date, published work is only that produced by Honess and Lintern.

Family Interaction Task
(Cooper, Grotevant & Condon, 1983 et seq.)

Theoretical Origins: (1A) Relational paradigm.

Focus: (2A) A measure of family structure through assessing how individual family members operate to sustain an ongoing family group interaction.

Subject Population: (3A) Adolescent and parents.

Format: (4D) The Family Interaction Task is an interactive problem-solving task which involves the family working together to plan a day-by-day itinerary for a fictional two week holiday. The task is held to be one in which the adolescent's interests and expertise are legitimate and can therefore contribute to the family's decisions. It takes approximately 20 minutes to complete. The family's discussion during the Family Interaction Task is recorded as the data source. The tape is transcribed and processed by content analysis. The first 300 utterances are analysed and each is assigned to one of fourteen categories which operationalise the dimension of individuation.

Validation and Use: The Family Interaction Task has not been widely used, but shares a number of attributes with other measures, such as the Reiss and Oliveri's (1987) card sort procedure. Convergent validity could most usefully be examined in respect of Type 4D (interactive) measures, as could the assumption that laboratory-type tasks do reflect mundane family functioning. Nevertheless, the measure has good face validity, and has produced useful data in the series of studies reported here.

Choice of Method (Level 4 Decision)

The choice of research measure (level 4) must depend on the particular research question. However, there are clear advantages and disadvantages with each measure which mean that some are more evidently suited to the relational paradigm. For example, family systems methods, such as the Family Interaction Task, have the clear advantage that they allow direct observation to the researcher and can generate material for process studies, e.g. in relation to conflict resolution. However, it should be noted that researchers using such methods assume that the family's core assumptions and beliefs will be made manifest in experimenter contrived tasks. However, this assumption is rarely tested (Costell & Reiss, 1982 is one of the few instances).

The major alternative research method of interviewing individuals about particular issues does allow particular contexts and different times (past and future) to be talked about, or "accounted for" by participants but cannot, of course, allow an external researcher perspective on the events under consideration. Interviews have been used by a number of researchers working within the family relations perspective. Typically, however, only one person is interviewed. Such data are necessarily silent on both partners' experience of the relationship, and cannot therefore allow a more systems-sensitive consideration of conflict, support and so on, and whether or not such relations are mutual or unidirectional. Interview studies, whether questionnaire based, or relatively open-ended should preferably involve more than one family member.

CONCLUSION

The literature review has identified convergence within the relational paradigm at a theoretical/conceptual level. This remains an important task in respect of building a unified theory, but it must go hand in hand with further empirical examination of the different measures that purport to operationalise these concepts.

Simple exhortations to investigators to attend to inter-relations between measures will, however, have little impact since the task of examining one's preferred method against the plethora that are available is too daunting. However a framework that provides a priori reasons for assuming convergence of measures should encourage such comparisons.

The framework offers a way of categorising different methods. It allows the researcher or practitioner to group together measures which fall under the same set of headings within each level. Such measures are prime candidates for the testing of "convergent validity", i.e. such measures should converge—be positively associated with each other—if they are measuring common concepts. Moreover, we should expect a greater degree of convergence the greater the number of level correspondences: from a complete lack of correspondence to correspondence at all four levels.

More generally, the framework may prove valuable for organising the findings and research methods from other arenas involving adolescent relationships, e.g. those with siblings or peers. This is theoretically consistent for a systems paradigm which emphasises that individual development takes place within a matrix of changing relationships: different contexts/people "call out" different behaviours (cf. the literature on "situated identities", e.g. Alexander and Wiley, 1981). Youniss and Smollar make a similar point when they discuss the way in which a focus on adolescent-parent relations alone can lead to a "stripping away" of the contexts of other relationships and, at a broader level, societal constraints.

CHAPTER FOUR

Variation in Maturational Timing and Adjustment in Adolescence

Rainer K. Silbereisen and Bärbel Kracke

Many adolescents are known to experience a difference between the timing of physical maturation and full psychosocial development. There is evidence that the gap between these two aspects of development is increasing as a result of the influence of modern living conditions. A consequence of this is that a growing number of young people are sexually mature, yet still have to live in economic dependency.

Imagine a picture of all the students in a classroom of, say, seventh graders. A huge variation in maturational status is evident. Is there any need to worry about it? Asynchronies between different facets of development are not a new phenomenon. For generations students have made changes within the school system at normative times, irrespective of the variation in maturational timing between and within genders. Furthermore, it may be that differences in the timing of developmental transitions are conducive to successful coping with the multitude of new challenges which occur during adolescence. Coleman and Hendry (1990) suggest that the young even attempt to space demands, and resolve them step by step and one at a time. Thus, synchronising the timing of social transitions with the pace of maturational growth is not necessarily an adaptive process. Not having to live with the burden of responsibilities for a family, for instance, is an advantage for those suffering from risks like economic hardship (Elder, 1986).

In a cultural climate favouring "precociousness", early sexual maturation may be seen as less problematic than in more traditional societal circumstances. Within the modern industrialised climate, a trend towards earlier occurrence of various forms of adolescent transition is taking place. Sport provides a good example of this phenomenon. As Zinnecker (1990) has pointed out, nowadays much younger age-groups are engaged in highly specialised exercise and training than was common in previous generations. One of the main reasons for this is the role of athletic achievement in providing an entry to adult privileges. Other domains like fashion and the media follow similar trends.

Despite these considerations, a major problem remains. Recent research has demonstrated that part of the variation in timing is an outcome of strains and malfunctions within the family (Moffitt, Caspi, Belsky & Silva, 1990) and that the genders differ in their vulnerability to atypical maturation. The latter is one of the results which emerged from the classical Berkeley, Oakland, and Fels growth studies. More specifically, early maturation seemed to be a greater social advantage for boys than for girls (Brooks-Gunn, Petersen & Eichhorn, 1985).

Some insight into the way biological processes influence social behaviour is provided by a seeming paradox in the relation between puberty and dating. During the last few decades, the age at which the first date takes place has decreased considerably, a trend which may well be related to the present-day acceleration in the timing of puberty. However, Dornbusch et al. (1981) have shown that, compared with chronological age, individual differences in maturational status have little influence upon dating. In interpreting this result, one has to regard age as a guide for social expectations concerning the appropriate time to begin dating. Such time-tabling does not need to be synchronised with the pace of sexual development. The reverse appears to be the case. Dornbusch et al. found that among females the association between maturational status and dating was weaker than among males, a finding which presumably indicates parental concerns about the risk of pregnancy. Thus, rather than directly effecting behaviours like dating, inter-individual differences in maturation influence behaviour indirectly through interaction with age-graded social expectations.

Gender differences in reactions to variations in the rate of maturation are the rule in this research area. Silbereisen and Kracke (1990) found that early-maturing adolescent boys reported receiving more warmth and acceptance and enjoying more psychological autonomy than did their on-time and late maturing age-mates. At later ages and for girls in general, no association between these variables and maturational timing was found. Bearing in mind the positive impact of authoritative parenting on adjustment and mental health (Baumrind, 1989), early-maturing young boys are presumably better off than most others.

The focus of this chapter is on previous research and recent analyses of the measurement, consequences and antecedents of maturational timing in adolescence. Results from our own work rely mostly on data gathered as part of the Berlin Youth Longitudinal Study (BYLS. See Silbereisen, Noack, & Schönpflug, in press). This study used a stratified random sampling procedure in more than 70 schools which were representative of schools in Berlin (West Germany, at the time of data collection) with regard to socio-economic status and educational level. Seven waves of measurement were conducted between 1982 and 1988. Three birth-cohorts were sampled with the oldest cohort born in 1967/68, the middle cohort in 1970/71 and the youngest in 1973/74. The oldest and youngest cohorts were followed for four years each and the middle cohort took part in the study for seven years. The results presented in this chapter are based on data from the middle and the youngest cohort, gathered at measurement points 3 through 6, when the middle cohort was between 13,6 and 16,6 and the youngest cohort between 11,6 and 13,6 years of age.

The remainder of the chapter is organised in three main sections. First, various issues related to the assessment of maturational timing are described. The emphasis is on self-rated differences in the pace of pubertal development compared to age-mates. Information on the validity of such measures is provided from the literature and from analyses conducted on the Berlin Youth Longitudinal Sample. Age-related changes and gender-differences are demonstrated in the association between maturational timing and body height and weight.

Second, consequences of maturational timing are discussed, exemplified by effects on the affective, relational and behavioural domains of adolescent development. Again, results are given from important previous research and recent analyses on the BYLS sample. Particular attention is given to the impact of maturational timing on self-evaluation, adaptive and maladaptive peer contacts and substance use in adolescence.

Third, antecedents of inter-individual variation in maturational timing are reported at some length. The finding that, on average, daughters of divorced families mature earlier, leads into a discussion of the recent debate on the relationship between maturational timing and strains within the family and in the parent-child relationship. Some preliminary information on the potential role of acculturative stress is given, based on an ongoing study of migrants to Germany.

ASSESSMENT OF MATURATIONAL VARIABLES

Two aspects of pubertal development have been the subject of particular attention: maturational status and maturational timing. Maturational status refers to the current level of physical development relative to the overall process of pubertal change, whereas maturational timing refers to whether the pubertal process occurs early, on-time, or late relative to a reference group such as age-mates or classmates (Dubas, Graber & Petersen, 1991). These aspects can be assessed in various ways, including objective measures and self-ratings. They can even be assessed in retrospect.

Retrospective data of certain pubertal events like age of menarche seem to be highly reliable. Bean at al. (1979) asked adults to recall the year of their menarche and found 90% of the reports concordant with medical information gathered up to 33 years earlier. The error margin was no more than one year. Despite this, one could argue that retrospective data are likely to be biased towards the population average. Stattin and Magnusson (1990) quote a Swedish growth study in which early-maturing girls did not report a later age nor late-maturing girls an earlier age of menarche. The correlation between menarcheal age reported in retrospect and actual menarcheal age recorded by nurses was 0.78. This correlation gives an important hint that maturational status relative to other girls was also reported correctly.

Maturational Status

Tanner (Marshall & Tanner, 1969; 1970) designed photographs to represent five stages in the development of primary and secondary sex characteristics during puberty. Stages of pubic hair development are depicted for both genders, as are breast development for females and genital growth for males. A major problem with this method is the need to undress the young person in order to allow assessment by a doctor. As a result, most researchers use self-report instruments. Duke et al. (1980) reported high concordances between physicians' ratings and self-assessments by the teenagers. Even classroom settings with group instruction were acceptable and indicated highly accurate self-perceptions.

Petersen et al. (1988) developed and validated a self-report questionnaire of pubertal development, the Pubertal Development Scale (PDS). Brooks-Gunn et al. (1987) compared ratings on this measure with physicians' and girls' ratings of the Tanner stages in early adolescence. The correlations between the two measures were fairly high (around the 0.6 level). Even higher correlations were obtained in mid-adolescence, because the PDS allows better classification of mid-pubertal status than of the pre- or early-pubertal stages.

Maturational Timing

Adolescence is a period of social comparisons. This means that maturational timing, rather than maturational status, is likely to have an impact upon psycho-social functioning.

A variety of researchers (e.g. Petersen & Crockett, 1985) have used estimates of age at peak height velocity in order to measure pubertal timing. Analysing data for boys and girls separately, Petersen and Crockett trichotomised the distributions of the measure into early (12.74 years), on-time (13.83 years) and late development (14.76 years). Another way to assess pubertal timing is based on the distribution of stage ratings at a given age. Alsaker (1990), for instance, defined subjects scoring 1 standard deviation below the mean as late-maturers and subjects scoring 1 standard deviation above the mean as early-maturers. Typically, the frame of reference is not a population statistic, but the maturational status distribution of the subjects' classmates or peer-group. Other studies, e.g. Duncan et al. (1985) made use of national norms to classify subjects.

When considering the impact of maturational timing on psycho-social functioning, the choice of frame of reference for relative maturational timing is of great importance. Using the immediate environment of the adolescents as a basis for forming timing groups, comes closer to a young person's actual experience of being faster or slower in development. General norms do not necessarily mean that in a specific environment the distribution of pubertal indices is similar to that of the population at large. This point is of particular importance because of the association between social class and nutrition (Eveleth & Tanner, 1976).

An alternative to the use of such computed measurements is to obtain direct subjective ratings of pubertal timing. Dubas, Graber, and Petersen (1991) gathered self-assessed timing at grades seven, eight and twelve. Half of the adolescents reported no changes across three occasions, a further 48% were consistent on two out of three occasions. Thus, perceived timing shows a moderate stability. The correlations with age at peak height velocity increased over time ($r = 0.56$ at grade 12) and accuracy was especially high for early-maturing boys and late-maturing girls. Moreover, retrospective self-assessments were even more valid than perceptions obtained during periods when the pubertal changes actually took place.

Self-assessed maturational timing is a measure which is subject to a complex of other factors including self-perceptions, social comparisons, personal attributes and aspirations. As both the person and the reference group are in the process of changing across adolescence, one might perceive oneself as faster one year and on-time the next, depending not only on one's maturational status but also on the mean status within the reference group. Furthermore, due to gender differences in the rate of maturation, males' compared to females' perceived timing may be based on different body attributes and, in turn, may differ in psychological meaning and stimulus value across and within age-groups.

The cues which are possibly related to perceived maturational timing can be illuminated by showing the latter's correspondence with age-related differences in body height and weight across adolescence. Using data from the Berlin Youth Longitudinal Study, Fig. 4.1 shows the correspondence between perceived maturational timing and body height, for males and females separately. Maturational timing was assessed by using adolescents' responses to a single item, namely, "Compared to my age-mates I develop slower (faster, as fast)." Height and weight were also assessed by self-report. For the present analyses, the data were organised as a series of consecutive one-year follow-ups between ages 11,6 and 13,6 for a younger cohort and between ages 13,6 and 16,6 for an older cohort. With both core longitudinal samples, subjects who dropped out were replaced by classmates. For the sake of brevity, only the first measurement of each follow-up is shown.

The general shape of the curves closely resembles previous findings concerning growth in height during adolescence (Marshall & Tanner, 1969; 1970). Girls approach their ultimate height earlier than boys (age 15 vs. 18

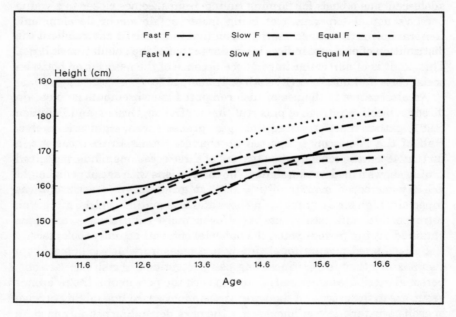

FIG. 4.1. Height and maturational timing. The Figure shows age-related increase in body height for males and females who perceived themselves as maturing faster, slower, or at the same pace, relative to classmates, together with average heights of cross-sectional samples, assessed at different ages. Sample sizes in the younger cohort (ages 11,6 and 12,6) were 114 and 105 for males and 101 and 108 for females; in the older cohort (ages 13,6 to 16,6) the totals for males were between 179 and 265, for females between 198 and 254. See text for further details.

approximately) and they also undergo the growth spurt earlier (age at peak height velocity is about 12 vs. 14 years).

Separate ANOVAs were conducted for each follow-up and gender, with maturational timing and time period as independent variables. Males and females showed significant differences between fast and slow maturation at almost all points in time, with the latter always reporting lower body height. While the differences diminished gradually for girls after age 12,6, differences for boys only began to emerge at about this time and did not start to decrease before 15,6 years of age. All of the F scores, except for those for the youngest males, were significant at $p < 0.05$ or less.

There was a significant increase at each follow-up (in most cases, $p < 0.001$). Some of the interactions with maturational timing were also significant, particularly among females. This occurred because of a steeper increase among the slow maturers. Thus, the observed height differences between maturational groups are presumably due to differences in the onset and slope of growth curves.

The latter effect emerged even more clearly from the subsequent longitudinal analyses. In Fig. 4.2, height change in succeeding years is shown for subjects who categorised themselves as fast, slow or on-time at ages 11,6 and 13,6, respectively. For convenience, the results of ANOVAs with maturational timing and repeated assessments as independent variables are given in Table 4.1.

Note the remarkable differences in the younger group. While fast-maturing girls were considerably taller than late- and on-time maturers, slow-maturing boys were considerably smaller than early- and on-time maturers. This pattern remained for the older male cohort, but was less clear for the older females. Nevertheless, particularly in early adolescence, a fast-maturing girl is much taller than her classmates, while in contrast, a late-maturing boy is much smaller than the majority. The Figure also shows that the height of subjects originally classified as faster, slower, or equal in rate gradually converged. This is due to the fact that the slower group caught up with the other two groups.

In further analyses of the 13,6-year-olds, their height at age 17,6, which was regarded as equivalent to the maximum achieved, was assessed. Height at 13,6 was then expressed as a percentage of this maximum and was divided into three groups, the top and bottom 14% and the middle 72% (Stattin & Magnusson, 1990). The contingency coefficient between percent maximum height and perceived maturational timing was 0.34 ($p < 0.001$), thus underscoring the likely role of the growth spurt in adolescents' self-rating of timing.

Where age-related differences in body weight are concerned, Fig. 4.3 shows stable differences between the maturational groups, with faster maturing girls always being considerably heavier than their slower

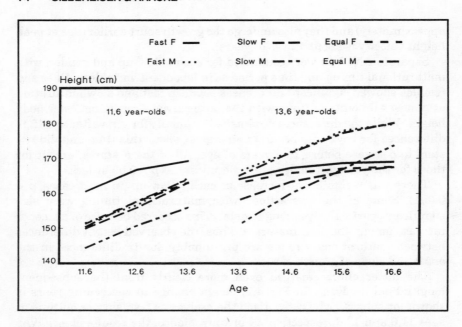

FIG. 4.2. Changes in height and maturational timing. The Figure shows the average increase in height among adolescents who categorised themselves as faster, slower, or equal in rate of maturation at ages 11,6 and 13,6 respectively. The longitudinal sample of the younger cohort comprised 66 males and 53 females; the older cohort consisted of 132 males and 152 females.

maturing age-mates. This was especially true for the youngest group. For boys, differences in weight began to emerge at about age 12,6. These gender differences fit in with expectations derived from normative data. Most of the F scores, except those for the youngest two groups, were significant at $p < 0.01$ or lower. Within each follow-up, the increase across the one-year periods was also significant. In contrast to height, however, the interaction was not significant except for females aged 13,6 to 14,6. Thus, the differences among the maturational groups were not paralleled by differences in the slope of weight increase.

For girls, weight changes in future years showed a pattern similar to that reported for height changes. Fast-maturing girls, particularly in the younger cohort, were heavier than slow- and on-time maturers. While no difference existed among the younger boys, slow-maturers in the older male cohort reported considerably lower weights than their classmates. The F scores and probability levels are shown in Table 4.1. As indicated by the significant interaction for the older females, slow-maturers eventually catch up in weight.

TABLE 4.1

ANOVAs on Height and Weight Increase in Two Cohorts of Adolescents
by Maturational Timing

	Cohorts							
	Age 11,6 to 13,6				Age 13,6 to 16,6			
	Height		Weight		Height		Weight	
Variable	F	p	F	p	F	p	F	p
Females								
Maturational timing	7.46	0.001	5.09	0.010	1.94	ns	9.82	<0.001
Longitudinal assessments	181.60	<0.001	115.95	<0.001	148.38	<0.001	124.16	<0.001
Interaction	2.79	0.030	1.06	ns	9.50	<0.001	2.56	0.019
n	53		49		152		138	
Males								
Maturational timing	1.91	ns	0.43	ns	11.61	<0.001	10.37	<0.001
Longitudinal assessments	116.34	<0.001	89.07	<0.001	273.12	<0.001	115.45	< 0.001
Interaction	0.76	ns	1.44	ns	5.11	<0.001	0.66	ns
n	66		68		132		128	

In sum, then, the data show that self-perceived maturational timing is meaningfully related to physical body attributes. Where magnitude of differences is concerned, weight seems to be a more impressive correlate than height.

Clinical research with growth-retarded adolescents has shown the deleterious effect of short stature for males (Apter et al. 1981). Since slowing of the growth-rate often accompanies delayed puberty and since the young are likely to have inadequate knowledge of the transitional nature of their body shape, lasting negative effects are likely. Indeed, Duncan et al. (1985) reported progressively less height satisfaction for objectively assessed early, on-time and late maturation in boys. Moreover, about two out of three early-maturing girls were dissatisfied with their greater weight. As the wish to be thinner tends to be normative among girls in Western countries, these early-maturers suffer in that they see themselves as being at a disadvantage earlier in life than do other girls of the same age.

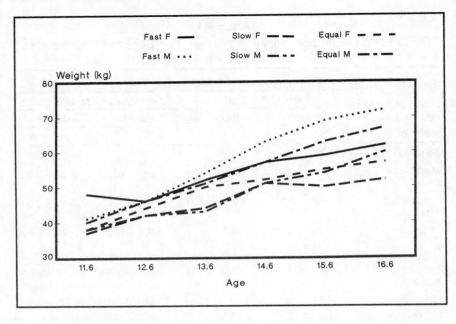

FIG. 4.3. Weight and maturational timing. The Figure shows age-related increase in body weight. Sample sizes were almost identical with those for height. For further explanation see Fig. 4.1.

CONSEQUENCES OF VARIATION IN MATURATIONAL TIMING

Physical appearance cues play a prominent role in adults' perceptions of adolescents' social maturity. Johnson and Collins (1988) found that when teachers and parents rated adolescents whom they knew, physical and social maturity were highly correlated. They also found that adults who were not previously acquainted with adolescent subjects, gave higher estimations of the age of those who were more mature-looking. Findings such as these indicate that given the impact of age-graded expectations on numerous aspects of life, in general, and on adolescent transition in particular, off-time maturers are likely to suffer from demands and experiences which are inappropriate to their actual social maturity.

Psychosocial Adjustment

Aro and Taipale (1987) examined the effects of age of menarche on psychosomatic symptoms such as headaches, excessive perspiration or heartburn in a group of girls who were investigated on three occasions between ages 14 and 16. As expected, early-maturers showed higher symptom scores than late-maturers. These effects disappeared for all except the 14-year-olds, however, when time since menarche was controlled. Thus, in older adolescents the differences in number of symptoms were associated with pubertal development, as such, rather than with timing. Although more of the early-maturers had already had a date and more of them reported use of alcohol during the previous month, factors such as these could not explain these girls' greater number of psychosomatic symptoms.

Some effects of pubertal timing seem to be related to the social stimulus value of the pubertal changes. While for females puberty means an increase in fatness, for males an increase in muscularity is prevalent. Western beauty standards for women demand slimness, so that at the end of puberty, more than 50% of adolescent females express the wish to be thinner. Consequently, these females experience the normal side-effects of sexual maturation as negative for their self-appreciation (Dornbusch et al. 1984). Similar results emerged from a study with a large Norwegian sample. Alsaker (1990) checked whether overweight (actually a measure of the deviation of a subjects' weight from the population average weight for a given height) might actually explain the relationship between perceived early maturation and low self-esteem in females. With the exception of those for the youngest group of sixth-graders, the results showed that a large portion of the timing effects could indeed be explained by being overweight relative to population norms.

Simmons et al. (1979) found more positive body images, indicated by higher satisfaction with weight and height and higher self-esteem for late-maturing girls. Among boys, however, more positive effects on the self were typical for early-maturers. Their findings were obtained from a North American sample and one might question whether they are generalisable to other countries. Elsewhere, factors such as more extensive sexual education may mean that side-effects of puberty (weight gains, for example) may be seen by young females as transitional and therefore less dramatic. However, Duke-Duncan et al. (1984; 1985) showed that even when information is provided about the course of normal development and special reference is made to weight gain, there was no change in girls' negative feelings about their weight.

Silbereisen et al. (1989) published analyses of German girls' self-derogation or negative self-evaluation ("I would like to change a lot concerning myself"; Kaplan, 1978), in which comparisons were made between groups who perceived themselves as developing faster, equally fast or slower than peers of the same age. At 11,6 years there was no association between self-evaluations and perceptions of change relative to others. Presumably this occurred because most of the girls were pre-pubertal or had just begun to mature. At age 14,6 however, fast-maturing girls reported less negative self-evaluations. This is quite the opposite of what was expected on the basis of previous research. One might remark, however, that the absence of negative self-evaluations is not necessarily equivalent to positive self-esteem.

Most of the existing research in this area has been conducted in the U.S., so that differences may result from the fact that in comparison with their American age-mates, German adolescents receive more information on sexual development within the normal school curriculum. Problems like adolescent pregnancy, which are usually seen as indicative of too little sex-education, are much less prevalent in West Germany than in the United States (Statistisches Bundesamt, 1984). Nevertheless, the evidence for this suggestion is not empirically based and systematic cross-cultural research is badly needed.

Brooks-Gunn and Warren (1989) conducted one of the few studies in which the behavioural impact of hormonal changes was compared with effects of changes in bodily appearance. It was expected that negative affect in girls in early adolescence would be more strongly associated with change in hormonal levels than with physical aspects, because affects are less likely than is self-esteem to depend on social-interaction experiences. It emerged that depressed-withdrawn affect was indeed highest at the time of the most rapid increases in the estradiol level, while maturational status (Tanner's measure, Marshall & Tanner, 1969), objective maturational timing and age at menarche showed no effect.

Interpersonal Relations

The majority of studies of interpersonal relations have investigated the effects of maturational timing on peer relations and friendship patterns. Most commonly, attention has been given to effects which increase the risk of status offences, i.e. acts such as under-age drinking, which are illegal because of the age of the offender. Kracke and Silbereisen (1990), however, reported on the association between age-adequate interpersonal relations and maturational timing at about age 14. While no differences were found in the portion of adolescents who belonged to a clique of peers, slow maturers were less likely than fast maturers to have a steady friend of the opposite sex (16% and 36%, respectively).

Magnusson, Stattin and Allen (1986) found early-maturing girls to be especially likely to have contacts with older male peers. They were more likely than late-maturing girls to have older friends, working friends, or experience with sexual relations. This, in turn, was seen as a mediating link to problem behaviour. Studies on the effects of maturational timing on boys' peer relations are scarce. Silbereisen and Kracke (1990) studied deviant peer contacts in two cohorts of male and female adolescents who were investigated annually between ages 11,6 and 13,6 and between 13,6 and 16,6. Separate ANOVAs were conducted for each follow-up and gender, with maturational timing and time-period as independent variables.

Concurrent analyses of females' perceived timing of maturation and contacts with deviant peers showed a clear pattern of associations. The results are shown in Fig. 4.4. From age 13,6 on, fast-maturing females reported more frequent contacts with deviant peers. The effects were significant at 13,6 ($F = 3.51, p < 0.05$) and 15,6 ($F = 2.80, p < 0.10$). Although the absolute frequency of such contacts was low (AM = 1.13, range 0 to 3), one should bear in mind the items included in the measure: friends who lie to parents, peers who stole something, friends who have trouble with adults. Thus, these girls seem to be involved with quite risky company.

With boys, maturational timing was related to deviant peer contacts in 14,6 year-olds only ($F = 3.75, p < 0.05$). In contrast to females, however, both fast and slow maturers showed more deviant contacts than adolescents who were equal to classmates in rate of maturation.

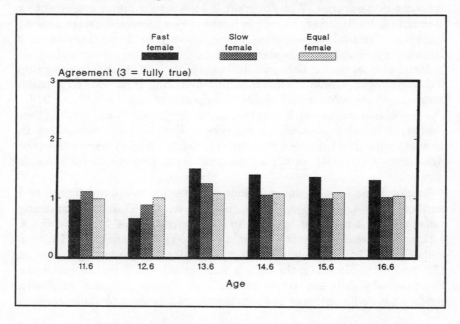

FIG. 4.4. Contacts with deviant peers and maturational timing. The Figure shows the average agreement to statements concerning the non-normative character of peer contacts among girls who categorised themselves as faster, slower, or equal in rate of maturation at ages 11,6 to 16,6. Girls at ages 11,6 and 12,6 belong to the younger cohort; girls between ages 13,6 and 16,6 belong to the older cohort. Sample sizes in the younger cohort were 84 at age 11,6 and 88 at age 12,6; sample sizes in the older cohort ranged from 199 to 222.

Contacts with deviant peers in early adolescence are most likely to be the result of prior problem behaviours, such as disobedience, status offences and delinquent acts (Patterson, DeBaryshe, & Ramsey, 1989; Maggs & Galambos, 1990). Thus, the concurrent association with maturational timing may be due to a shared variance with, for instance, higher alcohol use among fast maturers.

Using regression analyses, Silbereisen and Kracke (1990) also investigated factors influencing change in contacts with deviant peers across one-year periods between the ages 11,6 and 13,6, and between 13,6 and 16,6. At each follow-up, maturational timing, parental support and contacts with deviant peers in the previous year served as predictors. Concurrent and cross-lagged relations with parental support were small but significant (r values about -0.20). Regression weights were almost zero, however, a result which reflected the high stabilities of deviant contacts (b scores about 0.60). This result, obtained with both males and females, does not come as a surprise. While support is known to enhance competencies (Baumrind, 1989), it is not likely to function as a protective factor against deviance. Parental supervision is more likely to serve in this way (Patterson & Stouthamer-Loeber, 1984).

Maturational timing showed a different pattern of results. In the group of 15,6-year-old female adolescents, fast-maturing girls showed a small cross-lagged correlation with problematic peer contacts ($r = 0.15, p < 0.05$). The regression coefficient, however, was not significant ($b = 0.11$). All other groups of females showed no significant time-lagged correlations in contacts with deviant peers and the regression weights were either not significant or merely indicated substantively irrelevant suppression effects.

Among boys, time-lagged relations between maturational timing and contacts with deviant peers were observed at age 11,6. Fast-maturing males tended to report an increase in such contacts ($r = 0.21, p < 0.05$; $b = 0.21$, ns), whereas slow-maturing boys reported a decrease ($r = -0.13$, ns; $b = -0.35$, $p < 0.10$). In the older cohort, a similar pattern emerged at ages 13,6 and 14,6. However, the effects were small and failed to reach the conventional significance levels. In sum, fast-maturing adolescents of both genders showed a tendency towards more contacts with deviant peers.

Substance Use

Smoking and drinking below legal age are status offences. Following the notion that early maturation implies a risk of "precocious" transitions to adult-like behaviours, several studies have investigated the relation between maturational timing and substance use.

Petersen, Graber and Sullivan (1990) reported more frequent use of nicotine, alcohol and marijuana among males and females who judged their own development as being faster than that of their age-mates. While this effect of perceived maturation was found at ages 13/14, no difference was found for ages 17/18. Timing measured by age at peak height velocity, however, showed no effects of substance use.

Crockett, Silbereisen and Kracke (1990) also attempted to show the impact of maturational timing on adolescent substance use. Timing was assessed by asking participants whether they were developing slower, as fast, or faster than others of the same age. At the first measurement, subjects' average age was 13,6 years. Additional waves of assessment were carried out at ages 14,6 and 15,6. The use of three substances was assessed: cigarettes, beer/wine and hard liquor. In each case, lifetime use, use in the past year and frequency of use in the past year were reported. The association between perceived timing of maturation and whether the adolescent had ever used the substances was analysed by cross-tabulations conducted separately for each gender.

In Fig. 4.5, a breakdown of lifetime prevalences is shown for female adolescents aged 14,6. The lifetime prevalence was highest among fast maturers, followed by adolescents who perceived themselves as similar in timing to most of their classmates and finally slow maturers whose prevalence was closer to that of the on-time group. Results for the previous and the following year were similar, although the effects of maturational timing were generally less salient in the youngest age-group.

The associations between maturational timing and having ever smoked cigarettes or having ever tried hard liquor were significant for girls. With boys, however, no significant association between maturational timing and having ever used these substances emerged.

As cross-tabulations of substance use in the past year (annual prevalences) showed similar effects, maturational timing seems also to have an impact on current rates of use among female adolescents. In sum, the percentage of female users was highest among fast maturers and lowest among slow maturers. With boys, an association between maturational timing and use of alcohol only emerged at the 14,6 age-level. The pattern of association was similar to that reported for girls: fast maturers were over-represented among current users of beer/wine and hard liquor.

Finally, the impact of maturational timing on change in the frequency of substance use above and beyond previous use was assessed by means of regression analyses in which gender and within-cohort age were controlled. The categories of maturational timing were coded to contrast fast- with on-time and slow- with on-time maturers, i.e. those who perceived their rate of maturation as equal to classmates. Substance use in the previous year served as the other predictor.

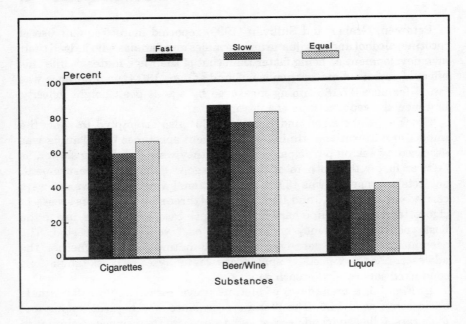

FIG. 4.5. Lifetime prevalence of smoking and drinking at age 14,6. The Figure shows the percentages of girls who have ever consumed cigarettes, beer/wine or hard liquor and who categorised themselves as faster, slower, or equal in rate of maturation at age 14,6. The sample comprised 364 girls; 72 of them categorised themselves as faster, 43 as slower and 249 as equal in rate of maturation.

The results differed depending on the substance analysed and the age-group studied. Effects of timing were only observed for the 14,6 to 15,6 follow-up. Furthermore, timing of maturation had no effect at all on smoking. With alcohol, however, a clear change in consumption frequency was found in the 14,6 to 15,6-year-olds. The unstandardised regression weights are provided in Table 4.2.

As the Table shows, consumption frequency in the previous year was the best predictor, with smoking showing the highest stabilities. Adolescents who matured faster increased their consumption of alcohol. When the analyses were conducted separately for males and females, the effects were similar for both genders.

Figure 4.6 shows the mean consumption frequencies separately for each timing group between ages 14,6 and 15,6. Fast maturers always showed the steepest increase in consumption frequency. On-time maturers also increased their consumption frequency, but in a more moderate way. Among slow maturers the pattern was less clear. There was an increase in consumption of light alcohol, but a decrease in the use of cigarettes and hard liquor.

TABLE 4.2

Regression Weights (b) in the Prediction of Change in Substance Use
Frequency for the 13,6–14,6 and 14,6–15,6 Follow-ups:
Gender, Age and Maturational Timing

| | Criteria | | | | | |
| | 13,6–14,6 Follow-up | | | 14,6–15,6 Follow-up | | |
Predictors	Cigarettes	Beer/Wine	Hard Liquor	Cigarettes	Beer/Wine	Hard Liquor
Substance Use Previous Year	0.60***	0.37***	0.50***	0.63***	0.48***	0.47***
Gender	0.13	0.18*	0.16	–0.14	–0.18*	–0.14
Age	0.22*	0.15*	0.01	–0.08	0.06	0.25**
Fast	0.10	0.13	0.15	0.19	0.30**	0.34**
Slow	0.18	0.11	0.47+	–0.27	0.12	–0.15
R2	0.43	0.16	0.25	0.39	0.24	0.37
n	160	338	96	206	369	117

+ $p < 0.10$,   *$p < 0.05$,   **$p < 0.01$,   ***$p < 0.001$

As mentioned earlier, Magnusson, Stattin & Allen (1986) reported the
role played by peers in mediating the effects of early maturation on
substance use. Kracke and Silbereisen (1990) used the 14,6 to 15,6 follow-
up to gain more insight into the impact of peer relations.

The regression analyses reported earlier were re-run with additional
predictors: contacts with deviant peers, clique membership and
engagement in a romantic friendship. While the first variable addressed
closeness to a peer context demonstrating opposition to adults, the latter
two addressed age-appropriate peer relations. The results for the 14,6 to
15,6 follow-up are shown in Table 4.3.

The Table shows that going steady with a boy-friend or girl-friend was
of no relevance for change in substance use. The increase in the
consumption of light alcohol and hard liquor was predicted by the two
peer-related variables. Adolescents whose friends opposed adult norms
were likely to increase their consumption frequency and those who
socialised with a clique of friends were also more likely to drink more often
than in the previous year. Both aspects were only slightly correlated (r
scores 0.18 for beer/wine, $p < 0.001$ and 0.13, $p < 0.10$ for hard liquor), a

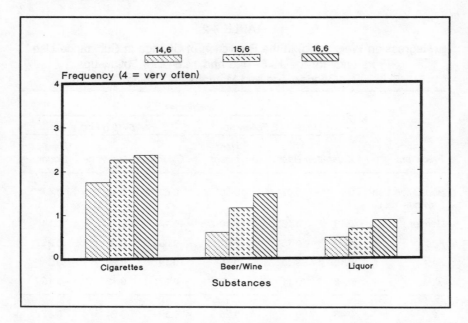

FIG. 4.6. Frequency of smoking and drinking between 14,6 and 15,6. The Figure shows the average increase in the consumption frequencies of cigarettes, beer/wine and hard liquor among adolescents who categorised themselves as faster, slower, or equal in rate of maturation at age 14,6. The longitudinal sample of consumers comprised 206 cigarette smokers, 269 beer/wine drinkers and 117 consumers of hard liquor.

result which may actually indicate different pathways into an increase of alcohol consumption. Above and beyond stability, only contact with deviant peers was related to change in smoking.

The peer-related variables did not diminish the effects of maturational timing. It seems therefore that these peer experiences do not mediate the impact of variation in the rate of maturation. In a nutshell, the results of the present study are in line with earlier research demonstrating that faster maturation implies the risk of an earlier transition to more adult-like behaviours such as substance use.

Long-term Effects of Maturational Timing

Using a retrospective interview technique, Ewert (1984) investigated perceived consequences at age 18 of growth spurt variations which occured with males when they were aged 13 to 14. Subjects were provided with a number of rating scales and asked to recollect how early and late maturing

TABLE 4.3

Regression Weights (b) in the Prediction of Change in Substance Use
Frequency for the 14,6–15,6 Follow-up:
Gender, Age, Maturational Timing and Peer Relations

	Criteria		
Predictors	Cigarettes	Beer/Wine	Hard Liquor
Substance Use Previous Year	0.64***	0.40**	0.45
Gender	−0.13	−0.19*	−0.19
Age	−0.12	0.07	0.23**
Deviant peers	0.22+	0.15*	0.23*
Clique	−0.19	0.28**	0.33**
Steady friend	0.06	−0.05	0.05
Fast	0.17	0.30**	0.34*
Slow	−0.26	0.10	−0.05
R2	0.42	0.26	0.48
n	193	348	110

$^+p < 0.10$, $^*p < 0.05$, $^{**}p < 0.01$, $^{***}p < 0.001$

classmates behaved at that time and how they would characterise the same classmates at present. Compared to late maturers, early maturers were described as physically more attractive, more self-assured and more adult-like in interpersonal interests and behaviours. Of these differences during puberty, one particular attribute remained at age 18. Those who were formerly early maturers still preferred to take initiative and responsibility and sometimes did so in a more aggressive than assertive way. In contrast, former late maturers were described as utilising more psychological strategies. They tried to understand the feelings of others or to adapt to majority opinions. In sum, while early maturation pointed to the development of a dominance-focused behavioural style, late maturers' behavioural repertoire was still characterised by more subtle methods of influencing others.

Duke et al. (1982) found that late-maturing males achieved less successfully at an academic level. The study involved several thousand adolescents who were representative of the young generation in the late 1960s in the U.S. Early and late maturers were defined as those youth, in each gender and age-group, whose Tanner stages were above the eightieth and below the twentieth percentile, respectively. In contrast to earlier research no differences were found for females, but late-maturing males, in particular, occupied a less advantageous position than the other groups of adolescents. Their educational aspirations and expectations were lower and parents and teachers shared this negative evaluation.

Compared to the pronounced disadvantage of late maturers, the advantage of early maturers was modest. The negative impact of late maturation even increased through adolescence and neither differences in intellectual functioning nor in family size could explain this pattern. Duke et al. speculated that parents' and teachers' stereotypic response to late maturers' smaller body size might have played a role in this by encouraging fewer challenges and lower expectations.

Other studies have focused on the relation between maturational timing and more problematic behaviour such as excessive drinking. Andersson and Magnusson (1990), for example, studied the impact of maturational timing in Swedish boys on alcohol consumption and its long-term consequences. Their maturation data relied on measurements of skeleton growth. The prevalence and frequency of drunkenness was assessed at ages 14,5 and 15,10. At 14,5, reported drunkenness was more prevalent and more frequent among both early and late maturers compared with the on-time group. The transitional nature of the difference seemed proven by the fact that all three groups were alike in their frequency of drunkenness at age 15,10.

For the late maturers, however, their early misconduct foreshadowed maladjustment which became manifest in mid-term perspective. In early adulthood, between ages 18 and 24, more than one third of them had committed alcohol-related offences. As with Ewert (1984), the Swedish authors interpret their results as stemming from late maturing boys' earlier attempts to gain prestige among age-mates by means of excessive drinking.

While we have no data on long-term consequences, we were also interested in whether our adolescent samples would reveal excessive drinking patterns among the late maturing boys. Using data on male users at ages 13,6 through 16,6, the monthly prevalence of drunkenness was compared across groups differing in maturational timing. The results are presented in Fig. 4.7. As can be seen, a smaller portion of the adolescents who were similar in rate of maturation reported experiencing drunkenness in the preceding month compared to faster and slower maturers. The difference is significant for the 13,6 year-olds ($p = < 0.04$, Fisher's test). Across age, the effects diminished gradually.

The next step was to correlate the data on annual consumption frequencies with the number of drunkenness episodes during the preceding

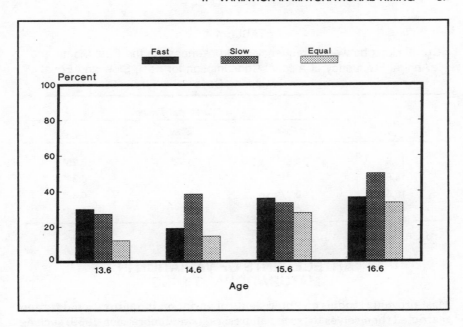

FIG. 4.7. Monthly prevalence of drunkenness in males. The Figure shows the percentages of boys who experienced at least one drunkenness episode in the month before the examination and who categorised themselves as faster, slower, or equal in rate of maturation at ages 13,6 through 16,6. The sample sizes were 98 boys at age 13,6, 102 boys at age 14,6, 120 boys at age 15,6 and 163 boys at age 16,6.

month. Following Andersson and Magnusson (1990), we predicted that the presumed excessiveness of late maturers' drinking would be revealed by a higher correlation, indicating a closer association between drinking as such and drunkenness. The results are given in Table 4.4.

Although all differences except one were in the expected direction, the mean correlation for slow maturers (0.54) did not differ greatly from that of fast maturers (0.46). Both differed, however, from the correlation between frequency of drinking and frequency of drunkenness (0.35) which was obtained for the equally maturing adolescents. Thus, being off-time seems to increase the risk of more excessive drinking patterns, at least in middle adolescence.

All of these studies have concentrated on maturational timing as a source of differences in adolescents' adjustment. The following section introduces a shift of perspective.

TABLE 4.4

Correlations between Frequency of Drunkenness in the Past Month and Annual Frequency of Alcohol Consumption for Fast, Slow and Equal Maturing Boys

| | Maturational Timing | | |
Age	Fast	Slow	Equal
13,6	0.67**	0.52*	0.25*
14,6	0.41*	0.59*	0.34*
15,6	0.37*	0.45	0.39*
16,6	0.40*	0.61**	0.43*

*p < 0.05,   **p < 0.01

ANTECEDENTS OF VARIATION IN MATURATIONAL TIMING

Most previous studies on antecedents of variation in maturational timing restricted themselves to "social addresses" (Bronfenbrenner, 1989) such as family size or social class. Until recently, research on genuine psychological mechanisms such as interpersonal stress has been largely non-existent.

Hereditary and Environmental Factors

Hamilton et al. (1988) demonstrated the effects of ballet training on menarcheal age. In dancers from both Chinese and American ballet companies, menarche was delayed by about six months for each year of premenarcheal training, up to a maximum of about two years above the respective population norms. In addition, Brooks-Gunn and Warren (1988) found a higher impact of training on maturational timing than of genetic influences as assessed by mothers' menarcheal age.

According to Surbey (1990), about 10% to 15% of the variability in the timing of menarche may be explained by genetic variation. Environmental influences, such as socio-economic status, family size and urbanisation may account for another 7% which presumably arises through differences in nutrition and health care. Factors such as exposure to sexual cues and psychological stress are also presumed to exercise an influence (Adams, 1981). Surbey (1990) studied effects of family composition and maturational timing. She compared girls whose father had been absent prior to menarche, with girls who had lived with both parents continuously. Father-absent girls matured four to five months earlier. This difference was even more pronounced when father-absence occurred before age 10, or when a stepfather lived at home. Even though the mothers had typically been early maturers—a finding which lent support to the idea of genetic influences—this effect could not account for the differences between the two groups of girls. Nor did making allowance for the higher stress experienced by father-absent girls lead to a substantial reduction in the relationship. There were also no differences between the groups in background variables such as social class or family size. Mekos (1991) confirmed Surbey's results on father absence. In particular, girls who had lost their fathers due to divorce and whose mothers had recently remarried, showed a greater increase in pubertal maturation. Among boys, however, the presence of a father at home accelerated pubertal growth. Thus, the consequences of father absence were in opposite directions, depending on gender.

Surbey's (1990) interest in family composition derived from Draper and Harpending's (1982) suggestion that humans utilise two alternative reproductive strategies both of which express attitudes towards males within families and are chosen on the basis of their adaptive function for different interpersonal climates. Girls who perceive early in life that males offer little and unreliable investment in parenting and consequently distrust them, adopt a reproductive strategy which involves early child-bearing without careful selection of a mate. Barkow (1984) expanded this hypothesis by suggesting that in addition to differing in their adoption of these behavioural strategies, father-absent and father-present girls should also differ in physical maturation. Specifically, he suggested that father-absent girls should mature earlier than father-present girls.

Recently, Maccoby (1991) has questioned whether the strategies proposed by Draper and Harpending (1982) are the only ones available. She argues that given scarce and unreliable resources from men, matrilineal patterns may prevail, whereby females rely on their mothers and sisters during child rearing. Additionally, they may pursue a strategy of restricted sexuality in order to establish a match between the resources available and the number of offspring. Thus, variation in the onset of puberty need not necessarily be seen as a response to negative experiences with regard to paternal investment.

Interpersonal Relations and Behaviours

There is an association between pubertal status and adolescent-parent conflicts, especially where these involve mothers (Steinberg, 1981; Savin-Williams & Small, 1986). Until recently, however, the direction of effects has not been at all clear.

In 1989, Steinberg described the results of a series of one-year follow-ups of teenage boys and girls. He used the same data set to analyse influences in both directions, thus implicitly assuming a reciprocal relation between physical maturation and adolescent-parent conflict. Young people perceived a relationship between pubertal status and level of conflict at home. For instance, the more advanced the adolescents' pubertal status in the preceding year, the greater the likelihood that both boys and girls would report an increase in conflicts with mothers and a decrease in closeness to fathers. The curvilinear trends indicate that the impact of pubertal changes seems to be especially intense during mid-puberty. Mekos (1991), however, found gender-specific effects. Girls who had been close to their fathers in the years prior to puberty, became more distant from them after puberty, while proximity to mothers increased as a function of low closeness before puberty. In contrast, boys showed increased tensions with their fathers but gained in closeness to their mothers.

When the relationship between closeness to parents in the previous year and change in pubertal status was examined, a different pattern emerged. Steinberg (1989) found effects for girls only: the greater the closeness of mothers to their daughters, the slower the rate of the latter's sexual maturation. These findings for girls were confirmed by Mekos (1991). She reported that among girls who showed higher levels of mother closeness before puberty, a higher proportion was still pre-menstrual after a period of two and a half years. Mekos found a similar result for boys; lower closeness with their mothers accelerated pubertal growth. With girls, Ellis (1991) found that higher degrees of self-governance, i.e. making decisions about important issues independent of parents, and higher peer orientation accelerated pubertal maturation compared to the past year. It is interesting to note in passing that the impact of the quality of social relations on female maturation finds a parallel in some non-human primates whose maturation is inhibited by the presence of mothers (Tardiff, 1984).

One possible interpretation of the mechanisms mediating this relation is the suggestion that stress may interfere with the hormonal activities involved in pubertal maturation (Whiting, 1965). Another, is to infer a pheromonal process which is known to function in synchronising menstrual cycles among women (Graham & McGrew, 1980). Still more provocative, however, is the evolutionary perspective offered by Steinberg (1989) and Belsky, Steinberg and Draper (1991a). They suggest that the heightened adolescent-parent conflict at mid-puberty is an influence which has evolved in the service of increased reproductive fitness.

In their view, the processes of affective and physical separation between parents and offspring which occur during puberty in non-human primates and which also occurred with our early ancestors, resemble present-day adolescent-parent conflict in humans. They suggest that further support for this view is provided by the institutionalised mechanisms which involved separating teenagers from their parents during puberty and which were still quite common in recent historical times. Steinberg quotes practices like the placing-out of youngsters who were sent to live with other families, or the removal of pubertal children to separate residences.

Surbey's (1990) study was retrospective and Steinberg (1989) was only able to rely on a one-year follow-up. In contrast, Moffitt, Caspi, Belsky and Silva (1990) utilised data from a long-term longitudinal study carried out in New Zealand. They attempted to predict the age of menarche by weight, behaviour problems and family conflict at age 7 and father absence for at least one year up to the age of 11. A higher percentage of the early maturers had experienced father absence before puberty than on-time and late maturers. Furthermore, an acceleration of about three months remained after controlling for pre-pubertal weight. Family conflict and father-absence in childhood had direct prospective effects on age at menarche, whereas behaviour problems and weight did not mediate the effects. The study can be seen as providing general support for Surbey's (1990) retrospective findings.

In response to criticism of their approach, Belsky, Steinberg and Draper (1991b) insisted on maintaining that early maturation as observed in father-absent families cannot be explained by concurrent factors like reduced monitoring, modelling, or perceived maternal attitudes about sexuality. Whether the evolutionary underpinnings raised by Draper and Harpending (1982) provide the right heuristic is a matter for discussion. Whatever the outcome of that discussion, a better understanding of contextual influences on the process of biological maturation is an important goal which requires serious attention (Gottlieb, 1991).

Finally, let us speculate on the role of maturational timing in a particular ecological transition. Acculturative stress due to immigration or other types of cultural association may increase family strains and lead to variations in maturational timing. Changes in health care or nutrition and cultural differences in developmental timetables (Feldman & Rosenthal, 1991) may also have bearing upon the timing of puberty. Silbereisen and Schmitt-Rodermund (1991) carried out pilot research on a particular set of immigrants to Germany. Their ancestors had emigrated to Russia, Poland and Romania, many years—sometimes centuries—ago. Because of the economic downturn in the East and the greater mobility resulting from political liberalisation, they decided to re-emigrate to Germany.

Preliminary analyses of in-depth interviews suggest that accelerated maturation in response to adaptive strains and acculturative stress may indeed take place. Of 36 families interviewed, 30 experienced no change in family cohesion. The parents reported that nine of the young people from the latter group of families were early developers and four were late. Two of the four families with increased strains, however, reported early development and none of the adolescents in this group was late. One of the two early maturers, for instance, left the family soon after immigration and went to live on his own. The two families with improved relations, reported one late developer and one as on-time. Thus, there was a greater degree of off-time maturation among families that reported a change in their family integration.

Another effect of acculturation emerged in the majority of the families. Irrespective of the reasons for variation in maturational timing, early developers had the advantage that their more adult-like physical appearance persuaded their parents that they should be given more leeway. In comparison with normal and late developers, for instance, they expected their children to go out partying on average one year earlier. A possible effect of such earlier autonomy is that it helps the young people concerned to catch up with the behaviours and privileges of the local German age-mates, thus easing their cultural integration.

In contrast, late developers were treated in a much more traditional way. As a result, they became isolated from the local German age-mates, accentuated traditional role expectations and ultimately preferred cultural affirmation over adaptation. One of the late-maturing females, for instance, did not go out, engaged in domestic roles and demonstrated opposition to the liberal attitudes of local German youths.

In sum, despite the risks of negative affect and self-esteem which early maturation can bring to girls (Alsaker, 1990; Brooks-Gunn & Warren, 1989), those maturing early in the acculturative context studied by Silbereisen and Schmitt-Rodermund (1991), may profit from a better goodness-of-fit (Lerner, 1985). In the specific circumstances of migration, they enjoyed a better match between the requirements of the local German social context and their physical and behavioural characteristics. This result on the impact of culture brings to mind an earlier research finding (Kimmel & Weiner, 1985). When Italian boys were compared with Italian-American boys, only the latter showed the well-known positive relation between early maturation and favourable self-appreciation.

OUTLOOK

This chapter has presented a broad overview of research on the antecedents and consequences of maturational timing during adolescence. Following the chronological order in which research perspectives were developed, we started with the sequelae of maturational timing and found that differences in the pace of pubertal maturation have consequences for adolescents' social relationships. Boys and girls who mature faster than their age-mates report more contacts with older adolescents and engage in intimate heterosexual contacts earlier than adolescents of the same age.

Relations with parents are also affected by maturational timing. In sum, maturational timing emerges as an important variable in understanding individual differences in adolescents' social behaviours.

Social stimulus value and selective peer affiliation were presented as the mechanisms linking maturational timing and problem behaviour. However, Caspi & Moffitt (1991) offer an alternative explanation for the findings concerning early-maturing girls. They suggest that stressful transitions such as early maturation serve to accentuate individual differences which already exist as a result of attempts to assimilate new experiences into one's behavioural repertoire. They argue that early pubertal growth has a magnifying effect on individual differences in emotional adaptation which can already be identified in late childhood. Caspi and Moffitt's ideas are provocative and require further study.

Next, we proceeded to discuss research on why adolescents differ in their pace of maturation. Since genetic influences account for differences in maturational timing to only a small extent, investigators have sought other explanations. Their findings suggest that maturational timing is influenced by social processes and especially by strains in the family context. Familial stress and the absence of the biological father were found to accelerate the pubertal development of girls. Research in this field has only recently started, however and investigators are far from a full understanding of the processes mediating between experiences in the family and maturational timing. Thus, although the female menstrual cycle is known to be influenced by stress, it is not yet appropriate to assume that physical effects of a similar nature occur during the period before females reach the reproductive stage.

Some recent research activities have been stimulated by ideas derived from socio-biological approaches. Early maturation, for instance, has been seen as a manifestation of a particular reproductive strategy, which typically occurs in situations where further emotional investment from parents seems unlikely to take place. Provocative though such ideas may be, they are perhaps less important than attempts to provide more detailed descriptions of the family processes which are likely to accelerate pubertal development. Recent findings concerning the gender-differential effect of father absence and the different impact of mother-son and father-daughter relations still need to be integrated within a common framework. The same is also true of findings concerning maturation and cultural context. There is evidence that effects of maturational timing on adolescents' psychological well-being and behaviour depend in part on the norms and opportunities within the prevailing cultural context. The sample case of re-emigrants to Germany suggests that early maturation may even serve as a protective factor by providing the adolescents concerned with behavioural opportunities similar to those available to their German classmates.

We have tried to show that pubertal development is an important source of individual differences in adolescent development. Since pace of maturation is related, at least in part, to processes which take place in childhood, we require prospective longitudinal research starting long before adolescence in order to understand the pattern of long-term adaptation and functioning. Such designs will allow analysis of the degree of reciprocity between maturational timing and the closeness of the parent-child relationship.

Developing such prospective studies is not the only possible research strategy. The re-analysis of existing data sets and further study of samples originally assessed in childhood may provide useful information on the relation between strains in childhood and the timing of puberty.

Recent work on the relationship between biological and social processes and the wider ecological and cultural context has already opened new horizons for further investigation. The evidence of reciprocal effects which has emerged from this research raises important questions concerning young people's adjustment to and integration within different social spheres.

CHAPTER FIVE

Dating and Interpersonal Relationships in Adolescence

Bruna Zani

Traditionally, adolescence is considered to be the age of sexual attraction and emergent love. During adolescence, youngsters become aware, probably for the first time, of their existential loneliness and unique individuality: sexual attraction and love help them break away from this isolation (Fromm, 1956) and begin to establish close intimate relationships. These processes run parallel to the cognitive transformations of adolescence which involve greater capacity for understanding oneself and the awareness of one's individuality.

Today, interest in members of the opposite sex outside the family is expressed in a general context which is rather different from that of a few decades ago. Research carried out in Europe and the United States indicates that important changes have occurred in relationships between the sexes and that these have also had an effect on the adolescent age-group. The habits of the adult world have altered, as have the ideas and expectations of many parents and adults about the sexual behaviour of their adolescent children (Allen, 1987; Bonini and Zani, 1991). As a result, one can now speak of a "new sexual morality" in which the attitudes of today's adolescents differ from those of 20 or 30 years ago in at least three important aspects: they are more open about sexual matters; they see sexual behaviour as a matter of private rather than public morality; they appear to be more conscious of the importance of associating sex with steady, long-term relationships (see Coleman and Hendry, 1990, p.141).

Two types of cultural and social influence play a major role in influencing the way in which people conceive of affectivity and heterosexual relationships. Through the mass-media, the wider culture or macrosystem propagates and imposes particular models and these combine with models presented by the microsystem in which the individual is located, i.e. the family and peer group.

It is particularly in the family that young people learn the rules about couple relations, assimilating the life-style of the parent couple and acquiring the relational rules about how affection and love are expressed. Often, they end up by adopting them in their own couple relationships, despite making an effort to differentiate themselves from the parent-linked model. Peer group affiliations also play an important role. They are essential to healthy identity development in adolescence and allow teenagers to explore interests and ideologies, to test their skills in forming intimate peer relationships and to abandon psychological dependence on parents. As Mitchell (1976) has noted, the need for intimacy is not satisfied in group settings nearly as efficiently as are the needs for recognition, belonging, and esteem. However, the group provides the initial meeting place, the trial ground, the experimental arena where tentatively formed bonds hopefully will lead to intimate exchange.

Inevitably, however, the new extra-family affective ties which the adolescent creates and the gradual focusing of affection on a single partner as a response to personal needs tend to lead to radical changes in the system of relationships with parents and friends. The analysis of such changes in the relational world of the adolescent is the topic of the first section in this chapter. Is a partner really so important for an adolescent? What meanings and functions does the couple relationship have in adolescence? Working within a psychoanalytic perspective, Blos (1962) has underlined the psychological importance of the love relationship. He argues that it helps the adolescent to become independent, contributing significantly to the emotive separation from parents and guaranteeing satisfaction of the need for security. According to Samet and Kelly (1987) and Silbereisen and Noack (1990), it also facilitates awareness of sexual self-identity, provides important confirmation of self-image, self-esteem and sex-role identity and helps achieve a synthesis between tenderness and sensuality, a characteristic of a mature genital relationship.

The literature concerning the role and meaning of partner and couple relationships in adolescence is certainly less rich than that on family relationships and the peer group. Nonetheless, researchers have shown a growing interest in this topic. The second section of the chapter will review the theoretical and empirical work which has been carried out.

The third section will be concerned with adolescent intimacy. The need for intimacy influences all adolescent patterns and habits—especially those relating to close friendship and romantic interests. It begins to manifest itself in the pre-adolescent years, when the desire for a personal confidant becomes central. It becomes stronger in middle and late adolescence, as the partial disintegration of the peer group and the tendency towards heterosexual pairing-up begin to take place. During this period, physical, cognitive and social changes contribute to the adolescent's increased capacity to be intimate. Deriving from Erikson's (1968) work, several authors have given particular attention to the interplay between identity and intimacy development: identity formation is seen as a major task of adolescence and intimate relationships serve as an important context for this self-development work (Paul and White, 1990). The discussion of this work will aim to highlight the most significant findings which have emerged.

CHANGES IN THE AFFECTIONAL WORLD OF ADOLESCENTS

The shift from childhood to adolescence, as authors from a range of different conceptual backgrounds have pointed out, is marked by changes in many aspects of social life and interpersonal relations. Adolescents begin to encounter many new demands and expectations in social situations and require different social interaction skills from those employed in the childhood years.

Family relations undergo remarkable alterations. The attainment of independence, one of the central themes in adolescent development, requires the renegotiation of relations with parents and movement from a situation characterised by compliance to one of greater mutuality between the parties. This occurs through the process of individuation (Youniss and Smollar, 1985, 1990; Grotevant and Cooper, 1986). Adolescents learn to express, rather than hide their ideas and to take responsibility for them when challenged by their parents. They start to assert themselves as individuals and parents begin to recognise them as such. At the same time, young people seek their parents' acceptance and respect for the new individuals they have become. It is important to note that this process of separation concerns not only the adolescent, but also the parents. They have to detach themselves from their children, accept their movement towards adulthood and help them achieve their independence. The way in which the parents cope with this detachment has effects on the process of growth and autonomy of their sons or daughters.

Peer relations also show development during adolescence. They become more intense and extensive and fulfil multiple functions such as socialisation into heterosexual behaviour, facilitation of identity development and organisation of status structures. Social interaction with peers also provides the opportunity to experience emotions and express feelings for age-mates of one sex or the other and to develop skills in dealing with and expressing such emotions (Coleman and Hendry, 1990).

Dunphy (1972) suggests that peer groups serve primarily to socialise adolescents into appropriate heterosexual interests and behaviour patterns. Peer groups evolve through several stages during adolescence. The isolated, unisexual cliques or pubertal groups (Meltzer, 1981) which are typical of early adolescence are succeeded by the fully developed crowds or heterosexual cliques in close association of mid-adolescence and these, in turn, lead to the relatively independent, heterosexual cliques or loosely associated groups of couples which emerge in later adolescence.

A study by Brown, Eicher and Petrie (1986), involving 1300 adolescents, supports the view that the importance of crowd affiliation declines across the teenage years. Younger adolescents generally attached great importance to group membership, viewing the group as a source of self-identification, a facilitation of social interactions, an aid in building reputation, image and status and as a source of emotional support. Older respondents laid more emphasis on the disadvantages of crowd affiliation. They expressed dissatisfaction with the conformity demands of the group and preference for the smaller and more intimate friendship networks in which they were involved.

According to the "focal model" of adolescent development (Coleman and Hendry, 1990), attitudes to all the relationships in which teenagers are involved (parents, peers, friends, partner) change as a function of age and, more importantly, concerns about different issues reach a peak at different stages in the adolescent process. From a situation where their main interest is in peer-orientated activities, adolescents tend to gravitate towards more exclusive patterns of relationship such as courting and romance, which gradually become central areas of interest.

In its turn, the presence of a partner brings radical changes to the network of relations in which the adolescent is involved. However, despite the extent of these changes, researchers have as yet given little attention to this topic.

More consideration has been addressed to the so-called "parent-peer issue", i.e. the question of the relative influence of parents and peers upon adolescents. It has been amply demonstrated that the peer group plays an important function in the adolescent's emergence from the family towards independence (Fend, 1990; Palmonari, Pombeni and Kirchler, 1989, 1990; see also Kirchler, Palmonari and Pombeni in this volume). Research has also shown that both parents and peers represent non-competitive sources of support: whether a particular issue is referred to parents or to peers depends on the type of issue which is involved.

Much less systematic attention has been given to how the introduction of a new element into the affective system of the adolescent (the presence of a steady partner, or even simple infatuation) leads to changes in relationships with the family and the peer group. In the next section, we will discuss the multiple significant functions which the partner relationship serves and the meanings it has. Attention will be given to the influence of a partner relationship on peer and family relations.

Group-partner Relationships

We have seen that there seems to be a uni-directional movement in which the adolescent joins a peer group and then breaks away as a closer and more involved couple relationship is established. The presence of steady couples in peer groups of Italian adolescents is generally very high. In research carried out in two towns in North Italy, in Bologna (Berti Ceroni, Bonini, Cerchierini and Zani, 1987) and Ferrara (Zani, Altieri and Signani, 1992), we asked teenagers if there were steady couples among the members of the group to which they belonged. More than 65% of adolescents answered positively. Given this percentage, it might be argued that the group is the ideal place for the development and acceptance of a close relationship. However, our findings show that the partner-group relation is not always easy. Let us examine the results in more detail.

Three main orientations were identified: a) the partner demands no change and the relationship with the group remains unaltered; b) the affectional relationship affects actual presence in the group, and conflict over the choice between group and partner is overcome in a variety of subjective ways, which often involve discomfort; c) the group loses its importance since the intimate relationship is given priority.

Major differences emerged according to the sex and level of schooling of the adolescents. Males tend to complain about having to make choices, since their young partners feel the need to spend much of their free time as a pair. Girls seem more concerned about forming intimate relationships of an exclusive nature while boys try much more to reconcile the formation of a steady couple and belonging to a group. In their opinion, the ideal situation is one in which the girl is a member of the group and it is not necessary to modify the frequency or venue places for meeting-up. The difficulty of having to make choices is clearly summed by one non-student boy who says: "It's different being with friends. It's interesting, fun. Especially at my age, you feel tied down because your girl-friend wants to be with you all the time, while sometimes you just want to be with your friends, playing around and enjoying yourself".

For males, therefore the affectional relationship is perceived as being important, though demanding and at times all-consuming. In contrast, the group has a liberatory function, free of responsibilities. This explains the importance attributed to belonging to a group and maintaining relationships with peers, even if one has a girl-friend.

Girls present a more differentiated pattern depending on level of schooling. For girls who have left school, it is not possible to "enter" or "leave" their heterosexual group on the grounds that they have or do not have a partner. The rule adopted by this kind of group allows them to have a partner only if they continue to participate in all group activities and do not disregard group life. Otherwise, they have to choose between the partner and the group. With high school groups, on the other hand, the partner is admitted, providing the couple behaves as though it were not a couple. Here too there is an implicit internal rule —"we are all equal". Affectionate behaviour directed towards one's partner is only permitted outside the group. Girls from vocational schools—i.e. schools which prepare students for a "low-qualification" profession and which are attended for 2 to 3 years after the end of compulsory education—tend to leave their groups generally because they have formed couples with adult partners. This often means entrance into a new group consisting of a small number of adult couples. These girls sometimes express feelings of regret at the loss of the "previous group" and the sensation of "feeling caged in". Becoming part of a steady couple seems almost to have forced these girls into a context which is precociously limited (Berti Ceroni et al., 1987).

To a certain extent the group represents an alternative to the couple relationship. Like some kind of grand partner it satisfies all the demands that arise within it, provided that faithfulness is guaranteed. Only intimate affairs which originate and develop inside the group are acceptable, since they do not interfere with meeting times and places or rules of interaction between the various members.

Given the importance of belonging to a peer group, we inquired whether young adolescent couples feel it necessary to plan their future and whether or not the peer group is the best place to help them make decisions. Respondents declared that they only rarely engaged in planning a future life with their partner. In cases where the relationship had been a steady one for a number of years, both males and females reported similar difficulties, independent of schooling. To admit to having plans for a life as a couple seems to indicate the assumption of responsibilities associated with entry into the adult world. Among those engaged in "short-lived affairs" nobody considered marriage with the partner involved. In fact, the nature of their affair did not allow it.

The extent to which an adolescent couple engages in future planning is inversely related to the level of schooling: the lower the level, the greater the emotional and affective investment in the partner. Where schooling lasts for longer, there is more resistance to becoming involved in close steady relationships and even to facing the idea of marriage.

Parental Reactions to a Dating Relationship

The formation of an emotional relationship outside the home has inevitable repercussions on the system of family relations. The established arrangements of the preceding phase of family life are brought into question and certain adjustments which affect all members of the family nucleus, become necessary.

Parents, in particular, must learn to accept an emotive distancing of their children and the development of an emotional relationship outside the family. They also have to accept a mixture of regressive and progressive tendencies, which are typically adolescent and manifest themselves in flights forward and sudden retreats back into childhood. Other difficulties arise from the changes in needs and preferences of the adolescent and how these link to the growing demands for independence from the family, a process which represents one of the final outcomes of adolescent development. Within this context, first love experiences are very important in that they allow adolescents to free themselves affectively from their parents and to put themselves on an equal footing with adults.

Research carried out in Bologna (Italy) on a sample group of parents investigated the strategies used in dealing with separation from their children (Bonini and Zani, 1991). We interviewed 43 fathers and 42 mothers from two different cultural levels (medium-high and medium-low) and who had male or female adolescent children. Results show that parents' reactions to their child's dating relationship differed as a function of the sex-composition of the parent-child dyad.

In general, mothers, whatever their cultural level, feel much more involved when the daughter, as opposed to the son, begins to distance herself affectively. Contradictory and ambivalent feelings are expressed indicating a situation which is seen as problematic, even for oneself: the breaking of well-established affective arrangements, the need to re-define intra-family relationships, the recognition of change. Reactions take on different connotations. Along with the joy of seeing their daughter happy, there is sometimes a feeling of jealousy and an awareness of having lost an exclusive position in relations with the daughter. This may be expressed in a sense of irritation towards the new relationship with the boy, who is often almost "imposed" on family members without much thought about disruption of affective arrangements. On other occasions a sense of guilt is expressed, a feeling of having failed to do something which might have pushed the daughter into finding a more satisfying affectional relationship elsewhere:

At the time I took it in my stride, even though it was all a bit sudden and she was still quite young. When I realised it was something serious I got a bit worried, mainly because it made me feel guilty because I thought she had developed this very close relationship out of a lack of affection on my part and that somehow she was trying to make up for it ... it is a question I still ask myself today (Bonini and Zani, 1991, p. 150).

When the son is involved in a couple relationship, mothers' responses follow different directions. In general they claim there has been no change in their attitudes and feelings, since what has happened is "a natural thing" and they are more than pleased since they consider it a positive experience for a boy. Other mothers however express more ambivalent feelings in that the satisfaction of seeing their son grow up and mature is tempered by the disturbing realisation that he is growing away from the family. This leads to feeling of being abandoned and consequently, of jealousy. One way of dealing with this jealousy is to transpose to the "other", the son's partner, certain aspects of her own role, in which, in a sort of idealised continuity the task of accomplishing what the mother had started is entrusted to the partner:

> I had a few big fits of jealousy but now I'm trying to get over it rationally, though I had hoped it would blow over by itself. Now I'd like him to find a pretty girl who loves him and tries to change him, or at any rate to have some influence over him where I couldn't (Bonini and Zani, 1991, p. 151).

Different ways of responding to the adolescent's new needs also emerged among the fathers. For one group of subjects (medium-high cultural level) the affective independence of their daughters is something expected and normal, it is part of the developmental process of the family and is helpful to the young person in this delicate period of growth. Strong feelings of ambivalence which has not been fully resolved, are also expressed. These include desire for and satisfaction at the "normality" of the new development coupled with fear and sadness at the prospect of imminent abandonment:

> I found it hard to accept my little girl becoming a young woman ... but I did so in the end. In fact, in a way it seemed right that she'd reached this stage of development, that physically speaking things were going like they were supposed to. At that particular point I wasn't struck in any negative way by her having a steady boyfriend. There might have been some doubt about her starting so soon, but then again it wasn't really soon ... because if she'd started it ... no, I don't suppose it was soon (Bonini and Zani, 1991, p. 152).

It is interesting to note that some of the fathers interviewed refer to the concept of "loyalty" (Boszormenyi-Nagy and Spark, 1973) defined as a commitment to the conservation of the group (in this case the family). This might be described as a kind of obligation on the adolescent to restore to the parents a part of the "availability" she had once enjoyed and for which she is indebted. At play here is the invisible network of expectations which govern the relations between members of the group: the establishment of a new relationship, the partner relationship for example, raises the issue of new pledges of loyalty. As always vertical pledges of loyalty (with regard to parents) tend to clash with horizontal ones (towards the partner):

> I'm happy if she has a steady boyfriend, we don't want to have a monopoly on her love; the fact is (and I told her so) that the relationships have to be well balanced ... I know it's right that kids should have relationships, but if that means excluding the family, then it's wrong (Bonini and Zani, 1991, p. 153).

Note that a similar problem may have emerged at an earlier stage with regard to peer associations. However, it is with the presence of a partner that the issue of loyalty emerges as crucial: parents and peers tend not to be seen as competing sources of advice and support (Palmonari et al., 1989; 1990), whereas the partner is considered to be more intrusive and more threatening to the balance of intra-family relationships.

The second group of fathers (the medium-low cultural level) express difficulty in calmly accepting the growing up of their daughters. They are concerned that they (the daughters) might be forced into choices which are not of their own making. It is almost as if they fear that having fewer cultural opportunities brings with it a greater risk of running up against adolescent developmental problems.

All of these reactions refer to relations with female children. Attitudes towards male affective development seem more superficial. It seems that the sons are not really expected to have an emotional life at all. In the first place, they are unlikely to be asked for any account of their affective affairs and further, it seems to be assumed that there is little room in "mens' talk" to discuss matters of the heart. Alongside the apparent lack of reaction concerning the new affectional situation of the son, jokes and witty remarks are often used as a means of facilitating communication in an area which is clearly experienced as embarrassing and difficult. Fathers, generally tend to speak to their sons about "women", or rather "not women, but dolls!" and always in a joking vein as if wanting to establish an atmosphere of complicity.

The partner, or future choice of partner, represents—especially for parents with daughters—a constant preoccupation in the imagination. If the daughters are still very young, the fears are vague and unclear. Very often the hope is expressed that "they don't make the wrong decision, get the wrong man", or else that they don't fall into a relationship which might leave scars; get involved with "someone who might make her suffer, where she might get burnt". If the daughters are older, the worry is more about marriage, "the fact that she might make a mistake she'll rue for the rest of her life", or else about the character of the partner that "he's got too big a place in her affections ... she'd do better going out with other boys to see ...". Fears are also expressed, though in a roundabout, indirect fashion, about sexual violence and abuse (Bonini and Zani, 1991).

Another issue addressed in the literature concerns the role the parents play in their children's selection of dating partners. The early work of Bates (1942) showed that parents are involved in such decisions to a greater extent than our "free will" norms of mate-selection might suggest. More recent researchers have presented evidence that young adults' dating involvement is associated with parental reaction, but the nature of this association varies across studies. Lewis (1973) and Parks, Stan and Eggert (1983), for example, found a positive relationship between dating partners' level of involvement in their romantic relationships and how supportive they perceived their parents to be. On the other hand, Driscoll, Davis and Lipetz (1972) found that romantic love was enhanced not by parental support, but by parental interference, the so-called "Romeo and Juliet effect". According to Leslie, Huston and Johnson (1986), this apparent contradiction may be partially due to the discrepancy between the theoretical basis for the questions and the empirical methods utilised. The different studies focus only on how parents influence children. They neglect the reciprocal nature of interpersonal influence.

In their own research involving students (mean age 19.9) at Pennsylvania State University, Leslie et al. (1986) analysed the reciprocal influence process occurring between parents and young adult children. Results indicate that the young adults' own attempts to influence parents increased with their stage of relationship involvement: the more committed the son/daughter to the relationship, the more likely he/she was to inform the parents of the relationship and to try to influence their opinion of it. Parents, in turn, were more likely to support relationships in which their offspring were highly involved. However the amount of support provided by parents seemed relatively unimportant where understanding changes in dating relationship were concerned. Two alternative explanations are offered. It is possible that parental approval, while not moving couples to higher levels of involvement, may allow (or be geared to allowing) the adolescent freedom to maintain the relationship at the level at which it is comfortable, or to evaluate it according to whatever criteria they consider important, without having to be concerned with parental disapproval. A second possibility is that parents' primary effect is indirect, in that adolescents hesitate to become involved in relationships of which their parents would not approve. Young people know their parents' views and may simply avoid informing their parents of a questionable relationship, thus blocking expected disapproval and its effect on the dating relationship (Leslie et al., 1986).

Another indirect way in which parents may influence their adolescent children is through their own example of how to live an affectional relationship. But is there evidence that the parental couple serve as a model for adolescent couples? Findings from the research mentioned earlier (Berti Ceroni et al., 1987) show that this influence is mediated by gender.

Girls proved very critical towards the parental couple. A few of them considered their parents a "good couple" and identified positive elements in their relationship which might be useful in their own case in a future couple relation. "Getting on well", "being balanced", "respect", and above all "loving each other" were repeatedly emphasised. These categories however were different from those which were generally sought after in their own couple relationship. Some other girls expressed categorical affirmations such as "I wouldn't use anyone as a model", even when emphasising positive aspects of their parents' relationship. One girl said:

"I think my parents are great as a couple, but I'm looking for a different relationship ... I wouldn't copy anything from their relationship". The majority of the girls judged the parental couple relationship in an utterly negative way: "My parents aren't a couple. If getting married means being like them, then I'd rather not get married" (Berti Ceroni et al., 1987, p. 122).

These answers should be seen in the light of other data which emerged from the research, namely differences between males and females regarding the parental relationship and the degree and quality of their communication with each other. The girls, to a much greater extent than the boys, considered the relationship to be difficult, conflictual and unsatisfactory.

Among the boys the majority considered their parents' relationship as "good". Many of them listed a series of parental qualities which they saw as desirable for their own future relationships. Only a few gave critical opinions, underlining the completely different nature of their experience due to the "uniqueness" of their own relationship. Some pointed to the "generation gap" as the obvious consequence of a different approach to various situations, including the affectional relationship. One boy said: "I wouldn't copy anything they do because I've got a completely different picture of what a couple should be like. They're old, too respectful, they never joke, they're a bit dead" (Berti Ceroni et al., 1987, p. 123).

Taken as a whole, the group of boys seemed very conservative with regard to both values and behavioural models and was less willing to expend energy in order to obtain change. This was the case even though they had found it less difficult to win those early concessions of freedom which had cost girls a good deal of effort and often given rise to "fights" with their parents. It appeared that "everything is OK" for boys and that to them, the family represented a very important reference model which could be imitated to the full, or at least in the more important aspects. Girls expressed more criticism and were generally more attentive in looking for changes in all aspects of their relational life, a situation which indicated new and different needs for their own future couple relationship.

THE MEANING OF THE DATING/LOVE RELATIONSHIP IN ADOLESCENCE

This section will first examine the functions served by the heterosexual, love/dating relationship in adolescence. It will then examine the impact of such a relationship on the self, the selection of a partner and the variables affecting the development of the dating relationship. Finally, attention will be focused upon the social competence necessary for successfully confronting the tasks and demands of a relationship with the opposite sex.

The Dating Process

Dating, i.e. the independent arrangement whereby a boy and girl arrange to meet alone or in a group at a specific place at a scheduled time, is a phenomenon of the twentieth century (Roche, 1986). Feinstein and Ardon (1973) argue that, even though the characteristics of the dating rituals have changed, the essential goal has remained the same; the achievement of a constant adult relationship model, through practice and experimentation in heterosexual relationships.

McCabe (1984) has suggested that as a result of the contemporary trend towards earlier commencement of dating and later entry into marriage, the date has become an end in itself; a social experience, and not just a part of the courtship process, as it was in the past.

Dating is recognisd as serving several important functions. In their classical analysis, Skipper and Nass (1966) identified four main functions: a) recreation, a source of entertainment and immediate enjoyment; b) socialisation, an opportunity for members of the opposite sex to learn co-operation, consideration, responsibility and to develop appropriate techniques for interacting with other people; c) status grading, a means of gaining status with one's peers by dating and being seen with persons rated as "highly desirable"; d) mate-selection/courtship, an opportunity to associate with others for the purpose of selecting a marriage partner.

McCabe (1984) and Rice (1984) identified three other reasons for dating: a) sexual experimentation, satisfaction or even exploitation; b) companionship, a means of interaction and shared activities in an opposite-sex relationship; c) intimacy, an opportunity to establish a unique, meaningful relationship with an individual of the opposite sex (Roscoe, Diana and Brooks, 1987). Paul and White (1990) pointed out that identity formation and individuation should be added to these lists, since dating can be considered as one of the forms of peer interaction which help adolescents clarify their identities and begin separating from their families of origin (see also Erikson, 1968; Sullivan, 1953).

Relatively few studies have focused on reasons for dating in adolescence. Roscoe, Diana and Brooks (1987) found that adolescents at different developmental stages (early, middle and late) have different reasons for dating. Early and middle adolescents (i.e. 6th to 11th graders from small towns in a mid-western American state) held an egocentric and immediate gratification orientation toward dating functions. They selected, in order of importance, recreation, intimacy and status as primary reasons. In contrast, late adolescents (college students) placed greater emphasis on reciprocal aspects in a relationship and referred more frequently to intimacy, companionship and socialisation as the major reasons.

Berti Ceroni et al. (1987) asked Italian adolescents (15-18) from different types of school to give reasons for the importance of a partner. The group who had already left school considered having a partner to be more important than did those at high school. The desire to find a partner was more consistent when the adolescent was in a position socially nearer to that of the adult. Where motivation to search for a partner was concerned, the largest percentage of answers referred to a need for affective support. The partner was seen as someone who can facilitate and protect the process of separation from parents, with whom one's intimate feelings can be shared. The second most frequent category referred to maturational needs. A partner was seen as someone who helps achieve self-realisation, increase personal self-esteem and resolve adolescent uneasiness. The needs of a sexual nature were of decidedly lower importance, confirming that adolescents usually separate affectivity from sexuality. Lower still in the percentage rates, were needs associated with exchange, i.e. where the other's needs are taken into consideration. Finally, came ideas associated with the need to project oneself into the future and make plans for a life together. Often these were expressed in romantic terms, with a need to believe in the "love story" of films. These motivations were mainly expressed by non-students who were inclined, to a greater extent than the other subjects, to plan for an immediate future (see also Zani, 1991).

These studies provide some evidence that dates and heterosexual relationships are not only an important part of young people's current social lives, but that they also seem to have a positive impact upon the expectations of young people about an ultimate marriage, even though it may still be regarded as a relatively distant event. As Long (1983; 1989) has emphasised, heterosexual involvement, especially in young women, offers different kinds of social satisfaction, including the attention and liking of male admirers, the approval of parents and friends, the respect of peers and the achievement of a higher social status. Such satisfaction is an important source of self-respect, so that greater heterosexual involvement may be associated with more favourable self-evaluation.

Support for this link between heterosexual involvement and self-evaluation has been obtained in studies carried out in different cultural contexts, with adolescents and young adults. Samet and Kelly (1987), for example, found a positive link between steady dating and the perception of self-esteem and sex role identity among Israeli high school students. Adolescents who had steady dates, compared to those who did not, were perceived by their peers as possessing higher self-esteem and higher correspondence to their gender identity.

College women in the USA (average age 19) who have a steady boyfriend were found to show higher self-esteem (Long, 1983). In a further study, Long (1989) tested undergraduate females (mean age of 17.7 at the onset of the study) on four occasions with an interval of one year between each testing. Those with greater heterosexual involvement, defined in terms of both commitment (having a steady boyfriend) and constancy (frequency of dating), were more serious about their boyfriends, showed higher self-evaluations, were more sure of marrying, and expected to marry at a younger age.

Complementary results were obtained from another study, which showed that American college students believed the break-up of dating relationships to be associated with a loss of self-esteem. This was particularly the case where the break-up involved rejection or loss to a rival (Mathes, Adams and Davis, 1985).

These studies show that the absence of a partner or the break-up of a dating relationship can be sources of problems for the young person. There are, however, a variety of effects of steady dating needs which require further consideration.

Though dating can be a positive and self-enhancing relationship, it can also have a range of negative effects. It may favour premature emotional involvement in the absence of sufficient emotional maturity (Sullivan, 1953). It may bring about peer pressures on those who fail to achieve the "norm" of dating (Brown, 1982) If it leads to a prematurely exclusive relationship, it may serve to create a premature crystallisation of identity, "hindering an actualisation of one's full potential with a variety of people" (Samet and Kelly, 1987, p.244).

Sequence of the Dating Relationship

While dating, the couple proceeds through a series of stages, each of which represents a change in the quality of the relationship (McCabe, 1984). Generally it begins with a period of casual outings, where both boy and girl may go out with other partners. Through time, the individual enters into a steady relationship with one partner. There is a greater commitment to one another than before and this close, intimate relationship may eventually lead to engagement and marriage, or to some form of permanent relationship.

Gender differences in these social patterns begin to emerge during mid-adolescence. Boys continue to participate in group activities whilst beginning to date girls. Girls, on the other hand, begin to discard youth club activities and prefer smaller networks, attending heterosexual meeting places and finally going steady with one boy (Coleman and Hendry, 1990). Roche (1986) showed that during the early stages of dating (dating with no particular affection, as opposed to dating with affection, but not love, or dating and being in love) males and females differ widely in their beliefs as to what is proper sexual behaviour. Males are more permissive and expect sexual intimacy sooner, while females tend to tie sexual intimacy to love and commitment. Similar findings emerge from other research (Schulz et al., 1977; Knox and Wilson, 1981). At later stages (dating one person only and being in love; becoming engaged), this "gender gap" virtually disappears (Roche, 1986). It is particularly in the early period of dating that male/female dissonance concerning their different reasons for dating and the asymmetry in what is considered proper sexual conduct can be a source of conflict and frustration. This may also explain why most dating relationships are so short-lived during the "practising stage" (Paul and White, 1990).

Why does the development of dating relationships follow different paths in males and females? Despite the political and ideological influence of the women's movement, traditional sex role orientations still seem to be powerful (Peplau, Rubin and Hill, 1977; Offer, Ostrov and Howard, 1981).

In the beginning, girls frequently seek a platonic, romantic love affair, while boys are more often attracted by sexuality alone. To a large extent, this pattern can be traced back to the process of socialisation. Boys learn social roles which lead them to desire physical intimacy from the dating relationship and to use love and affection for bargaining purposes, while girls strive for greater commitment from the relationship and so exchange sex for promises of love and marriage (Maddock, 1973). McCandless (1970) suggested that males approach the dating relationship from a psycho-biological standpoint while females approach it from a psycho-affectional perspective. There is some evidence that traditional role-playing persists, with males being more concerned with encouraging intercourse and females with avoiding it. Sexual intercourse has traditionally had different meanings for the two sexes. For women love provides both the justification and meaning for sex, while men, in contrast, have traditionally been permitted a greater variety of sexual meanings. In casual relationships men can emphasise experimentation and sex for "fun"; in a committed relationship, sex is associated with love (Peplau, Rubin and Hill, 1977).

Similar results have recently been reported by Juhasz and Sonnenshein-Schneider (1987). Adolescent males saw sexual intercourse as a means of self-enhancement and hence were more oriented toward sexual-impulse gratification. For females, intimacy considerations regarding sexual intercourse were more important and the relationship aspects of sexual behaviour were stressed.

These different patterns can be attributed in part to the role played by biological maturation and the physiological changes of puberty. However, other major forces influencing dating orientation have also to be taken into account. These include social influences (family socialisation; peer group pressures) and the personal meanings placed on these forces (McCabe, 1984). She argues that familial influences in the child-rearing process lead to the development of an individual's sex role. Traditional socialisation results in the development of a sex-typed role and a more egalitarian approach results in the development of an androgynous sex role. Where dating orientation is concerned, a masculine sex role type leads to a sexual orientation and an androgynous sex role leads to an orientation which is both sexual and affectional (McCabe and Collins, 1979). Peer group pressures may emphasise the sexual aspects of dating, although for androgynous and feminine individuals this sexual aspect may be incorporated within a caring relationship. Other social factors which influence dating attitudes and behaviours include religion, church attendance and the type of school attended.

Selection of Dating Partner

Relatively few studies have focused on factors influencing adolescents' choice of partner (Hansen, 1977; Roscoe, Diana and Brooks, 1987; Berti Ceroni et al., 1987). Hansen (1977) analysed senior high school students' views about characteristics considered important in dating partner selection. She found that personality variables such as being pleasant, cheerful, dependable, honest and affectionate were more important than prestige factors such as popularity with opposite sex or having a car.

Ten years later, Roscoe, Diana and Brooks (1987) obtained the same results, but with one important addition. Adolescents at different developmental stages (early, middle, and late, i.e. 6th graders, 11th graders and college students) differed in the level of importance they placed on personal/prestige characteristics possessed by potential dating partners. Early adolescents emphasised status-seeking and dependence upon others and tended to give more weight to superficial features (e.g. fashionable clothes) and approval by others (e.g. approval by parents; well-liked by many people) than late adolescents. Late adolescents placed more stress on independence and future orientation in their dating concerns (e.g. dating partner has set goals for the future; someday will have a good job). Another important aspect of their findings concerned the differences between males and females. Males were more interested in the appearance and sexual activity of dating partners, while females placed greater importance on personality and behaviour traits. Roscoe et al. (op. cit.) point out that, in the light of prevailing socialisation practices, these differences between the sexes are not surprising. Historical influences and cultural pressures such as peers and the media have taught males that they should be the initiators of sexual activity and that to be sexually active is a highly valued status. Females, in contrast, have been prepared to be nurturant and caring, and the recipient of sexual interactions.

Research in Italy (Berti Ceroni et al., 1987) provides a somewhat different picture. Ambivalent and apparently contradictory feelings emerged, as if, alongside the persistence of sex-role stereotypes, there was a desire to find new ways of defining the relationship with the other sex. The choice of partner was mainly influenced by personality factors, but there were important differences between males and females. Boys claimed to be attracted by aesthetic characteristics to a greater extent than girls. They also looked for psychological and moral qualities, as well as cognitive attributes. A girl should be cheerful, serious, able to joke, intelligent and, above all, not "empty inside". Girls, because of their propensity to look for a romantic partner, tended to seek a wide range of attitudes and behaviour of a psychological and affective nature. Despite striving to obtain more autonomy and emancipation, they often underlined the importance of a protective partner, who would be older, who would know how to look after them and protect them. They almost appeared to hope that it might be possible to prolong the path towards individuation in time, without having to take on too many responsibilities.

Social Competence

Some authors have also considered which social skills, or more generally, types of social competence are necessary to deal successfully with the tasks and demands required by opposite-sex relationships. Activities such as asking an individual for a date, together with the appropriate social behaviours to exhibit when on a date, involve new skills which have to be acquired during adolescence (Coleman and Hendry, 1990). These skills involve complex behaviour patterns which are not part of most adolescents' repertoires and can be a source of anxiety for many teenagers (Arkowitz et al., 1978).

In her recent analysis of adolescents' transition from same-sex peer relations to opposite-sex peer relations, Miller (1990) found that there was a relation between same-sex and opposite-sex measures of characteristics such as cognitive skills, popularity, and perceived social competence. These three variables have been shown to be important indicators of adolescents' healthy interactions with peers. However, Miller's findings suggest that this relation may be different for boys than for girls. Both same-sex and opposite-sex popularity were more strongly related for boys than for girls. Adolescent boys who were involved in opposite-sex relationships, gained status in their same-sex peer groups from their abilities in interacting with girls. Girls, on the other hand, experienced more conflicts in same-sex peer relationships when they engaged in opposite-sex relationships, because of competition and jealousy from other girls.

Further research is required in order to study the differences between teenagers in the responses they make and the coping strategies they use, when confronted with the specific developmental task represented by dating behaviour. Another area which merits research concerns the effect upon self-concept of lack of social skills in heterosexual relationships. Despite their importance, thus far these issues have received little attention.

IDENTITY AND INTIMACY

One of the central concepts in the analysis of the affectional world in adolescence is that of intimacy. Authors have long asserted that it is during adolescence that individuals need intimate relationships and begin to develop the capacity to be intimate (Erikson, 1968; Sullivan, 1953). According to Berndt (1982), intimacy develops as a result of the physical, cognitive, and social changes experienced of adolescence. At the physical level, puberty and the changes in sexual impulses which it brings, raise new issues and concerns requiring intimate discussion (Maddock, 1973; Steinberg, 1985). Cognitive development enables adolescents to establish and maintain more mature relations, evidence of which is shown by advanced levels of empathy, self-disclosure and responsiveness to another's experiences (Hill and Palmquist, 1978). Changes in social roles result from increased levels of independence and provide greater opportunities for teenagers to be alone with their friends. Taken together, these three factors increase the adolescent's need, capacity and opportunity for intimacy (Roscoe, Kennedy and Pope, 1987).

A review of the theoretical and empirical work on this topic indicates that researchers have defined intimacy in a variety of ways. Most studies of intimacy have addressed the relationship between identity and intimacy as contiguous constructs. Much of the relevant work has been derived from Erikson's conceptualisation of the adolescent identity crisis and young adult intimacy crisis. In his theory of psycho-social development, identity resolution inevitably precedes intimacy resolution. Identity includes a personal interpretation of early identification and subsequent relationships with significant others. It also includes commitment to a personal ideology which integrates self-definition, sex-role identification, accepted group standards and the meaning of life.

Intimacy is defined as "the capacity to commit (oneself) to concrete affiliations and partnerships and to develop the ethical strength to abide by such commitments even though they may call for significant sacrifices and compromises" (Erikson, 1968, p.263). The main elements of Erikson's definition of intimacy include: openness, sharing, mutual trust, self-abandon, and commitment. In his framework, an individual without a firm sense of self will be unable to commit himself to another person. Thus, fulfilment of intimacy requires a sense of shared identities.

Several studies have provided tentative and indirect support for Erikson's sequential assumptions by revealing that persons with more advanced identities are also likely to have achieved a more advanced level of intimacy (Marcia, 1966; Orlofsky, Marcia and Lesser, 1973; Tesch and Whitbourne, 1982). Most studies of intimacy have used Orlofsky et al.'s operationalisation, which identifies three major criteria for determining intimacy status: a) the extent of the individual's involvement with male and female friends; b) presence or absence of a committed heterosexual relationship; c) the degree of depth and quality of the individual's friendships and dating or love relationship. Using these criteria, Orlofsky defines five intimacy statuses: intimate (characterised by deep, enduring, committed love relationships); pre-intimate (deep relationship, but with ambivalence about commitment); pseudo-intimate (relationships lacking closeness and depth, but committed); stereotyped (superficial and conventional relationships, limited in closeness and communication); and isolate (absence of enduring personal relations).

In a later study, Orlofsky and Ginsburg (1981) showed that intimacy with others is associated with openness to and ability to conceptualise affective experience. Through self-disclosure the self is revealed not only to the other person (permitting greater intimacy), but also to oneself. Mutual disclosure of feelings between intimate partners allows each to achieve greater emotional differentiation and self-awareness. The authors conclude by suggesting that "the increased ability to experience, conceptualise and articulate feelings, in its turn, facilitates further disclosure and intimacy" (p. 99). Mitchell (1976) regards intimacy as a need for deep involvement with another person at a meaningful level. The most essential attribute is honesty; in fact, authentic self-disclosure requires that the individual shows himself as he is, without pretence or facade. In line with Erikson's view (Erikson, 1968), Mitchell states that genuine intimacy rarely takes hold in an insecure or immature personality because it requires more than receiving affection from others. It demands selfless giving and genuine sharing. Although moments of intimacy are experienced during middle and early adolescence, it is not until late adolescence and early adulthood that durable intimacy occurs (Mitchell, 1976).

Roscoe, Kennedy and Pope (1987) examined how late adolescents define intimate relations as distinguished from non-intimate ones. They show that, twenty five years after Erikson, adolescents' definitions are still consistent with his original description of intimacy, as being characterised by openness, sharing and trust. There were, however, three important differences: adolescents (and especially males) included physical/sexual interaction as a critical component. Very few included self-abandon and commitment as necessary elements of an intimate relationship.

The authors refer to the dramatic changes in free sexual expression which have occurred in the past 25 years, as possible explanations for these discrepancies. They suggest that they have led to uncertainty "as to the extent one can give and still maintain an intact sense of 'self'. It is possible that as identity is more clearly attained, one may be better able to experience what Erikson has labelled 'self-abandon'" (Roscoe et al., 1987, p. 515).

Eriksonian theory and its sequential assumptions about the relation between identity and intimacy have been subjected to many criticisms. On the one hand, it has been criticised as being primarily a theory of male development (Gilligan, 1982). It has also been pointed out that in emphasising identity and its precursors, Erikson failed to provide an adequate conceptual foundation for intimacy (Franz and White, 1985).

As many authors (Douvan and Adelson, 1966; Gilligan, 1982; Josselson, 1987) have argued, girls' identity development appears to be fused with intimacy formation. Thus, while boys may focus on ideological and autonomy issues of identity development, girls may tend to focus more upon its interpersonal and social role aspects (Craig-Bray, Adams and Dobson, 1988; Dyk and Adams, 1990). The importance of relationships for adolescent females is such, that some researchers have speculated that intimacy development may occur simultaneously, or even precede, identity development. Josselson (1987) has also underlined the fact that theories of development have emphasised separation and autonomy, instead of connection and relationships. She suggests that "a central aspect of identity is the commitment to a self-in-relation rather than to a self that stands alone facing an abstract world" (p.22). When conceptualised in this way, women's life stages may be different from men's, but unfortunately, these gender distinctions remain somewhat ambiguously stated.

Dyk and Adams (1990) provide an initial investigation of the identity/intimacy association during late adolescence which is based upon different theoretical perspectives. Their findings suggest that sex-role orientation may be an important factor in understanding the relationship between identity and intimacy. For females, a masculine orientation is associated with a pattern similar to that observed for either masculine- or feminine-oriented males. Females with a feminine orientation show a closer connection between identity and intimacy. They provide evidence to partially confirm Erikson's assumption that identity predicts intimacy in development and Gilligan's suggestion that there are at least two developmental patterns or "voices". A male voice (comprising all males, regardless of sex-role orientation, and females with a masculine sex-role orientation) defines identity more in the context of individual achievement and goals (instrumental role) and focuses on the role of separation. A female voice, expressed by females with a feminine sex-role orientation, defines identity in the context of relationship (expressive role) with a focus on the ongoing process of attachment (Dyk and Adams, 1990). However, the explanations offered for these differences are neither convincing nor conclusive and more clarification is needed if we are better to understand the interplay between sex-role orientation, biological factors and psycho-social factors.

The work of White and her associates (White, Speisman, Jackson, Bartis and Costos, 1986; White, Speisman, Costos and Smith, 1987; Franz and White, 1985; Paul and White, 1990) suggests one possible direction for achieving this goal. They formulated a theory of relationship maturity which provides a useful framework for examining close interpersonal relationships in late adolescent and young adult years. In the first paper of the series, Franz and White (1985) argued that individuation and attachment are both central to the development of males and females: identity and intimacy are developmental tasks of the late adolescent transitional period and progress towards mature identity and mature intimacy takes place concurrently. They suggest that three levels of relationship maturity can be identified: self-focused, role-focused and individuated-connected. Each of these describes a different degree of maturity brought to a relationship with a close partner, in areas such as orientation (perspective taking), communication (self-disclosure, initiating, listening, and responding), commitment, concern/caring, and mature sexuality.

The self-focused level involves unilateral self-involvement and a small capacity for concern for other persons. The individual's own wishes and plans overshadow those of others. Where sexuality is concerned, there is scant understanding of mutuality or consideration of another's sexual needs.

Individuals at role-focused level begin to recognise that acknowledging and respecting another is part of being a good friend or romantic partner. Commitment to a person is not articulated, however and while some sharing of feeling occurs, this is unlikely to be fully expressed.

At the individuated-connected level, individuals exhibit active understanding of themselves and others and commitment to a specific person with whom they share a relationship. Concern and caring involve role-appropriate activities as well as emotional support. With sexual behaviour, there is evidence of a comfortable expression of tenderness and affect, as well as acceptance of occasional frustration.

Within the framework, the self-focused process of identity and intimacy development serves as a foundation for a later, more mature capacity for intimate relationships (Paul and White, 1990, pp. 378-379). Paul and White (op. cit.) use a review of the literature on the development of friendships, romantic dating, sexual relationships, etc. in adolescence, to support their developmental model of intimacy maturity. They point out, however, that further research is needed if we are better to understand the specific functions of these various dyadic relationships and the role they play in the movement towards intimacy maturity.

CONCLUSIONS

One of the major developmental accomplishments of adolescence is acquiring new and more mature relations with age-mates of both sexes and entering a committed, mutual sexual relationship with a particular close partner. In view of this, an understanding of the life space of adolescence appears incomplete without an understanding of the social organisation of the dating process and of the role played by love relationships.

It is clear that adolescents spend a good deal of time thinking about relationships with the opposite sex and give them a high priority in their lives. Their involvement in heterosexual/dating relationships can be seen as providing not only the opportunity to develop a firmer sense of self, but also the romantic context in which to further test one's ability to relate interpersonally (Cate and Koval, 1983).

In this chapter attention has focused on three major issues which have emerged as particularly relevant: i) the changes a partner relationship brings to the whole relational system of the adolescent, i.e. parents and peer group; ii) the functions and the meanings of dating/love relationships; iii) the process of identity and intimacy development in adolescence. The research findings indicate that the partner generally responds to the need to satisfy the affectional and maturative needs of an adolescent. He or she expedites, guards and protects the process of separation from the parental figures and, at the same time, facilitates self-realisation and an increase in personal self-esteem. The complex process of elaborating identity therefore seems to be helped by the presence of a partner.

Analysis of the literature in this area reveals that research work is somewhat fragmentary; it is concerned with limited aspects and often lacks an unifying conceptual framework for understanding the processes involved. Gender differences in identity and intimacy development remain inadequately charted and many of the constructs used require clearer definition. Many topics are still neglected and need further study. As a result, hardly anything is known of the consequences for adult life of different patterns of teenage sex, in particular, the effects of early premarital sexual relations on psychological maturation (Coleman and Hendry, 1990). Furthermore, relatively little information is available on topics such as sexual difficulties in adolescence, the psychological consequences of abortion, the problem of handicapped adolescents, adolescent parenthood.

Two topics have not been dealt with in this chapter: adolescent homosexual relationships and problems linked to AIDS. To date, the former has received scant attention in the psychological literature reviewed in this chapter. It is only recently that homosexuality has ceased to be regarded in terms of "deviancy" or "illness" and become a phenomenon that is tolerated, even if not yet accepted (at least in the Catholic countries). For this reason, perhaps, it is still difficult to find psychological research on homosexuality in adolescence. It is a topic which urgently requires further study. Parallel studies to those on heterosexual relationships and their developmental implications could serve as a useful starting point.

Where AIDS is concerned, it is clear that the dating and sexual behaviour of the present generation of adolescents will have to take account of the problem. During the last few years it has become an important public health issue for many countries across the world. Government health campaigns have tried to inform people about AIDS so that they can protect themselves from the disease and the subject has been the focus of much media attention. Even if researchers begin to pay attention to the multifaceted nature of AIDS in different cultural contexts (see for example, the Special Issue on "Social Dimensions of AIDS" in the *Journal of Community and Applied Social Psychology*, vol.1, 1991), it is still too early to know whether this will lead eventually to a substantial and general shift in teenagers' approach to sexual behaviour. Changing behaviour is far more complicated than merely changing knowledge and beliefs. One might anticipate that health-enhancing knowledge and beliefs help to support safer behaviour, and this should be further examined.

Information concerning the influences of the macrosystem on the beginning and modalities of adolescent dating remains an important requirement. It would be useful to analyse in more detail the influence of the mass-media in creating and inculcating behaviour patterns in heterosexual relations. In this context, one might think of the possible influence of the endless TV "soaps" which propagate life styles, sexual role models, rules and norms of behaviour which are typical in another country. To what extent, if any, do these have an impact on the expectations and/or behaviour of teenagers?

It is also important to emphasise the need for cross-cultural research. As will have been apparent from my review of research, the data generally refer to a specific adolescent population in a particular country at a particular time. The findings are often limited to a population represented by white, urban, middle-class, student adolescents. Despite this, researchers often appear to be ready to make generalisations to adolescence itself, independent of context. Studies with a clear cross-cultural approach are few and far between. It remains important to underline the fact that concepts concerning the development of heterosexual relationships in adolescence need to be developed not only within cultures, but also across cultures. This is particularly important in a situation where societies are becoming multi-ethnic with a wide range of diverse cultures. A perspective is needed which takes account of the different meanings assigned to obtaining/having a partner, to the affectional relationship in different contexts and to the social factors which can affect the dating process.

There are a variety of important issues concerning the relation between features of the current socio-cultural context and changes in intimacy in the middle and late adolescent years which require further research. How, for example, does the transition from an established social network such as (high) school, to a situation such as university, with its increased opportunities for developing other relations, affect intimate relationships? Similarly, it would be useful to analyse the meaning of the dating process for adolescents with different levels of schooling and for those who have moved out of the educational setting.

Some authors (Coleman and Hendry, 1990; Paul and White, 1990) have pointed out that the earlier onset of puberty and a more general societal expectation of more adult behaviour mean that there are increased social pressures on adolescents to grow up faster. How do such pressures affect intimacy development? We also need to know more about the varied effects, positive and negative, of steady dating on the development of self.

We have seen that research often distinguishes between different age-periods in adolescence. For example, early, middle and late adolescence are often differentiated and reference is sometimes made to young adults.

There is a need to set out more clearly the "boundaries" of adolescence in order to try to arrive at a shared definition of what these boundaries are. However, the question of age is not simply a question of terminology or semantics: age, whether considered in its own right, or alongside other variables such as sex, economic condition, professional status (student or worker) has an enormous effect on all aspects of affective development and dating behaviour. There are many questions in this context which require research attention. What, for example, are the consequences of beginning dating behaviour at a particular age? Why do some individuals (male or female) begin dating earlier than others? What are the differences, if any, between early and late daters? To what extent does biological maturation play a role in the dating process? Is there a relationship between the social skills available to adolescents at an earlier age-level and those that come into play at the beginning of dating?

Swedish studies have shown that biological maturity is related to social adjustment processes via the characteristics of one's circle of peers (Magnusson, Stattin and Allen, 1985; see also Silbereisen and Kracke, this vol.). Early maturing girls are more at risk of deviant behaviour and have more negative long-term prospects within the educational domain than on-time or late-maturing girls. They tend to devote more time to steady contacts with boys, engage earlier in intimate sexual relations, and wish to bring up their own children. Compared to late-developers, they are more likely to aspire to activities such as family life than to progress towards higher education.

These studies, together with other work reported in the present chapter, have important implications for future research in that they emphasise the need for a longitudinal perspective. Achievement of a better understanding of the psycho-social processes involved in the development of adolescent affectional relationships requires an approach in which the same individuals are followed over a considerable period of time.

CHAPTER SIX

Adolescents' Relationships with Grandparents: Characteristics and Developmental Transformations

Maria Tyszkowa

Adolescents grow up in a social world which embraces younger children, age-mates and adults of various ages. Grandparents are a part of the world of grown-ups. They represent the oldest generation in the family and, parents aside, they are most likely to be the only adults who have accompanied the individual from earliest development onwards.

To date, the analysis of relationships between youth and adults, and of the latter's role with regard to psychic and social development in adolescence has concentrated mainly on relations between children and parents (see Youniss 1980). Both the role of the oldest generation in the family and relationships between grandchildren and their grandparents have been neglected for a long time. The family, a primary context of the development of the individual (Bronfenbrenner 1979), has been treated as a nuclear, two-generational unit. As Troll, Bengtson and McFerland (1979, p. 151) point out, however, "almost all surveys find that the oldest generation is an integral and active part of the family structure". Following their review, a number of studies of grandparenthood appeared (see Smith 1991). Problems of the role of grandparents in the family and of their relationships with grandchildren were approached by sociologists, social psychologists, psychoanalysts and developmental psychologists from within their respective viewpoints. Studies of the relationships between grandchildren and grandparents were conducted from the perspective of both grandparents (using a life-span approach) and that of grandchildren. In this chapter we will be primarily concerned with the latter.

Relationships between grandchildren and grandparents first became an object of research interest in the 70s and since then, this interest has blossomed (e.g. Kahana and Kahana 1970; Robertson 1975, 1976; Hartshorne and Manaster 1982; Kivett 1985; Eisenberg 1988; Sticker 1991; Werner 1991; Tyszkowa 1991; Delestre 1991). A smaller number of studies of the influence of grandparents on the development of grandchildren have also appeared.

The relationship between grandchildren and grandparents has attracted attention, not only because of the large age and generation difference, but also because of the mediating role fulfilled by the middle generation, i.e. the grandchildren's parents and grandparents' children. Parents are described as mediators (Robertson 1975) and the grandchild-grandparent relationship as contingent (Troll 1980). The mediating role of parents seems to be especially important in the childhood years, when they are able to control contacts between children and grandparents and can influence thereby the development of more or less permanent ties between them. Nevertheless, where contact occurs, grandchildren-grandparents relationships can be and indeed usually are direct and do not always require parental mediation (Hurme 1988, 1989; Sticker 1991; Werner 1991; Tyszkowa 1991). This means that Matthews and Sprey's conclusion (1985, p. 621) that "conceptualising the grandparent-grandchild tie as indirect is clearly appropriate" does not hold, at least where adolescent grandchildren are concerned.

Research also shows that the frequency and quality of contacts between children or young people and their grandparents is a fundamental feature of the relationship. The relationship is particularistic, i.e. is connected with a given grandparent and influenced by his/her characteristics, rather than with the grandparent role as such (Matthews and Sprey 1985).

A further factor which is of similar importance is line of kinship, i.e. whether the linking parent is a mother or a father. Some studies on inter-generational relationships in families have revealed strong emotional bonds between maternal grandmothers and their daughters' families (Cohler and Grunebaum 1980; Hurme 1988).

Interpersonal relations are also formed by social norms, expectations and stereotypes (Stone and Farberman 1970; Ziolkowski 1981). Troll, Bengtson, and McFerland (1979) in their analysis of intergenerational relations in the family, suggest that the problem of the effect of ontogenetic developmental processes upon interpersonal bonds should become one of the major questions for further research analysis. Even at an early stage, studies reported that children of different ages emphasise different aspects of grandparent-grandchild relationships (Kahana and Kahana, 1970). Despite this, very little has yet been done to take account of developmental changes in grandparent-grandchild relationships between childhood and adolescence. Some studies have analysed relationships between adolescent and young adult grandchildren and their grandparents. Matthews and Sprey (1985) found that a high percentage of adolescent grandchildren have rather frequent contacts and close relationships with grandparents, especially with maternal grandmothers (MGMs) (60%). On the basis of their research, they concluded that adolescents' relationships with their grandparents are perceived as a continuation of the earlier childhood ones. This finding has been supported by further research results (e.g. Sticker 1991; Tyszkowa 1991). However, while accepting that mutual attachment can be maintained, it is rather difficult to agree with Matthews and Sprey's conclusion that grandchild-grandparent relationship remains "unchanged through time" (op. cit. 1985, p. 625).

From the cognitive point of view, attachment is seen as "a social relationship involving reciprocal role interactions in which complementary role transactions determine development of interpersonal emotional ties" (Schultz 1980). These relationships are supposed to undergo developmental transformation (see Hurme 1986), i.e. to change with time. What appears to be a more tenable position is taken by Kahana and Kahana (1970) and by some psychoanalytical writers who argue that the relationship evolves in time according to the age of the grandchild (Cavallero et al. 1981, after Battiselli and Farneti 1991, p. 146).

The dynamics of the grandparent-grandchild relationship has been shown clearly in the study by Battiselli and Farneti (1991) who approached the issue from a psychoanalytic perspective. The authors asked 475 subjects from three age groups: 8-9, 12-13, and 16-17 years old, to complete a questionnaire in which one item was a list of four pairs of adjectives (one positive, one negative). Subjects were asked to choose one of the adjectives from each pair in order to describe each of their four grandparents. Taking as a point of departure the psychoanalytical concepts of an Oedipal period in childhood and a separation process in adolescence the authors expected "the place that grandparents have in their grandchildren's world to become more and more limited" (p. 148). The results of their investigation did not confirm this expectation. However, significant changes in the grandchild-grandparent relationship in childhood and in adolescence did emerge. The main trend of this change was "a progressive levelling-out" of the place of maternal and paternal grandparents and an "increasingly less positive judgment" (p. 153). The authors link this process with the dynamics of the relationships between child, parents and grandparents in childhood and adolescence, suggesting that it is a product of transformations in attachment to parents (adults) in the Oedipal period and of separation from parents in adolescence. Their findings are interesting, even though their interpretation seems to be one-sided.

As this brief review of the literature has shown, the nature of the relationships between adolescents and their grandparents as well as the position of the latter in the world of the former, is not clear. Kahana and Kahana (1970) refer to developmental changes which can be expected in this relationship as the grandchildren grow older. However, opinions concerning the very existence of such changes (see Matthews and Sprey 1985), their origin and nature are contradictory (see Robertson 1976; Battiselli and Farneti 1991). Neither the main characteristics, nor the trends of developmental transformation of the relationship have been satisfactorily recognised. As Sroufe and Fleeson (1986, p.52) have pointed out "The child brings forward only an organisation of feelings, needs, attitudes, expectations, cognitions and behaviour; that is, only the relationship history as processed and integrated by the developing individual."

These uncertainties about the nature of adolescents' relationships with grandparents led to the present study. It aimed to clarify the nature of adolescent-grandparent relationships within a developmental psychology context.

AIM AND ASSUMPTIONS

The present study set out to examine the position of grandparents in the social world of their adolescent grandchildren and to compare adolescent relationships with their grandparents with those of children at the late childhood stage. In doing so, it aimed to reveal the main developmental transformations which were thought to occur in these relationships.

Adolescence is a period of physical maturation and, thus, of changing self-perception of the individual as he/she becomes more adult-like. Adolescence is also a period of intensive identity formation (see Erikson 1968; Bosma 1985, and others) and a time when an individual must make decisions of life-long importance, is exposed to challenges and threats of different kinds and must learn how to cope with them (see Bosma and Jackson 1990). Thanks to developmental achievements in both social and cognitive development (see Youniss 1980; Youniss and Smollar 1985; Inhelder and Piaget 1970) the adolescent also develops a greater ability to decentrate in relations with others. In the context of these deep developmental transformations in the inner and social world of adolescents, it seems likely that relationships with their grandparents also undergo qualitative changes. Probably these changes bear upon all of the main dimensions of the grandchild-grandparent relationship. This assumption is based on the changes which have been perceived in adolescents' relationships with parents and peers (see Youniss and Smollar 1985; Czikszentmihaly et al. 1977).

Youniss (1980) suggests that developmental transformations in which a sense of ongoing ties is maintained, express themselves in three main ways. A growing interaction and mutuality of the relations occurs, perceptions of adults alter as they come to be perceived not only as figures from the world of adults, but as individuals having their own characteristics, virtues and vices and, finally, there is a growing sensitivity to the needs and experience of adults. These characteristics correspond to those found in research on grandchild-grandparent relationships (Battiselli and Farneti 1991). Generally speaking, adolescent-adult relations gradually take on the form of a personal relationship of more symmetric character.

Grandparents are older than grandchildren by two generations and their position in the family is specific and different from that of parents. Studies have already shown that grandparents continue to play an important role in the life and development of adolescent grandchildren (Tyszkowa 1991). Questions remain, however, concerning: the structure and dynamics of relationships between adolescent grandchildren and their grandparents; the extent to which transformations in these relations during adolescence reflect the overall pattern of developmental changes in the adolescent-adult relationship; and their specificity to relationships with grandparents. With such questions in mind, the present chapter sets out to describe relationships between grandchildren and grandparents and compare their characteristics in childhood and at two stages of adolescence It also aims to examine the developmental transformation—if any—of these relationships which takes place during this period of individual development.

The description and analysis of interpersonal relations means that a number of basic dimensions need to be considered. Following Hinde (1979; 1988), we have focused upon the content, diversity, and quality of the interaction, the mutuality and intimacy of the relationship and the perception of the partner.

Relationships between adolescent grandchildren and grandparents have their own history which reaches back to the early childhood of the former. They are entangled in a wider context of interpersonal relations and exist within the broader system of the family. Research (Kornhaber and Woodward 1985; Kivnick 1982; Stueve 1982) shows that they belong to the most significant relationships in the extended family system. An interpersonal relationship can emerge only when two individuals are in a position to enter into an interaction with each other. As Hinde has pointed out "relationship involves a series of interactions between two individuals, each interaction being relatively limited in duration but affected by past interactions between the same individuals and affecting future ones" (Hinde 1988, p. 1).

In setting out to analyse the structure of grandchild-grandparent relationships and the changes which occur with development, we began by posing a series of specific questions. How frequent is the contact between grandchildren at different age-levels and their grandparents? What is the emotional tone of the grandchildren's opinions on and attitudes towards their grandparents? Which activities do they share? How do adolescent grandchildren at different age-levels perceive grandparents and their position in their own life?

Frequency of contact is seen as the basis for interaction, and thus, for maintenance and development of the relationships between grandchildren and grandparents. In the light of previous research findings (Hurme 1988; Sticker 1991; Delestre 1991), it is important to see whether frequency of contact changes as grandchildren grow older. In analysing the relationship, it is also important to describe the content of these interactions—what kind of activities do grandchildren perform together with their grandparents. This will make it possible to evaluate the potential value of these interactions for adolescents. Analysis of the emotional tone of the adolescents' opinions of their grandparents will, in turn, provide information concerning the emotional dimension of the relationship under study. As previously stated, the perception of a partner is one of the main dimensions of a relationship. It seems likely that grandchildren's perceptions of grandparents will evolve over time as both partners in the relationship grow older and as the young person's social contacts and involvement with peers increase. With this in mind, it is important to examine the changes—if any—which occur in perceptions of grandparents in the pre-adolescent period and at different stages during adolescence.

Relationships between adolescents and their grandparents are viewed here as a consequence of interactions and thus as a developmental phenomenon. They are influenced by past experiences with grandparents as well as by current interactions (see Tyszkowa 1986b; Hurme 1986). Hence, we set out to collect information concerning social facts (contact frequency, common activities with grandparents), subjects' feelings and attitudes towards grandparents and their subjective evaluations of their grandparents as persons. The focus was on the perspective of the grandchild and how it changes with development into and through adolescence.

SUBJECTS AND METHODS

The total sample consisted of 255 grandchildren comprising 58 children aged 7-11 (27 boys and 31 girls) and two sub-groups of adolescents. The younger of these sub-groups was aged 12-15 ($N=100$; 51 boys and 49 girls) and the older one comprised 97 subjects—47 boys and 50 girls aged 16-19. Participation was voluntary. In 12 cases either parents (7) or subjects themselves did not agree to participate in the study.

A greater proportion of adolescents was included in the study because of the likelihood that adolescents will have fewer living grandparents than children. Data were collected by means of a variety of research techniques which were adapted to the different age-levels of the subjects. The youngest sub-group of subjects was interviewed by means of a semi-structured questionnaire carried out while the individual child was busy drawing family and grandparents (results of the analysis of these drawings will be reported elsewhere). They were asked to describe each of their living grandparents and those who were already dead, if they could remember them. They were asked questions such as: How often do you visit this grandmother/father? How often does s(h)e visit you? What do you do together? The interviews were tape-recorded.

The two older sub-groups were asked to write compositions on the theme "My Grandparents and I" during a class which took place on Grandmother's/Grandfather's day. The composition was written under the supervision of the class teacher. Pupils were asked to name all of the grandparents whom they knew, to describe them and to give details of their current contacts and relationship with them. They were also asked to try to describe the significance of grandparents (or of a given grandparent) in their life. While the use of compositions as a method of data collecting is well known in developmental psychology, it tends to produce a wide range of material. In view of this, the main variables were determined using content analysis procedures based on a pre-defined set of categories. Only some of these variables will be considered in this chapter.

Where compositions failed to include important information, an interview was carried out in order to obtain the information, or to clarify points which were unclear. These interviews were not tape-recorded, subjects' answers were noted directly. All subjects also completed a Test of Uncompleted Sentences (TUS). This test was designed to explore the subject's relations with each grandparent and was carried out orally with the youngest age-group. Subjects' answers were noted immediately on a form. Older subjects completed the test in the classroom. The TUS was based upon the list dealing with parent-child relations designed by Sachs and Levy (1952). Examples of the material include: "My grandma and I...", "I like my grandpa but...", "My grandpa/grandma doesn't like me to...", etc. The test contained 14 incomplete sentences. In this chapter, data collected with the TUS will only be used for illustrative purposes.

The main set of data (from the interviews with 7-11-year-olds and the compositions) was analysed in two stages. First, each subject's material was analysed in order to examine the character of information it contained, the completeness of answers, duration of the interview, length of composition, etc. Subjects' personal data (age, sex, school grade, etc.) were also determined, together with the number and type of grandparents who were described. Second, the data were analysed by means of categories such as tone used when describing a given grandparent, frequency of contacts, subjective evaluation of these contacts, content of relations (common activities, interpersonal communication, exchange of information, or just sitting and doing nothing; gifts taken and given etc.). Following this analysis, a further quantitative and qualitative analysis was carried out. We will only consider selected results of this analysis here: those concerning the main dimensions of grandchild-grandparent relationships; those involving anticipated differences between age-groups; those dealing with developmental aspects of the relationship under study.

RESEARCH RESULTS

Numbers and Categories of Grandparents
Mentioned by Children and Adolescents

Table 6.1 gives details of the number of different grandparents mentioned by children and adolescents in the interviews or compositions.

In total, the 255 subjects named and described 439 grandparents out of a potential maximum 1020 (255×4), i.e. only about 40% of all grandparents (living and deceased) were referred to by the grandchildren. Of the 439, 395 were still alive. Children below 12 years of age referred only to living grandparents or to grandparents who had died within the previous two years. In general, if a grandparent had died before the grandchild was about 9-years-old, the latter had no memory of him or her. When asked

TABLE 6.1

Number of Grandparents of Different Types Mentioned by the Subjects

	Categories of Grandparents								
	MGM		MGF		PGM		PGF		
Age of Ss	alive	dead	alive	dead	alive	dead	alive	dead	Total
7–11	54	1	40	2	50	0	31	0	178
12–15	62	3	27	0	25	2	26	1	146
16–19	32	8	16	9	19	10	13	8	115
Total	148	12	83	11	94	12	70	9	439

MGM = maternal grandmother; MGF = maternal grandfather. PGM = paternal grandmother; PGF = paternal grandfather about their other grandparents, i.e. grandparents who were not spontaneously referred to, subjects usually stated that they did not know them (they died before the grandchild's birth or during his/her early childhood). In three cases other reasons were given; loss of contact with grandparents as a result of parental divorce, emigration or change of religious affiliation.

The distribution of living grandparents among the three age groups was not even. On average, the youngest subjects had about 3 living grandparents per person, the younger teenagers 1.4, while the older ones had only 0.8 per person.

Children's and Adolescents' Contacts with Grandparents

Table 6.2 provides information on the occurrence and frequency of contact between children of various ages and their grandparents. As can be seen in the Table, a significant majority of children and adolescents has contact with grandparents. Subjects reported a lack of contact with 36 living grandparents—9% of the total. Contact with 34.5% of the grandparents was frequent, and very frequent with 18.2%.

TABLE 6.2
Number of Contacts with Living Grandparents

Age Groups of Ss	Frequency of Contacts with GPs of Different Categories																			
	MGM					MGF					PGM					PGF				
	0	1	2	3	4	0	1	2	3	4	0	1	2	3	4	0	1	2	3	4
7–11	2	3	10	17	12	3	6	11	14	6	3	4	12	26	5	1	10	9	11	0
12–15	6	8	11	21	16	5	2	7	10	3	4	3	5	9	4	3	5	4	9	5
16–19	6	7	3	8	8	3	1	6	5	1	2	6	3	3	5	1	6	3	2	1
Total	14	18	24	36	34	11	9	27	29	10	9	13	20	38	14	5	21	16	22	6

0 = no contacts or no mentioning of them
1 = seldom – 1 to 3 times a year
2 = rather often – about once a month
3 = frequent contacts – at least once a week
4 = very frequent contacts – almost every day (or daily)

The data show that frequency of contacts tended to decrease as the age of the grandchildren increased. They also demonstrate differences in the frequency of contacts with grandparents of various types. For the youngest sub-group, this tendency is closest to the pattern which is found elsewhere in the literature (Smith 1991), i.e. MGM>MGF>PGM>PGF. With the older subject group, the frequency of contacts with various types of grandparents tended to decrease and to level out. This tendency did not hold, however, for maternal grandfathers. Here, the order of frequency of contact is MGF>MGM>PGM>PGF. Since the total number of living grandparents for this group was low, however, it is difficult to know how far the result reflects a general pattern.

Frequency of contacts between grandchildren and grandparents is also influenced by distance between places of residence. A small distance apart—less than 60 minutes travel time—favours frequent contacts in both later childhood and adolescence. Contacts and interactions may be initiated either by grandparents (or parents) or by grandchildren. The most common frequency of contact with grandparents of all four types is once a week, including customary family visits at weekends. The content analyses of compositions and interviews indicate that the majority (about 67%) of the two younger groups takes part in such visits. Older adolescents, on the other hand, seem to prefer individual contacts with a given grandparent, which they themselves initiate. Sixty-three (65.5%) of the 97 adolescents aged 16-19 and a smaller number (37, i.e. 37%) of those aged 12-15 referred to such contacts in their compositions. This can be seen as an indication of a qualitative developmental transformation in grandchild-grandparent contacts in adolescence.

Grandchildren's Emotional Attitude to Grandparents

Analyses of the emotional tone of the subject's descriptions of grandparents provided information concerning subjects' attitudes towards specific grandparents and the nature of the interpersonal relationship involved. Utterances of different emotional colouring emerged, ranging from words of love, attachment and admiration for grandmother or grandfather, through neutral descriptions, down to expressions of dislike and disapproval, and occasionally even of hostility.

Four categories of subjective ratings of grandparents were differentiated and used in analysing the data from the interviews and compositions. These were: (1) negative—for instance, utterances like "She always nags me, is aggressive", "He is unpleasant. I don't like him", "I don't like her for she didn't do anything for us" or "A lazy, old egoist"; (2) neutral—neither positive nor negative, dispassionate descriptions with equal numbers of positive and negative adjectives used in description of a grandparent and the subject's relations with him/her; (3) positive—description of positive features of a given grandparent prevails and positive adjectives used by the subjects are more numerous then negative ones; utterances like "She is nice and most often generous to me", "My grandpa is good for me, he likes me and I also like him" or "My grandpa and I are two fine buddies"; (4) very positive—descriptions in which only very positive adjectives are used, utterances expressing a very positive emotional attitude towards a given grandparent ("My grandma is the best person in the world", "She is always nice and smiling, like an angel in our family", "She is very wise" or "Wonderful person", "My grandpa is the most knowledgeable man I have ever met").

The frequency of occurrence of each of these different categories of emotional reactions is shown in Table 6.3.

Analysis of the data focused upon subjects' attitudes to grandparents in general and to the particular grandparent categories. It also examined group differences in the distribution of data on grandchildren's relations and more specifically on age-related aspects of the emotional dimension of their relationships with grandparents.

Across age-groups, grandchildren's attitudes towards grandparents were largely positive or very positive. The percentages of subjects in the different groups who expressed a positive or very positive attitude to grandparents was 64.5% for the child group and 68.41% and 65.63% for the two adolescent groups. Negative attitudes appeared infrequently—1.6% in the youngest subgroup and 5.2% in the oldest. Neutral descriptions were more numerous and tended to increase slightly with age (youngest group—34.3%, young adolescents—28.1%, older adolescents—39.1%).

No significant age-related differences emerged in the distribution of these attitudes towards grandparents χ^2=5.23; df=2; $p < 0.80$). This result can be interpreted as confirming the thesis that the grandchild-grandparent relationship remains unchanged with age (Matthews and Sprey 1985). However, this result holds true only for the emotional dimension of this relationship.

With earlier research findings in mind (e.g. Cohler and Grunebaum 1980; Hurme 1988), it was expected that the emotional tone in the descriptions of grandmothers (especially MGMs) would more often be positive than in descriptions of grandfathers. It was also anticipated that attitudes towards maternal grandparents would more often be positive than those concerning paternal grandparents.

These expectations were examined by analysing the data in Table 6.3. Calculations using χ^2 provide only slight support for these expectations. We tested the results concerning the pairs MGM-MGF and PGM-PGF in the particular age groups. Significant differences were only obtained with regard to emotional attitudes to PGM and PGF for the children's group

TABLE 6.3

Emotional Atittude of Grandchildren to their Grandparents

Emotional Tone in Age Groups of Ss	Number of Utterances Concerning a Given Category of Grandparents					
	MGM	MGF	PGM	PGF	N	%
7–11						
1	1	1	1	0	3	1.5
2	17	18	11	14	60	30.3
3	29	19	36	15	99	58.8
4	8	4	2	2	16	8.0
12–15						
1	1	0	1	3	5	3.4
2	13	13	6	9	41	28.1
3	49	14	18	15	96	65.7
4	2	0	2	0	4	2.7
16–19						
1	4	0	1	1	6	5.2
2	13	7	16	9	45	39.1
3	15	14	8	9	46	40.0
4	8	4	4	2	18	15.6
Total	160	94	106	79	439	

1 = negative emotional tone
2 = neutral, neither positive nor negative
3 = positive
4 = very positive

(χ^2=4.66; df=1; $p < 0.05$) and for the younger adolescent group (χ^2=4.37; df=1; $p < 0.05$). The data on the emotional attitude to MGM and MGF showed no significant differences for any of the different age-groups. However, grandchildren's emotional attitude to maternal grandparents taken together (MGM and MGF) and paternal grandparents (PGM and PGF) varied significantly in the youngest (7-11 yrs old) age group (χ^2=4.11; df=1; $p < 0.05$). This finding indicates that in late childhood, grandchildren's attitude to maternal grandparents (MGPs) is more often positive than with paternal grandparents (PGPs). However, this result did not hold for the adolescent groups: 12-15 year-olds χ^2=3.23; df=1; $p < 0.05$; 16-19 year-olds χ^2=3.14; df=1; $p < 0.05$. None of the age-groups showed any significant differences in emotional attitude to maternal and paternal grandmothers ($p < 0.80$ and < 0.50).

The data also show that girls of all age-groups described both grandmothers and grandfathers more positively than did boys. In the two adolescent sub-groups, girls' descriptions of grandfathers had a more positive tone than their descriptions of grandmothers. In contrast, boys' description of grandmothers became more positive with age while their descriptions of grandfathers became less positive. The least positive descriptions of grandparents of both sexes by both girls and boys emerged from the compositions written by the younger adolescents.

Content and Diversity of Adolescents' Interactions with Grandparents

Subjects described 856 actions and activities which they performed together with their grandmothers and grandfathers. The average number of shared activities decreases as the grandchildren grow older. Subjects aged 7-11 mentioned 5.21 different activities on average per person, while younger adolescents named only 2.92 and the older adolescents 2.7.

Table 6.4 shows that the most common shared activities were conversations, walks and table games (also in childhood—plays). The first place held by conversation is particularly noteworthy. Nearly every subject mentioned this activity (average 0.98 times per person). Conversations with grandparents (often while taking a walk together) were liked by grandchildren. They were seen as showing the grandparents' interest and involvement in the grandchild's problems, goodwill and friendliness. The content analysis of the compositions revealed that adolescents saw this as important for several reasons. Hardworking and busy parents rarely have enough time to talk with children about matters which are important to them. Parents are too eager to carry out tasks of socialisation and enforce their own point of view. Grandchildren are linked to grandparents by close ties, but these are of a different nature from their ties with parents—there is more independence despite the age difference. This means that the young person can talk with grandparents about topics, or even secrets, which they would not like to disclose to parents. Thus, a 17-year-old grandson writes that he likes to talk with his grandmother because "... she's patient and understanding. She can persuade and dissuade". A 14-year-old granddaughter observes: "with grandma you can talk about anything".

Other activities performed together involve housekeeping, shopping and, above all, recreation and introducing grandchildren to family

TABLE 6.4
Activities Performed by Grandchildren of Different Ages with Grandparents

| | Age of Grandchildren | | | | | |
| | 7–11 | | 12–15 | | 16–19 | |
Kind of Activity	N	%	N	%	N	%
1. Conversation	99	31.9	78	41.5	72	52.2
2. Walks	48	15.5	52	24.3	33	23.9
3. Plays/games	42	13.5	36	15.2	42	13.5
4. Cooking	17	5.5	21	9.6	13	9.4
5. Housework	22	7.1	23	7.4	13	9.4
6. Gardening	18	5.8	16	4.1	11	8.0
7. Shopping	13	4.2	17	5.4	10	7.2
8. Family photos	6	1.9	6	2.8	10	7.2
9. Fancy work	10	3.2	12	3.8	9	6.8
10. Excursions	7	2.3	9	3.1	9	6.8
11. Party activities	3	0.9	4	1.4	8	6.5
12. Music	0	0.0	1	0.3	8	6.5
13. Reading	4	1.3	0	0.0	7	5.0
14. Visiting	1	0.3	0	0.0	6	4.3
15. Fishing/baking etc.	4	1.2	6	2.8	5	3.6
16. Caring for pets	0	0.0	2	0.6	4	3.0
17. Religion	1	0.3	3	0.9	2	1.4
18. Watching TV	2	0.6	3	0.9	0	0.0
19. Sports	1	0.3	0	0.0	0	0.0
20. Stamp collecting	2	0.6	3	0.9	0	0.0
21. Drawing	2	0.6	0	0.0	0	0.0

tradition. This last activity (looking at photographs and other family tokens) is mentioned more often by adolescents then by younger schoolchildren. Grandparents may start introducing grandchildren into the family tradition only after the latter have reached a certain stage of development or alternatively, this information may become relevant to grandchildren only after they have reached a certain level of psychic maturity.

There are good reasons to think that the subjective importance of messages communicating family tradition increases with the formation of the so-called permanent self (cf. Lewin 1954; Tyszkowa 1986b) and development of identity (Bosma 1985; Erikson 1968; Bosma and Jackson 1990). The building of one's self-image in the context of the past can be seen as including the family past, i.e. what might be called a pre-history of individual existence. Information about one's own past and that of the family serves as material for the process of identity formation. First signs of this process can be observed at about 12 years of age. The reasons for the increase in interest in looking at family souvenirs as subjects get older may be rooted in this developmental process.

Activities performed together change slightly with the age of the grandchildren. Adolescents tend to carry out practical jobs such as clearing up, cooking or shopping with their grandparents. They go on trips more often. Conversations, walks and games remain on nearly the same level. Time devoted to conversations approaches the same levels as with peers (Czikszentmihaly et al. 1977). However, important changes occur in topics of conversation. Children talk with grandparents mainly about family and school (68%), television programmes (26%), and heroes of books. They talk less frequently about other matters such as the past, church or religion and only occasionally—as one 8-year-old boy put it—"about life". In adolescence, on the other hand, it is the conversations "about life" which take on the highest position and become increasingly frequent. Adolescents with close contact with grandparents talk with them about matters such as friendship and moral problems (37% in both age sub-groups), choosing a future career (62%) and making other important decisions with regard to their interests, or even to their sexual life. Conversations more often take the form of exchange of opinions, not just the provision of one-sided information.

Many references illustrate this trend. Younger subjects usually stress the fact that conversations with grandparents take place and emphasise what they can take out of them. For instance, a 10-year-old girl says: "With this grandma (PGM), we like to talk. She tells me about the past, how things were when she was young—that there were no television sets at home ...". A 11-year old boy states: "Grandpa knows a lot about fish. He tells me what kinds of fish are in the lake, and what in the sea". Another 11-year old girl relates that with MGM "We discuss clothes. She is a good dressmaker. We also talk about school, what grades I got and such things".

Older subjects, on the other hand, emphasise exchange of ideas and discussion of problems during conversations with grandparents. For instance, a 13-year-old girl writes about her contacts with MGM: "When I come to her we drink tea and talk. I tell her about what is going on at school, what kind of friends I have, about my problems with them and she tells me about her school years, too. She helps me to solve my problems". The reciprocity of communication exchange is stressed even more strongly in the following opinion of a 13-year-old girl on her relations with PGM: "I like to talk with my grandmother. She can listen to me and usually tries to understand my problems" and a 16-year-old girl about her relations with PGM: "We used to go for a walk. We discuss different problems. I can tell her about everything". In some cases, the problems which adolescents have talked about with their grandparents are described. They most often concern interpersonal relations with other family members (parents 15 times and siblings in 4 cases) and with peers (12 cases). Talks with grandparents help adolescents better to understand their own position and to clarify points of confusion in relations with parents. This suggests that conversations with grandparents may play a therapeutic role similar to that performed by conversations with peers (Czikszentmihaly et al. 1977; Youniss and Smollar 1990).

Other problems discussed with grandparents are connected with the processes of physical and social maturation and the new position of adolescents in the social world. For instance, an 18-year-old girl wrote about her MGM: "She was the person who told me how to be a woman" and a 17-year-old boy about his MGF: "With my grandpa we discuss usually technical problems. But sometimes some other problems, too. He told me how one may refuse to drink alcohol with other boys" (adding that it is something which is difficult to do). Another 16-year-old boy wrote that his MGM "... is the only person with whom I can discuss my problems".

Sometimes, however, discussions on problems lead to conflicts with a given grandparent. A 17-year-old boy said of his relations with MGM: "She is good and mindful. We can talk about everything except religion. I cannot stand her devotion and hypocrisy and we quarrel about it often". Adolescents (and to some extent children as well) know what topics they should not discuss with a given grandmother or grandfather and they try to avoid such conflict-generating issues. In general, however, conversations with grandparents tended to be valued highly by young people.

The frequency with which interactions of this kind are rated positively, increases with the age of the subjects. No data on this topic were collected when interviewing the youngest group of subjects. However, 32% of the utterances identified in the compositions written by the younger adolescents indicated the importance given to such interactions with grandparents. Similar statements were also found in 56 out of the 97 compositions (57.7%) written by the older adolescents. Adolescents sometimes search for contact with a given grandparent and initiate conversation on the problems they are facing. The following utterance illustrates such situation well: "I often drop in to her after school just to tell her what I'm thinking" (a 17-year-old boy about his MGM).

Not only the selection, but also the character of various kinds of common activities changes during adolescence. They tend to assume a more co-operative character. Grandchildren more often engage in activities to satisfy their grandparents' needs and not just their own. This tendency can be seen in such utterances as the following: "I help my grandma in the kitchen because she likes me to do so" (a 14-year-old girl) or "Grandpa and I like to go for excursions with a tent. I carry the tent for he is not so strong anymore" (a 15-year-old boy about his MGF). Such comments indicate a greater mutuality in the grandchild-grandparent relationship and seem to be connected with changes in the way in which grandparents are perceived.

PERCEPTION OF GRANDPARENTS: DEVELOPMENTAL TRANSFORMATIONS

Changes in adolescents' relationships with adults, including grandparents, involve transformations in the way in which people are perceived. In the analysis of our empirical data, we observed differences in the perception of grandparents by grandchildren in their late childhood and adolescence.

Children under 12 perceive grandparents as somewhat older adults who belong to a different world as regards their role and position in the family system. When describing them, children refer to external features (short, fat, tall, has grey hair, etc.) and to ways in which attitudes to themselves are manifested (good to me, kind, super, gentle, shouts at me or never shouts). They value grandparents' kind and gentle attitude, their care and interest for them. The majority of the children in the study described grandparents' personalities by using one or two (less often three) adjectives, e.g. "good", "fine", "kind" etc. On the other hand, only a minority (12.5% of cases) was able to name a grandfather's or grandmother's job, irrespective of whether this was performed in the past or in the present. Where they were able to do so, this occurred where they found the profession interesting, or where they were especially proud of their grandmother's or grandfather's achievements. A 9-year-old boy, for example, said: "My grandad used to be a fireman. He still works in the hotel..." and a 10-year-old girl: "My grandma is a psychologist. She helps children in trouble. And my grandfather is a professor of biochemistry. He got a state prize for his works last month. I went to Warsaw with him".

Children, on the other hand, mentioned individual features (including external ones) only when they wanted to compare grandparents with each other or with parents. They rarely referred spontaneously to grandparents' individual needs, though they were willing to help them if told that help was required. Adolescents, however, begin to perceive grandparents as persons with individual qualities. The first sign of a changing perception of other family members is through reference to the grandparents' age and to symptoms of ageing. This takes place towards the end of childhood. Obviously, as the years pass by, the process of ageing becomes more advanced, but children's perception of this in their grandparents depends more on their own age than on that of their grandparents. Following this, they start to notice grandparents' individual needs and in some measure to take them into account. The possibility of helping a grandparent, or of pleasing them by giving them a nice surprise becomes a source of personal satisfaction. Thanks to this process, adolescents' relationships with grandparents come to acquire a certain mutuality. This change appears to be rooted in emotional ties formed earlier in life and in a sense of obligation and gratefulness for the grandparents' care, concern and love. For instance, one 12-year-old grandson writes: "I help grandma because she's old and weak and she took care of me when I was little. She pushed me in a pram and fed me...". Adolescents also begin to be attentive to grandparents' personal experience, show them sympathy and support in suffering. A 13-year-old grand-daughter writes: "I often visit grandma and even stay overnight because she's lonely and she cries after grandpa's death. I read to her, we watch television together and this helps her". They also become more aware of grandparents' individual traits (from 20% in the children's group to 72% of the subjects aged 15-19). At the latter stage, their descriptions of grandparents contain more expressions referring to individual physical and psychological characteristics. Adolescent grandchildren's positive evaluation of grandparents is expressed in references to features such as friendliness towards others, honesty, courage, intelligence, knowledge, interests, resourcefulness, wisdom, reliability, diligence, sense of dignity and people's respect, etc.

Some grandchildren express sharp criticism of grandparents (5.8%). Adolescent grandchildren do not tolerate prying and are not prepared simply to do what they are told. However, some of them voluntarily give way to their grandparents and control negative feelings by expressing their empathy. "I usually listen to grandma because I love and respect her though sometimes she's unbearable" writes a 16-year-old grandson. Another 18-year-old girl tries to explain her grandma's aggressive behaviour writing that "...she has become such, due to the hard conditions she had to live in". The range of positive features which grandchildren perceive in their grandparents serves both as an indicator of how adolescents' perception of adults changes with development and of the emotional attitudes adopted towards grandparental figures. The number of positive features mentioned by subjects in their descriptions of grandparents is relatively low in childhood (1.3 per person on average) for both boys and girls. With girls, this number increases gradually with age and reaches 3.2 per person on average in the subgroup of older adolescents. The number of positive features provided by boys in early adolescence drops to an average of 0.8 per person and then increases in older adolescence to the same level as with girls. Adolescents of both sexes refer to positive characteristics which are of a more personal character than those mentioned by children. This seems to indicate a change whereby adolescents perceive grandparents more as individuals than previously. Weakness as a result of age or illness, or financial dependence on adult children (parents) mean that the grandparent's position may be quite similar to that of adolescents themselves. Where illness occurs (18 subjects referred to it), young people may participate in nursing and caring activities.

About 30% of the compositions indicated that adolescents begin to understand more deeply that grandparents went through the same stages of individual development which they themselves are now experiencing, i.e. they begin to recognise that they were young in the past. This provides a good basis for moving closer to grandparents and leads to awareness of the differences and similarities between them. This strengthens and extends the intimacy with grandparents which had been established in earlier years. In childhood this closeness is expressed in caresses and physical signs of tenderness. In adolescence, the intimacy of the relationship with grandparents assumes the form of self-revelation based on trust. Nearly 60% of the adolescents talked with their grandparents about their own problems and 28% entrusted them with secrets which they would not like to have revealed to their parents. This emerges in sentences such as: "With grandma I can talk about my problems" (a 17-year-old girl), "Grandma will always understand and advise me" (a 16-year-old boy), "With grandpa I can talk about anything. We have our best times talking when going fishing or taking a walk" (a 15-year-old boy). Sharing of experiences and thoughts brings a new form of intimacy into the grandchild-grandparent relationship in adolescence.

The content analysis of the compositions showed that grandchildren's ideas of grandparents include characteristics such as protectiveness and readiness to be of help to the younger generations in the family, sacrifice, modest needs and a cheerful spirit, friendliness towards others and goodness. If grandparents' behaviour and personality features are perceived as complying with this stereotype, they evoke gratefulness and a sense of obligation. The majority of subjects perceived their grandparents positively, as persons who met these expectations (58.0%, 65.7% and 55.6% according to age). Such grandparents are regarded as being worthy of love. In cases where grandparents depart from this "ideal", their behaviour arouses surprise, disapproval and dislike in grandchildren. Grandparents are expected to act in accordance with social stereotypes by children and the same is true, though to a slightly lower extent, for adolescents. In the Incomplete Sentences Test, for instance, a 9-year-old girl completes the sentence "My mum doesn't like it when grandma ..." with " ...still goes to work", and an 8-year-old grand-daughter finishes the sentence "I would most like my grandma to..." with "...retire". Another 7-year-old boy expressed his expectations towards MGM more openly by finishing the same sentence with "...stayed with me at home".

Adolescents, being more independent of adult care, are also less dependent on social stereotypes in their perception of and feelings towards grandparents. A 16-year-old girl writes about her grandmother (MGM): "My grandma is not a typical grandmother. She never took care of us when we were little. She is a doctor and always busy. We only see her on Sundays and not every Sunday at that. Still, we love each other very much". The "still" shows both the functioning of the stereotype and a sense of incompatibility with it, despite a close emotional link. Children perceive grandparents and particularly grandmothers mainly as care-givers. In contrast, adolescents begin to perceive them as conversation partners; as persons introducing them to family traditions; as a source of emotional support; as individuals in their own right.

CONCLUSIONS AND DISCUSSION

This study set out to describe the characteristics of relationships with grandparents in adolescence and—through comparison with those in late childhood—to examine the developmental transformations which occur in this relationship.

The results indicate that the majority of this Polish sample had rather frequent contact with their grandparents. The frequency of these contacts corresponds with that found in a French study (Delestre 1991) but differs from results obtained elsewhere (Matthews and Sprey 1985; Kahana and Kahana 1970). These contradictory findings may reflect differences between different cultures or may stem from more general shifts in family life. As Patricia Minuchin writes (1988, p. 23) "...families show increasing contact between generations" and it appears that this is a tendency which covers contacts with grandparents. In spite of this general finding, it should be noted that the frequency of contacts with grandparents tends to decrease slightly during adolescence. This finding is congruent with other research results (Kahana and Kahana 1970; Matthews and Sprey 1985; Sticker 1991).

Generally speaking, adolescents' relationships with their grandparents seem to acquire a new quality and a new meaning. This new quality is revealed in all main dimensions of the grandchild-grandparent relationship. First of all, contacts with grandparents are more often initiated by adolescents themselves and thus are less dependent on parental mediation or initiative than in childhood. The present findings suggest that the conceptualisation of grandchild-grandparent relationships as indirect (Matthews and Sprey 1985) and contingent (Troll 1980) does not hold in adolescence. In cases where the relationship remains close, it can be viewed as a continuation of ties established in childhood. This continuity is restricted to the emotional dimension, however and is an expression of a relatively stable interpersonal attachment.

As development into adolescence takes place, young people more often meet their grandparents at an individual level—i.e. without parents being present. Such dyadic contacts provide an opportunity for deepening interactions with grandparents and lead to greater intimacy.

The percentage ratios of positive and very positive attitude at different age-levels suggest that little change occurs in the emotional dimension of the grandchild-grandparent relationship with increasing age. There was a slight increase in the number of both neutral and negative descriptions of grandparents in the early adolescent group. Taken overall however, our findings do not confirm the thesis advanced by Battiselli and Farneti (1991, p. 153) that changes in the grandchild-grandparent relationship lead to "increasingly less positive judgements" and attitudes towards grandparents. This pattern failed to emerge from our analyses and this was especially true of the older adolescents. Conversations with grandparents are the most frequently named joint activities referred to by both children (31.9%) and adolescents (52.2%). In adolescence, conversations with grandparents reach a position close to that which they occupy in relationships with peers (Czikszentmihaly et al. 1977). This can be viewed as a manifestation of a developmental trend towards increased symmetry in interactions with grandparents. A feature of this is that topics discussed between adolescents and grandparents involve increasing exchange of opinions, thoughts and ideas.

Topics may include important problems which young people are currently experiencing. For a high percentage of adolescents (37% in the younger group and 62% in the older), grandparents are the adults to whom life problems and secrets can be entrusted. Such conversations seem to be gratifying and helpful for adolescents and lend additional significance to their relationships with grandparents. Such exchanges of opinions and thoughts help adolescents to elaborate their new life experiences. This elaboration can occur more easily in an externalised form, i.e. in an interpersonal relationship with a given grandparent (see Tyszkowa 1986a,b). Coupled with this, details of the family history and information about the grandparents themselves seem to play an important role in the processes involved in identity formation in adolescence (Erikson 1968). Discussions of this sort also help the young person to acquire effective strategies for coping with new commitments (Bosma 1985) and for dealing with developmental tasks (Olbrich 1984; Bosma and Jackson 1990). Such intergenerational transmission of individual experience may also be of some help in building up images of one's personal future. The relevance of these conversations probably explains the high value which adolescents give to them. Thirty-two percent of the younger adolescents referred to such coversations and 57% of the older group. With the exception of Sticker (1991), the role of grandparents as discussion partners for adolescents has received no attention in the research literature. It is a topic which requires further investigation and analysis.

Perceptions of grandparents evolve from the superficial, role-related view taken by children, towards an increased recognition of them as individuals with their own characteristics, problems, feelings and life experiences. As a result, adolescents are better able to understand their grandparents' situation and to empathise with them. This means that more often, they are able to provide grandparents with help and emotional support.

In summary, the results of this study indicate that in the majority of cases, adolescents' relationships with their grandparents remain close and personally important. In the adolescent's social world, grandparents occupy a specific role which is different from that of parents and other adults. They are persons with whom adolescents are familiar from their earliest childhood—persons close to them, older by two generations and yet without the authority of parents.

The results suggest that grandparents and grandchildren generally remain close and need each other during the latter's adolescence. For adolescents, the relationship serves to maintain close contact with family tradition, gives social and psychological support and provides the opportunity to gather important experiences concerning the older generation. Grandparents hand down heritage and transmit life experience to the younger generation and, in doing so, satisfy needs associated with generativity (see Erikson 1980).

A developmental transformation occurs in relationships with grandparents between childhood and adolescence. This influences the interactions, quality, intimacy reciprocity and emotional closeness of the relationship. The main changes involve a movement from:

- indirect and contingent contacts in childhood towards more direct, grandchild-initiated contacts in adolescence
- great diversity of common activities towards co-operation, partnership, and self-involvement
- physical (kisses, embracing, etc.) towards psychological intimacy (self-revelation)
- perception of grandparents as figures, performing given social roles in the family (adults, old people, care-givers) towards perceiving them as individuals and persons with their own qualities, needs, experiences, etc., and as partners (especially as conversation partners)

- asymmetric, submissive relations in childhood towards more reciprocal, mutual and symmetric relationships in adolescence.

Relationships with grandparents extend the social experience of adolescents. They provide experience of persons who differ in age and possibly in social class and subculture. Such experience is very important for young people's social development (Coleman 1972).

This study has examined adolescents' relationships with grandparents from the perspective of adolescents. However a relationship involves two partners. A more comprehensive analysis of the relationships between adolescents and their grandparents requires data collected from both partners.

Ideally, it would go further than this and examine them in the context of the family system. It would be of interest, for example, to compare transformations in adolescents'relationships with grandparents with their relationships with their parents.

Further research on relationships between adolescents and grandparents needs to take variables such as the age and sex of grandparents into consideration. In the present study, no attention was given to possible variations in relationships arising from the age of the grandparent. Similarly, little attention was given to possible variations in relationship pattern arising from the gender composition of the relationship.

Finally let us consider some of the methodological issues which arise from this study. It has shown that compositions are a useful method of collecting data from adolescents. They provide the researcher with an insight into the young person's inner world and yield information on the ways in which adolescents perceive themselves, others and the relationships they share. The data obtained do not lend themselves to interpersonal comparisons and require very careful content-analysis. This shortcoming might be overcome by using compositions in combination with a more structured technique such as a focused interview.

Comparison of the present research findings with other work (Sticker 1991; Hurme 1988; Matthews and Sprey 1985; Delestre 1991) indicates that the grandchild-grandparent relationship in both childhood and adolescence is strongly influenced by the life-conditions, cultural norms and expectations concerning family roles and relations within a given society. Individual development in adolescence is also affected by socio-historical and cultural factors (Erikson 1968, 1980; Schaie 1984). Taking both of these influences into account suggests the need for more attention to cross-national studies of relationships between grandparents and adolescents.

CHAPTER SEVEN

Developmental Tasks and Adolescents' Relationships with their Peers and their Family

Erich Kirchler,[1] Augusto Palmonari and
Maria Luisa Pombeni

Today the period of adolescence is no longer seen as a period of "Sturm und Drang". In the past, adolescence was often perceived as a stormy period accompanied by painful crises and stressful disturbances (Hall, 1904; for a review see Miller, 1989). Recent research presents a view of adolescence as a period of transition which demands new forms of adjustment, a period during which the individual is confronted with new problems and unfamiliar tasks. Contrary to the idea that adolescents are often unable to solve their developmental problems productively, recent studies paint a picture of teenagers as remarkably competent decision makers (Olbrich, 1990, Coleman and Hendry, 1990; etc.).

One of the scholars who contributed most to the understanding of problems arising during adolescence is Havighurst (1948; 1953). Almost 40 years ago, he defined developmental tasks as problems which arise at certain periods in an individual's life. He hypothesised that successful achievement of these tasks leads to happiness and greater probability of success with future tasks; whereas failure leads to unhappiness, societal disapproval, and difficulty with later developmental tasks. He suggested that developmental tasks arise from different sources, namely physical maturation, cultural pressures or societal expectations, and individual aspirations or values. This means that developmental tasks differ from culture to culture and may vary from one social stratum to another. Furthermore, developmental tasks are related to the age of the individual and vary in the course of time. Finally, they are interdependent, that is, coping with one task may give rise to another.

Havighurst presents a fair picture of the major developmental tasks which teenagers encounter between 12 and 18 years of age. The tasks to be achieved by the individual are: (a) accepting one's physical make-up and acquiring a masculine or feminine sex role; (b) developing appropriate relations with age mates of both sexes; (c) becoming emotionally independent of parents and other adults; (d) achieving the assurance that one will become economically independent; (e) determining and preparing for a career and entering the job market; (f) developing the cognitive skills and concepts necessary for social competence; (g) understanding and achieving socially responsible behaviour; (h) preparing for marriage and family; (i) acquiring values and an ethical system of beliefs that form the basis of one's behaviour and become the subject's ideology. Even though Havighurst described these tasks as early as the 1940s, they seem to be equally valid for today's adolescents (Dreher and Dreher, 1985).

Adolescence may not necessarily involve crisis and distress and developmental tasks are not necessarily conflicts and troublesome problems. In this perspective, adolescence in itself may not involve turmoil but rather define a period in which new specific problems are faced (e. g. Coleman and Hendry, 1990; Olbrich, 1985; Petersen, 1988). It is these problems which are usually called developmental tasks and the most popular scientific approach to adolescence studies the way adolescents face their tasks. Olbrich (1984), for instance, suggests that adolescence should be seen as a period of coping with new requirements. In this chapter, the terms "developmental tasks", "problems" and "difficulties" are used as synonymous terms referring to adolescents' new requirements and demands to adjust to them.

Besides troubles at school, some of the major problems are located in social relationships. Family-adolescent interactions are perceived as changing and as often stressful for both the parents and the child. Affiliation with peers and integration into a group of age-mates requires social competence and self assertion which adolescents do not always possess. For example, teenagers do not always act in a socially efficient way or overcome the shyness which is typical of the age period (Zimbardo, 1977; see also de Armas and Kelly, 1989). Engel and Hurrelmann (1989) report that 82% of German teenagers between 12 and 16 years have problems with requirements at school, 51% suffer from problems with their parents and 43% have troubles in finding friends and age mates.

Successful coping with developmental tasks has often been perceived as being mainly dependent on the personality characteristics of the individual (see Bosma and Jackson, 1990). While many studies contribute to a better understanding of the relationship between individual personality and coping strategies, we are convinced that other important variables need to be studied in order to understand adolescents' problems and resolution processes. We hold that, besides depending on personality characteristics, adaptability to new requirements depends on youngsters' interpersonal activities. Participation in social and interpersonal relationships helps to provide the resources for successfully coping with developmental tasks. In a series of studies we have tried to shed some light on this idea (Palmonari, Pombeni and Kirchler, 1989, 1990; Pombeni, Kirchler and Palmonari, 1990; Kirchler, Pombeni and Palmonari, 1991; Palmonari, Kirchler and Pombeni, 1991). Starting from a social-psychological approach, we have concentrated our attention on the importance of peer-groups as sources of support for young people.

In the following section, peer-groups as a social reference point are discussed. Various types of peer-groups in the Italian adolescent population are distinguished and the influence of these types of groups on adolescents' coping with developmental tasks are analysed. Attention then focuses on the relationship between adolescents and their groups: the closer the relationship the higher the adolescents' identification with their groups will be and the more fruitful the interactions with peers. Empirical studies will be presented which show the importance of identification with peer-group and of identification with the family. The chapter ends by concluding that coping with developmental tasks depends heavily on adolescents' identification with their peers and their families.

PEER-GROUPS AS A SOCIAL REFERENCE POINT

During adolescence, young people need to re-define their relationships with significant social entities, such as the family, and to initiate new forms of contact with peers. Establishing new contacts, developing a larger range of contacts with peers and participating in social activities with them is important. Peers are highly significant for adolescents; their importance has increased steadily since the 1950s (Kreutz, 1988). The peer-group can be thought of as a laboratory where one can try out one's role as a young adult (Sherif and Sherif, 1964). A group of age-mates represents a forum within which one can talk about one's problems. Such groups serve mainly to socialise adolescents into appropriate heterosexual interests and behaviour. As Sherif and Sherif (1965a, p. 286f) emphasise, the self-image of the adolescent consists "in large part, of his ties with his reference group and the yardsticks it provides. The continuity of his ego identity from day to day depends to a large extent on the stability of his ties with members and their consistency in appraising him according to the patterned relationships and norms shared in common. They are among the stable anchorages in his world." Peers are crucial normative and comparative reference points for adolescents (Engel and Hurrelmann, 1989).

The peer-group offers the adolescents multiple opportunities for witnessing the strategies others use to cope with similar problems, and for observing how effective these are. It offers an area for learning to present oneself in society and for accounting for one's behaviour. It allows the adolescent to explore autonomy without the control of adults and parents (Olbrich, 1985; Weinstein, 1973; Youniss and Smollar, 1990). Adolescents perceive their peers as providing support in defining identity, interests, abilities and personality, in building reputations and in developing a balance between individuality and conformity. The peer-group is also perceived as providing instrumental and emotional support, as offering the opportunity to build and maintain friendships and as a place where a variety of activities takes place (Brown, Eicher and Petrie, 1986). Adolescents who do not participate in social activities with peers are presumed to feel lonely and insecure (Brennan, 1982).

Several authors emphasise that the quality of interactions with the peers, rather than the frequency of social activities with them, favours the transition process into adulthood (de Armas and Kelly, 1989). Jones (1981) found that students who describe themselves as lonely, report that their interactions with peers are less warm and friendly.

In this chapter, the peer-group is conceived of as a small group of similarly aged, fairly close friends, sharing the same activities. This conception is slightly narrower than that which appears in the broader literature where "peer-group" often features in a much more general sense, referring to adolescents within the culture who are of roughly the same age as a given individual. Engel and Hurrelmann (1989), for instance, conceive of peers as age-mates, most often as friends in the same class at school, rather than as a group of adolescents sharing similar interests and performing the same activities.

There is a variety of places where adolescents frequently meet and where they engage in a range of activities. In Italy, they most often join others at street-corners for entertainment (Amerio, Boggi Cavallo, Palmonari and Pombeni, 1990). Many teenagers also belong to peer-groups which are focused upon sports, religious programmes or ideological and political activities, art performances or other structured activities. Teenagers usually belong to a variety of groups of friends but there is often one specific peer-group which they conceive of as being the most important to them and in which they most often participate.

The Sherifs make a distinction between artificial or laboratory groups and natural groups, and hold that adolescents' reference groups are formed in a spontaneous and natural way (Sherif and Sherif, 1965a). Palmonari and his colleagues found that most of the adolescents who join a group do indeed choose a group of peers which meets at street corners and other places in the city and which forms spontaneously for no specific reasons apart for amusement and discussions about personal and social issues (Palmonari et al., 1989; 1990). Other groups meet at members' homes for entertainment. Palmonari and his colleagues described groups meeting at street corners or members' homes as informal peer-groups. In their research they distinguish between informal and formal peer-groups. Like informal groups, formal groups consist of about 5 to 15 persons, though sometimes they may be even larger. Unlike informal peer-groups, formal ones are committed to a specific project (sport groups, religious groups, political groups, groups performing arts etc.). They are well structured and often supervised by one or more adults.

Palmonari and his colleagues report that more than 90% of Italian adolescents join an informal or formal peer-group fairly regularly (97.6% of boys, 92.2% of girls). This result largely confirms the Sherifs' (1964) findings, indicating that the majority of adolescents join one or more peer-groups. It is interesting to note that in a study of 363 Austrian adolescents, Schün (1990) found that only 80% of the respondents joined a peer-group. Although peer-groups are important for adolescents in Italy and Austria, the difference may indicate that experiences with peers are culture-specific and the results which will be reported in the following pages, while valid for Italian teenagers, may not be readily generalisable to adolescents living in other European countries.

More than 75% of the adolescents who participated in the studies met with informal groups (53% joined groups meeting in squares and streets of the cities, whereas 26% met at peers' homes); the remaining 21% joined more or less formal groups (11% met with sports groups, whereas 10% joined groups committed to religious programmes; almost no adolescents joined political groups or groups engaged in artistic programs such as drama, choirs etc.; Palmonari et al., 1990). The low interest in political activities was also encountered by Engel and Hurrelmann (1989): only 3% of the teenagers in their survey reported participating in political activities. In the Austrian sample (Schün, 1990), 50.6% of the respondents indicated meeting an informal group; 21.1% joined sports groups, 21.1% met with religious groups; 6.7% met with a group engaged in artistic programs and less than 1% joined a political group. It should be emphasised here that adolescents often meet with various peer-groups. In such cases Palmonari et al. asked the respondents to indicate the peer-group which was most important to them and which they would not be prepared to give up. The subjects were asked to refer to their experiences with their specific peer-group rather than with groups in general.

Palmonari and his colleagues (1989; 1990) found that the main reason for being in an informal or formal peer-group was to enjoy oneself (38.8% of the respondents reported that enjoyment was the main purpose for meeting their group). But the group was also seen as an opportunity for meeting friends (20.5%), sharing meaningful experiences (19.6%) and maturing (13.3%). A small percentage (7.8%) considered group life as an alternative to loneliness. Some sex-differences emerged. Males generally met their peers for amusement, whereas girls more often than boys reported that the main reason for joining their group was to have social contacts. The reasons for participating in a group did not vary between students and those adolescents who were already working. While it is true that adolescents spent most of the time with their peers for amusement, leisure and fun, they reported that talking about one's problems is the most important activity.

TYPE OF GROUP AND DEVELOPMENTAL TASKS

Commonsense holds that formal groups are a better means for leading teenagers through the often conflicting years of adolescence. A common general assumption is that public adolescents meeting with peers on street corners for amusement risk being influenced negatively by drug abusing age-mates, delinquent individuals etc. From a social psychological point of view it may be hypothesised that formal groups, as compared with informal groups, are more structured and tend to bind the members closer together. Moreover, they are engaged with specific projects, led by adults, and therefore supposed to be better able to provide the requested emotional and informational support to their members than informal groups. Additionally, since formal groups spend more time on organised activities than informal groups, they are able to present their members with a clear "universe of symbols", that is, with values and norms. Adolescents may learn to understand and accept the peers' values and imitate the models which the group displays. In other words, formal groups seem to present a more clear-cut point of reference to their members than do informal groups. Therefore, formal groups could be a more fruitful source of support than informal groups and adolescents joining informal groups should have fewer problems in adapting to their new requirements than others.

Palmonari and his colleagues carried out a series of studies which tried to analyse the significance of the nature of the group for coping with developmental tasks. They asked 600 adolescents aged 16 to 18, from Bologna in Italy to complete a questionnaire, consisting of three parts: first, the adolescents were asked whether they participated fairly regularly in an informal or formal peer-group, where the group met, who the group members were, what the group aims were, which activities the members performed in the group and to what extent the group interacted with adults. Second, the respondents were asked to describe themselves and their peer-group as well as two groups of adolescents which they considered to be different from their group. The third part of the questionnaire dealt with developmental tasks which were derived from interviews with adolescents belonging to the same population as the participants in our studies. The interviewees evaluated the importance of and difficulty of coping with (a) overcoming restlessness, (b) accepting one's body after the changes linked to development, (c) acquiring autonomy as regards the choices to be fulfilled, (d) developing self-awareness, (e) finding reference values, (f) coping successfully with different situations of everyday life, (g) building up stable relationships with a group of friends, (h) establishing positive relationships with the age-mates of the other sex, (i) successfully completing one's schooling, (j) preparing oneself for integration into a work environment, (k) achieving economic independence, and (l) preparing oneself for the responsibility of having one's own family.

Factor analysis of the results showed that developmental tasks can be summarised into three clusters: relational problems (relationships with friends of the same and opposite sex), personal problems (overcoming restlessness, accepting oneself, autonomy, self-awareness, reference values, coping with everyday life) and socio-institutional problems (school, work, economic independence, responsibility for creating a family). These clusters of problems are important to the adolescents and they often find them difficult to resolve. The most important and difficult were found to be socio-institutional tasks, especially where these concerned school and employment. These results correspond with Engel and Hurrelmann's (1989) finding that the school is the most crucial source of difficulties for most teenagers in Germany. It should be mentioned here that socio-institutional tasks are defined as problems which adolescents may have with their teachers and other adults representing norms, values and duties which characterise school and working place. Tyszkowa (1990a) analyses difficult school situations in detail, by focusing on a variety of interpersonal aspects and also on other requirements at school.

Surprisingly enough, the type of the peer-group, informal or formal, which the adolescents joined was of minor importance. Analyses of variance with the type of peer-group as independent variable and the importance and difficulty of the three developmental tasks as repeated dependent variables revealed a highly significant difference between the task types. No significant differences between the group types were obtained. It was found that socio-institutional tasks were the most important and difficult tasks to resolve for adolescents from both formal and informal groups. Personal problems and relational requirements were perceived as far less difficult.

At first glance, the results of this study seem to be rather disappointing since they contradict what appears to be common sense. Despite failing to find support for our hypothesis on differences between formal and informal groups, however, the results encouraged us to have a closer look at the importance of peer-groups for adolescents. We found, that there is a high variance between the participants in the similarity of self-descriptions and descriptions of their group on adjective scales. While some adolescents perceived themselves as highly similar to their peers others described themselves as highly different. These differences were especially true of teenagers joining informal groups.

Turner and colleagues (1987) used similarity of self-descriptions and descriptions of one's own peer-group as an indicator of identification with the own group. Looked at from this point of view, our results suggest that some adolescents feel close to their group and identify highly with it, whereas others do not. In a follow up study Palmonari et al. (1990) set out to analyse the importance of identification with the peer-group for developmental tasks.

IDENTIFICATION WITH THE PEER-GROUP AND IMPORTANCE OF DEVELOPMENTAL TASKS

In a study designed to assess social categorisation processes in groups and the importance of developmental tasks, 3744 adolescents from the Regione Emilia Romagna, Italy, were contacted by a research assistant at vocational centres and various high schools and invited to respond to the same questionnaire as had been used in the former study. Again, participants saw socio-institutional problems as far more important and difficult to resolve than other developmental tasks, concerning personal and relational problems. This finding was true irrespective of the type of group (formal or informal) in which the subjects participated. All subjects also perceived socio-institutional tasks as problematic for their age-mates.

In this study, the degree of identification with one's own peer-group played an important role. Identification was operationalised as the difference between self descriptions and descriptions of one's own peer-group. The sample was split on the median of the difference-index into two sub-samples, one consisting of adolescents identifying highly with the peers, the other consisting of participants with low identification. As Figure 7.1 shows, highly identified adolescents found personal and relational problems much less important and difficult to resolve than low identifiers. Where socio-institutional problems were concerned, there was no difference between high and low identifiers. When asked about their peers' opinions concerning developmental tasks, high identifiers reported that their peers found socio-institutional problems highly important. Low identifiers found that their group gave considerably less attention to these problems. Where the importance given by the group to personal and relational tasks was concerned no differences between high and low identified youngsters emerged. Figure 7.1 shows that the distances between high identifiers' judgments of importance of tasks and the importance which their group assigned to these tasks were much smaller than the respective distances for low identifiers. Since the highly identifying adolescents perceived that their peer-group assigned importance to those problems which were also important to them individually, we may assume that highly identifying members have less difficulty in disclosing their problems to their peers, are more easily understood by them than low identifiers and consequently receive more informative, emotional, and perhaps instrumental support from their peer-group. The fact that low identifiers perceived their individual

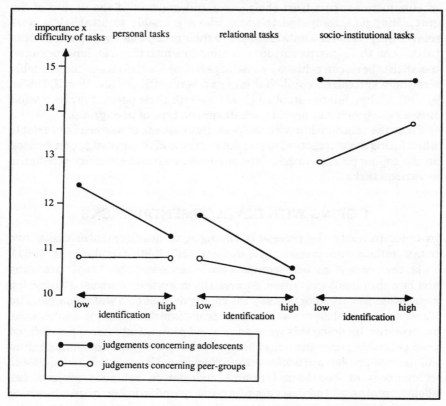

FIG. 7.1. Importance and difficulty of developmental tasks as perceived by low and high identifiers and their peer-groups. Importance was ranked from 1 (not important) to 5 (important), and difficulty from 1 (not difficult) to 5 (difficult). The two variables were merged.

problems as much less important to their peers than to themselves, suggests that they may have considerable problems in talking about their situation and in getting the necessary assistance from their peers.

These results are striking: it should be remembered that the type of group the adolescents joined had no impact on their perception of either the importance of or the difficulties in coping with developmental tasks. It was the relationship which the adolescents were able to establish with their peer-group, operationalised as identification with the group, which played a major role. It appears that whether a teenager joins a street group, a religious group or a group engaged in a sport programme, has little bearing on his or her success in adapting to new developmental requirements. If youngsters are able to create a close relationship with their peers then they receive more support from their peers, independent of the nature of the group they join, compared to those who are unable to establish a close relationship. If adolescents feel close to their group and their group accepts them, then their group provides a context in which they can have personal ties with others, can achieve a sense of personal worth in ways not available elsewhere and can accomplish things as a person (Sherif and Sherif, 1965a, p. 286). If they fail to establish close ties with their peers, they lack what only a peer-group can provide, whatever the type of peer-group.

Since the relationship with the peer-group seems to be a crucial variable when facing developmental tasks, the next step of the investigation focused on the coping process rather than on importance and difficulty attributed to various tasks.

COPING WITH DEVELOPMENTAL TASKS

In order to study the process of coping with developmental tasks, two investigations were carried out (Pombeni et al., 1990; Kirchler et al., 1991). First, members of six peer-groups were interviewed about their problems and how they dealt with these. Second, the interviews were used to develop a questionnaire in order to study the coping process on a wider sample. The interviews served to derive a list of tasks which represent adolescents' experiences. By doing this we tried to avoid presenting a list of pre-defined problems which runs the risk of being much more explicit and definite than are the real problems of adolescents (Silbereisen, Noack and Eyferth, 1986).

Members of two formal groups engaged in religious projects (22 adolescents) and 53 adolescents who participated in informal groups which met mainly for entertainment at street corners, completed a questionnaire on demographic characteristics (sex, age, occupational status, father's profession) and on identification with the peer-group. We presented 12 adjectives derived from a pre-testing (Palmonari et al., 1990) and the subjects rated themselves and their peer-group on 5-point scales. As in the first two studies (Palmonari et al., 1989; 1990), the Euclidean distance between the two resulting profiles of self and peer-group was taken as the index of identification. Second, Brown's (1988) Group-Identification Scale, consisting of ten items, was presented (5-point rating scales). A principal components analysis derived from pre-testing of the items revealed two factors. Only the first factor was taken as index of identification. In other words, identification was measured here by the following items: "My group is very important to me", "I identify with my peer-group", "I have a strong relationship with my group", "I am happy to be with my group", and "I consider myself a member of my group".

As in the previous studies, the sample of adolescents was split at the medians of identification indexes into two sub-samples, one highly identifying with their peers, the other with low identification indexes. The two identification indexes were significantly correlated ($r = 0.41; p < 0.01$). In cases where the two indices gave conflicting classifications, Brown's index was taken as splitting criterion. The decision to take Brown's index seemed reasonable given its high reliability (alpha = 0.89). Moreover, since in previous studies the Euclidean distance between self descriptions and group evaluations was applied, the decision to take Brown's index made it possible to test whether identification with the group still proves to be a significant variable if operationalised in a different way.

A pre-structured interview was carried out. First, the subjects were asked to imagine three critical incidents. These were selected from three situations from each of the three clusters of relational, personal and socio-institutional problems. If an adolescent had never had to cope with the problem presented by the interviewer, another critical incident out of the respective cluster of problems was presented. The aim of this procedure was to obtain information from each individual on three different types of incident. The incidents, presented in random order, read as follows:

Relational problems:

(1) Do you have a steady boy-friend or girl-friend. If so, have you ever had a serious problem with him or her?

(2) Imagine being with your best friends. Can you think of any serious problems you have had with them?

(3) Imagine being together with your colleagues at work or class-mates at school. Can you think of any serious problems you have had with them?

Personal problems:

(4) Imagine yourself in a state of depression. Have you ever been depressed due to loneliness and isolation?

(5) Imagine yourself in a state of depression. Have you ever been depressed because you felt you had nothing to believe in, no real values worth fighting for?

(6) Imagine yourself in a state of depression. Have you ever been depressed because you wanted to make decisions, such as buying something, against the wishes of others?

Socio-institutional tasks:
(7) Do you remember moments of high tension at school? Perhaps you were frustrated with school, felt unable to fulfil the requested duties or thought of leaving the school.
(8) If you have a job, you will probably remember moments of high tension at work. On such occasions did you think you would not be able to fulfil the required tasks?
(9) Can you remember situations where you acted against the law? Using drugs, for example.

After having presented the critical events the subjects were asked to (a) describe precisely the situation and how they had behaved, (b) to describe their emotional state and (c) to indicate whether other members of their group had faced similar situations. They were then asked (d) whether they had asked somebody for support, (e) what the reaction of the other was, (f) whether anyone had spontaneously offered support, and (g) whether they had accepted or rejected the offer. The interview contained questions concerning (h) whom the adolescent talked to, (i) whether the mood was positive, indifferent, or negative during the talk, (j) whether the outcome of the talk was positive or negative, and (k) what the outcome was in terms of emotional tone. The interview ended with questions about (l) whether the problem was finally solved and who found the solution for the problem, and (m) how the problem and solution process affected the adolescent's mood and behaviour in the long run.

Each adolescent was asked to report on three problems, one out of each of the three clusters, which they had experienced in the past. In sum, 50 adolescents reported about three issues and 25 talked about two problems only. Six different types of problems were disclosed most often: concerning social relationships, the problems were conflicts with an intimate partner (12.0% of the cases) or misunderstandings in interactions with friends and colleagues (15.5%). The personal sphere encompassed feelings of loneliness or social isolation (13.5%) and loss of values or experiences of an existential vacuum and loss of orientation (17.0%). The remaining two problems, concerning school and work (26.5%) or minor criminal acts (12.5%), were problems with the society and law or institutions. A few cases were reported where the problem concerned a purchase decision against others' wishes (3.0%).

Where the process of coping with these problems is concerned, the study revealed that teenagers often feel rather alone with their problems. However, there were important differences between high and low identifiers. Especially when the problems concerned school or work, high identifiers when compared with low identifiers less often felt a lack of self-esteem and more often experienced bad mood and a need to talk to somebody. High identifiers asked somebody for support more often, and more often obtained positive answers from others than did low identifiers. They were also more likely to receive offers of support from others and to accept those offers than were low identifiers. Adolescents who were close to their group reported more often that the discussion with somebody was fruitful and that it had lead to a solution. They thought that they had found a way out of their problem thanks especially to the assistance of their peers and their family. Low identifiers, on the other hand, were often unable to resolve a task and felt release only some time later. After having resolved their problem, high identifiers tended to express gratitude to others and reported that what had happened had contributed to their maturation. Adolescents with a rather loose relationship with their peers, thought much less frequently that the problem which had arisen had contributed to behaviour changes or to their maturation.

These results confirm that peers are a source of help for adolescents. If teenagers feel close to their peer-group, it seems indeed to help in defining their identity, interests, abilities, and personality, in building their reputations, in developing a balance between individuality and conformity, in providing instrumental and emotional support and finally, in providing a situation for building and maintaining friendships (Brown et al., 1986). If identification with the group is low, adolescents risk losing these advantages.

Since the sample size in this study was small, a further investigation on 770 adolescents was conducted (Kirchler, et al., 1991). The participants answered a questionnaire on identification with their peer-group and several questions concerning the process of coping with various developmental tasks. Again, the results confirm a significant difference between high and low identifiers. Adolescents who had established a close relationship with their peers talked more often to the peers about problems with their best friend than those with low identification. They judged the talks more positively and more often reported maturation as a long term effect of the problem. Where the problem concerned friends in general, high identifiers more often than others sought support from their peers, judged the talks favourably and reported that the event had led to maturation. The coping process with personal problems, such as feelings of loneliness or lack of life values, was also affected by identification with the group. High identifiers disclosed their personal problems more often to their peers than did low identifiers and were more satisfied with the results. If socio-institutional conflicts had occurred, high identifiers were found to reveal their problem more often to their peers than did low identifiers and, if the discussion with others was positive, high identifiers took more advantage of this than low identifiers. Delinquent adolescents emerged as feeling rather lonely and unable to find solutions. In this area, identification with the peers had no effect on the coping process.

Problems with the family, especially with the parents, were also presented as a critical situation during adolescence in this study. If the peer-group represents a challenge to the family, i.e. if those adolescents who join their peers regularly have less time for their parents and are less interested in their parents' opinions, then high identification with the peers should negatively affect the process of coping with parental conflicts. However, the results show again that high identifiers had less difficulties in coping with such problems than low identifiers.

In conclusion, our studies show that adolescents who are able to establish a close relationship with their peers have significant advantages. "Muddling through the troubles of adolescent years" may not only depend on the capability to identify with age-mates, but also on the possibility to be close to other social entities, such as their own family. In a further study the impact of identification with peers and the family on coping processes was analysed.

IDENTIFICATION WITH THE PEER-GROUP AND THE FAMILY

During adolescence, young people need to re-define their relationships with their family and with significant other social entities and to initiate contacts with peers. Re-definition of social relations can lead to conflict. The initiation of relationships with peers and friends has often been conceived as a challenge to the adolescents' relationships with their parents and as the cause of a fundamental gap between the generations. The notion of a serious divergence of attitudes and beliefs between teenagers and parents has encouraged the assumption that increased involvement with the peer-group inevitably leads to a rejection of parental values. There are several reasons why adolescents may risk breaking positive relations with their parents or suffer from inadequate relationships with them. Social conflicts at home are a source of risk because the family, as a crucial social reference point, may fail to provide the necessary emotional, informative, and financial support which the adolescent needs in order to cope with certain developmental tasks. This is especially true of future-oriented domains with regard to school, work or future aspirations (Coleman and Hendry, 1990; Hunter, 1985; Kandel and Lesser, 1972; Larsen, 1972; Seiffge-Krenke, 1985). The family provides significant support to adolescents, and connectedness with the family was found to be favourable for adolescent development (Seiffge-Krenke and Olbrich, 1982).

In a study of 1600 adolescents from three cities in Italy, Palmonari et al. (1991) found that identification with the peer-group and identification with the family are significantly correlated (the correlation between identification indexes amounted to $r = 0.22; p < 0.01$). Although significant, the correlation is not very high and indicates that there are many youngsters who either identify highly with both social entities or do not identify with the peers and the family, but there are also many who identify with one entity highly, but not with the other. Being interested in difficulties with developmental tasks, we split the sample into four sub-samples on the medians of identification with the family and the peer-group. This gave us one sub-sample of adolescents who identify highly with both family and peers; one sample identifying highly with family, but not with peers; one identifying highly with peers but not with family; and one having difficulties with identification with both family and peers.

The results show that those youngsters who did not feel close to either their family or to their peers talked least often about their problems to others. The person to whom the adolescents disclosed their problems was most often their best friend (41% of the cases). Overall, in 18% of the cases the problems were disclosed to parents, 14% of the cases to peers, 6% of the cases to other adults, and in 23% of the cases the adolescents did not talk to anybody about their stressful experiences. These general results can be compared with those from a study of more than 1700 German teenagers, ages 12 to 16 years (Engel and Hurrelmann, 1989). German teenagers were most likely to talk to their parents or to a friend if they had a personal problem or difficulties at school. Disclosure of problems to grand parents, teachers and other persons was found to be rather rare. The peer-group as a social entity with which to share one's one problems was not mentioned. Perhaps, in this study, friends and peers were used as interchangeable terms.

Further examination of our results showed that those teenagers who identified highly with their family talked more often to their parents than others. On the other hand, those adolescents who identified highly with their peers talked more often to their peer-group than did the others. Table 7.1 displays relative frequencies of talking to somebody by high versus low identification with family and peers.

In general, the adolescents judged talking to somebody in rather positive terms. Except where the problem concerns delinquency, teenagers express relief after having disclosed their problem to somebody. Again, high identifiers reported more positive reactions than low identifiers. The type of group in which the teenagers participated again had no effect. Positive effects increased with closer identification with the family or the peer-group and was highest if the adolescents were willing and able to identify with both entities (see Figure 7.2).

TABLE 7.1

Relative Frequency of Talking to Somebody by High versus Low
Identification with the Family and Peer-group

Identification with	Discussion Partners					total absolute frequency
	peer-group	best friend	family	other persons	nobody	
Family: low						
peers: low	0.11 –	0.42	0.14 –	0.07	0.27 +	1725
peers: high	0.17 +	0.45 +	0.10 –	0.06	0.22	1291
Family: high						
peers: low	0.10 –	0.36 –	0.27 +	0.06	0.21	1135
peers: high	0.12	0.40	0.22 +	0.06	0.21 –	1614

Note: The signs "+" and "–" indicate significant differences between observed and expected frequencies: "+" indicates that the observed frequency is higher than expected; "–" indicates that the observed frequency is smaller than expected.

Except for family conflicts and delinquency, most of the youngsters reported finding a solution to their problems. Overall, a solution was found in 76% of the cases. Low identifiers more often reported not having found a solution for their problems (27%) than those adolescents who either identified with their peers, their family or with both the family and the peers (22%) and this was especially so if conflicts with the family or personal problems were at stake (28% versus 21%). In comparison with teenagers who identified highly with their peers, low identifiers claimed lack of support from their peers when the problem concerned a conflict with a best friend, social isolation or feelings of no values in their lives (high identifiers reported support from their peers in 14% of the cases, whereas low identifiers only reported having received any support in 5% of the cases). Low identifiers also missed the help of their family, when the problem concerned intra-family conflicts (high identifiers reported support from their parents in 16% of the cases, whereas low identifiers reported having received support in only 9% of the cases). Also, adolescents with high identification with peers but low identification with the family were often unable to resolve intra-family conflicts (32% as compared to 20% of those identifying highly with their family). In general, they missed support from the family (while high identifiers obtained support from their family in 16% of the cases, low identifiers reported support from their family in only 6% of the cases). Those teenagers identifying highly with their family but not identifying with their peer-group, received help from their family

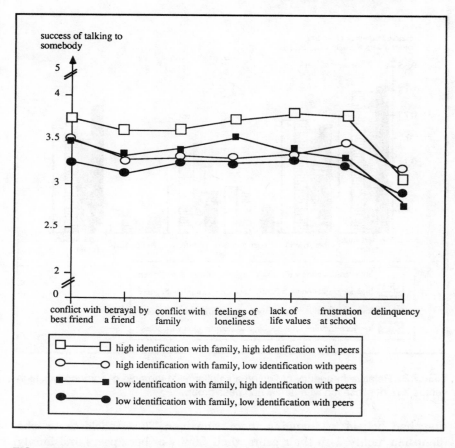

FIG. 7.2. Success of talking to somebody (1 = negative, 5 = positive) × high versus low identification with peers and family and problem type (conflict with best friend, betrayal by a friend, conflict with family, feelings of loneliness, lack of life values, frustration at school, delinquency).

in resolving problems with the best friend (18%), with the family itself (18%), the school (46%), and illegal acts (11%). High identifiers had the advantage of receiving support both from the family (especially if the problem concerned family relationships [15%] or feelings of loneliness [13%]) and the peer-group (especially if the problem was a serious conflict with the best friend [14%] or lack of values [17%]). Figure 7.3 shows the relative frequencies of support provided by various social entities by high versus low identification with the family and peer-group

When asked whether the respective problems had had a long term effect on their transition into adulthood, the teenagers most often reported that

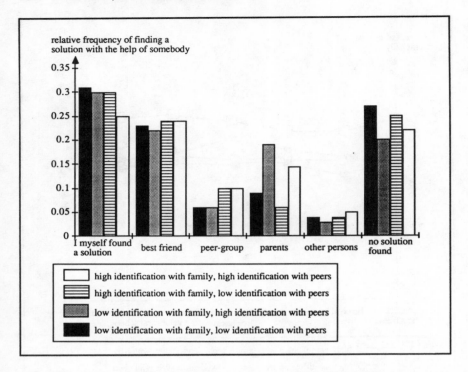

FIG. 7.3. Relative frequency of finding a solution with the help of somebody × high versus low identification with family and peer-group.

they had helped in changing their behaviour. Those adolescents who identified highly with their peers, their family or both peers and family reported more often that the resolution of a stressful event helped them to mature (55%) rather than leading merely to a change of mood or behaviour (45%). Low identifiers more often reported a change of mood or behaviour (53%) rather than maturation (47%). With increasing identification with both the family and the peer-group the probability of a successful resolution of the problems increased. Adolescents who were unable to identify with both, showed less positive effects than those identifying with one or both entities.

Palmonari et al. (1991) conducted a separate path analysis for each type of problem. Figures 7.4 and 7.5 provide examples. These analyses represent a summary of the stress-coping paradigms which were elaborated by the authors. The process of coping was perceived as moving from awareness of a problem to the need to talk to somebody, the outcomes of the talk, a solution of the problem and long term effects. The sex of the respondents, the type of group they joined (informal versus formal), and the degree of

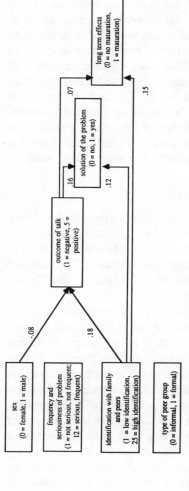

FIG. 7.4. Process of coping with difficulties within the family.

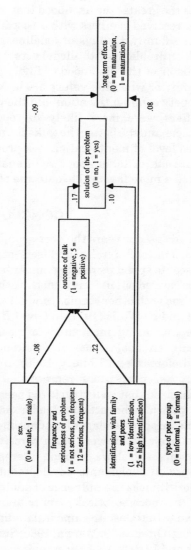

FIG. 7.5. Process of coping with a lack of life-values.

identification with the family and the peer-group (combined factor) were considered as antecedent variables which affect the coping process.

The analyses confirm that the type of group is largely irrelevant, whereas identification with both the family and the peers, is of great importance in the coping process. The higher the identification with both entities the greater the likelihood that adolescents reported maturation after having resolved conflicts with a best friend, betrayal by a friend, conflicts with the family, feelings of loneliness, lack of life-values, frustration at school, or problems with illegal acts. Identification was also important as a predictor of the likelihood of finding a solution in conflict situations in the family or when life-values are lacking. The most significant path was found between identification and the outcome of talks to somebody. High identifiers were more likely to report a positive outcome than low identifiers and the better the talks the more profitable the long term effects. Besides level of identification, sex proved to be an important predictor of the outcome of talks about relational and personal problems. Females reported a more favourable outcome of talking to somebody than males.

CONCLUSIONS

In the adolescent years the peer-group provides the opportunity for trying out various social roles and sets standards for adolescent behaviour. Adolescents spend increasing amounts of time with their peers. A series of studies carried out in Italy underline the significance of peers. The findings are in line with other studies conducted by the Sherifs (1964) in the United States and by Willis (1977) in Great Britain.

The increasing importance of peers results in an increase in their influence on adolescents' self-concept development (Sherif and Sherif, 1964; Coleman and Hendry, 1990). In the past, this has often led to the assumption that peers represent a challenge to the family. It was hypothesised that well structured peer-groups, which are influenced by an adult person who acts as leader and defines and organises common projects, support teenagers in adapting to new requirements. Other groups, on the other hand, were often perceived as small, tightly knit groups of youngsters who share common interests, but who tend to have a negative influence on adolescents' development. The less structured a peer-group, the more it lacks the influence of adult persons and the vaguer its common aims, the more sceptical parents and researchers tended to be about its positive value. Despite empirical findings which have failed to support this view (e.g. Offer, 1969; Marcia, 1980; Smith, 1976; Salmon, 1979; Greenberg, Siegel and Leitch, 1983), it remains very much alive in parents' and other adults' cognitive representations of the teenager's world (Amerio et al., 1990).

Our studies have shown that during adolescence, the peer-group becomes important but not omnipotent and that the family remains highly influential. Peer-group and parents fulfil different needs for the adolescents. Parents provide guidance where necessary, skills-training and a forum to discuss future-related problems, such as school and work. The peer-group provides recreational outlets, age-mates share developmental tasks with the individual, and the group represents a context in which to try out adult behaviour (cf. Burke and Weir, 1978; Offer and Offer, 1975; Brown et al., 1986). Our studies have also shown that the type of peer-group an adolescent joins is of subordinate importance. Formal groups are not a better source of support than informal groups. It is the type of relationship that the adolescent is able to establish with the group which significantly affects the developmental process. The higher the identification the more emotional, instrumental and informative support the teenager can expect from his or her group.

Identification was defined as similarity between individual and group characteristics and as importance of group to the individual. High identifiers may be conceived as being close to their group or in the "centre of the group"; low identifiers, on the other hand, may be located at the "border of the group". Engel and Hurrelmann (1989) found that adolescents who are at the margins of their group have more severe problems with self-esteem than those who are in the centre of their group. These results seem to confirm our findings about the support which individuals derive from their groups.

Identification with peers was found to be correlated with identification with the family, school mates, and best friend (Kirchler et al., 1991). It can, thus, be assumed that those adolescents who are close to others and identify with them are able to make use of this in different situations and so may have less serious problems on their way to adulthood. Depending on the type of problem, they get the necessary instrumental and emotional support from the source which is able to provide it. Once a positive relationship with one or other social entity has been established it has to be maintained. The instrumental and emotional support provided by a positive relationship may not only be continued to the period of transition into adulthood but also continue into adulthood. Adolescence can be perceived as the period during which the individual needs to learn to structure his or her social environment, to establish meaningful relationships, to reveal his or her problems, to share them with others, and to maintain the social relationships which may move more and more towards long-term friendships which remain important into adulthood.

Up to now we have mainly concentrated on high identifiers and their approaches to developmental tasks. Where low identifiers are concerned, we observed that they are on the "margin of the group" and are also often not closely connected with their family, class mates and others (cf. Smith, 1976; Iacovetta, 1975). The reasons for adolescents' problems with identification are unknown and require detailed study. Personal characteristics may hinder individuals from identifying with their peers, but there may also be a variety of intra-familial and social circumstances which present serious obstacles for contacting peers and maintaining friendship.

In conclusion let us repeat that the peer-group in adolescence fills a vacuum rather than provoking a conflict between parents and teenagers (Coleman, 1980). Adaptation within modern societies demands responding to several social entities and not just to one. Apart from the family, adolescents need to socialise with peers, establish contact with class-mates, etc. In the past, the peer-group may have had a compensatory role for children of broken families (Bronfenbrenner, 1974). It can be seen as an additional point of reference. As Marcia (1980) maintains, a good relationship with family and peers is important for a positive self-concept. Greenberg et al. (1983) found that support from both parents and peers is important during the high school years. The closer the youngster feels to his or her significant "social reference points", the family and the peer-group, the more advantages he or she derives from the relationship. We should emphasise that, rather than being a source of distress, the family can provide significant support to adolescents in reorganising intra-familial relationships. Closeness to the family is favourable for adolescent development. However, the family needs to leave the adolescent enough "space" for the development of his or her individuality (Grotevant and Cooper, 1985). If the parents allow for individuation in the family context, i.e. a balance between connectedness and individuality, they positively affect the process of transition in adolescence. If, however, the parents observe with fear the changes occurring in their sons or daughters, are shaken and insecure about the needs for autonomy, or are too norm-oriented, then they act as an obstacle. It seems likely that the same is true of the peer-group and that it needs to leave enough "space" for its members to develop as individuals. While high identification is important and useful for adapting to new situations, groups that tightly knit their members together, claim full identification with the groups' interests and do not allow for individuality (e. g. religious sects, delinquent gangs, circles of drug abusing teenagers, etc.) may represent an obstacle for individual teenagers rather than a helpful source of support. Sherif and Sherif (1965) repeatedly emphasised the importance of joining the peer group. They underlined the significance of latitude of involvement in the peer-group, holding that sharing some activities and fields of interests with peers is significant, but that it is also important to share other activities and areas of interests with other people, parents, brothers and sisters, class-mates, etc. In sum, relationships with neither the family nor the group should become the exclusive "yardstick" for the young persons' success or failure in accomplishing developmental tasks. The family provides a point of reference for some areas (e.g. school, work), the peer-group may be important for other relevant fields of interest (e. g. social contacts, intimate relationships; Sherif and Sherif, 1965a, 1965b). Identification with these social entities and acceptance by them is important in order to provide teenagers with support in responding to the varied demands and tasks of adolescence. The young person needs to identify with social entities, not to be absorbed by them.

NOTE

1. Much of the work on this manuscript was carried out while the first author was on study leave at the University of Bologna, Italy.

CHAPTER EIGHT

Stress, Coping and Relationships in Adolescence

Inge Seiffge-Krenke and Shmuel Shulman

The past two decades have seen a dramatic increase in research examining the relationship between coping and stressful life events in adults (e.g. Dohrenwend & Dohrenwend, 1974). Recently, this research has extended to younger age-groups and increasing attention has been given to coping behaviour in adolescence and to the social resources available to young people at this age group (see summaries by: Siddique & D'Arcy, 1984; Seiffge-Krenke, 1986; Compas, 1987). Two of the key concepts in all of this work are "life-stressors" and "social resources" (Lazarus & Folkman, 1984).

Several factors should be considered when examining how stress relates to coping strategies used by adolescents. These factors include: the specific nature of the stressor, the individual appraisal of the stressor and the availability of personal resources, such as family support (Folkman & Lazarus, 1980; Patterson & McCubbin, 1987). It appears that the nature of stressors and their association with symptomatology during adolescence may differ in some fundamental ways from what happens during adulthood. Furthermore, due to the specific developmental dynamics of this phase, relationships with parents and peers may not only constitute a stress buffering factor, they may also act as an additional source of stress (Glynn, 1981; Barrera, 1981). Social support has been described as an important mediating variable in the relation between psychosocial stress and psychological and somatic symptoms (see reviews by Cohen & Wills). However, in spite of a large body of empirical research pointing to the importance of social support in managing stress, some fundamental conceptual and methodological questions have remained largely unaddressed (Monroe, 1983). The problem of confounding social support and psychological distress, for example, was raised by Slavin and Compas (1989), who pointed to an overlap in contents and methods of social support and symptoms. Researchers and clinicians need better indices for life stressors and social resources in order to describe adolescents' life contexts more adequately, to explain individual differences in the impact of events with respect to social resources, to predict adaptive and maladaptive outcome and finally, to develop intervention programmes in case of severe stressors.

In discussing coping from a developmental perspective it is important to distinguish between coping as an effort to respond to stress and overall adaptation, a question first addressed by Murphy and Moriarty (1976). Coping is frequently equated with successful adaptation. However, the effectiveness of a particular coping strategy cannot be determined independent of the context within which it occurs. A strategy which is adaptive in one situation may not be adaptive elsewhere. Furthermore, empirical support for equating coping with successful adaptation would require examination of cross-situational consistency or variability in adolescent coping and/or prospective studies of the coping process. Studies of this sort have rarely been carried out.

The focus of this chapter is on stress and coping during adolescence. The main emphasis will be placed on three topics: events or conflicts which are considered as "stressful"; factors which determine the stressfulness of events; and finally, the way of coping with normative and non-normative stressors. A full understanding of how adolescents respond to stress requires consideration of the relationship between the context in which stress occurs and the personal coping resources of the individual. Thanks to refinements in operationalisations and the development of new measurement procedures including the use of several informants, such an approach promises to provide new and more complex answers. Although research conducted from a variety of different traditions has been concerned with these issues, discussion here will be limited mainly to studies which focus on interpersonal stress and coping.

THE RELATIONSHIP BETWEEN STRESS AND COPING

The field of stress research has been strongly and justifiably criticised for its failure adequately to define the concept of stress (Compas & Phares, 1986) The same holds true for coping, which appears to be a comparable "umbrella construct". Despite these failures, research on the relationship between stressful life events and coping in adults remains an area of undiminished interest. Comparable work with adolescents, however, has been far less extensive. A review of existing research, analysed according to age-groups, revealed that only 7% of all studies carried out in the past 20 years dealt specifically with adolescent coping (see for a summary Seiffge-Krenke, 1986). Until recently, research activity has been very restricted and limited to certain specific issues. For example, two-thirds of the studies investigated responses to traumatic events and critical life events. The typical approach involves studying the reactions of small homogeneous groups of adolescents to an extremely stressful, non-normative event such as kidnapping, rape, death of friends or family members, or contracting a serious illness. This narrow approach has led to examination of a great many defence strategies, but little attention to coping behaviour. Thus, the operational definition and measurement of coping has been heavily dominated by defence aspects. For example, eleven of the twelve "coping dimensions" in the instrument developed by Houston (1977) were in fact defence mechanisms such as denial, suppression or reaction formation.

In recent years, a clear change of approach has taken place. More refined methods for investigating stress and coping in adolescence have been developed (Compas, 1987; Daniels & Moos, 1990; Seiffge-Krenke, 1990a), as have new models for integrating different types of stressors (Wagner, Compas & Howell, 1988). Longitudinal studies involving large representative samples have increasingly been used. The interest in assessing how adolescents cope with developmental stressors has also served to focus attention on coping with normative events, with everyday problems and with developmental tasks.

Some of the attempts to conceptualise coping during adolescence have drawn on broader theoretical models (Murphy & Moriarty, 1976). Our own research on stress and coping in adolescents has drawn extensively on the conceptual framework of Lazarus and Folkman (1984). Their approach is appealing because of the emphasis they place on the interdependence between the two constructs. Stress is defined as "a particular relationship between the person and the environment that is appraised by the person as taxing or exceeding his or her resources and endangering his or her well-being" (Lazarus & Folkman, 1984, p. 19). Coping is defined as "problem-solving efforts made by an individual, when the demands he/she faces are highly relevant ... and tax his/her adaptive resources" (Lazarus et al., 1974, p. 250). Thus, whether one perceives oneself to be faced with a stressful situation or not, depends, in part, on one's appraisal of coping resources. This approach to coping provides a useful conceptual basis for research on adolescence, because of the enormous adaptational demands experienced by the young person during this phase of development.

Effective adaptation to stressful events entails a complex interplay among several different factors. The latter include the nature of the event itself, the individuals' appraisal of the event, personal and social coping resources available to the individual and the actual coping strategy which the person employs (Lazarus & Folkman, 1984).

COPING WITH DIFFERENT STRESSORS

Developmental Tasks, Normative Demands and Critical Life Events

Adolescence is a developmental period in which the individual is not only confronted with a dramatic change in bodily contours, but has also to master a series of complex and inter-related developmental tasks. The young person's way of coping with these normative demands is of special relevance. According to Havighurst (1972) adolescents have to accept their own body, learn a masculine or feminine social role, prepare for an occupation, achieve independence from parents and establish a personal scale of values and ethical system. Similar lists of adaptive demands have been provided by other researchers on adolescence. Sroufe (1979), for instance, describes "salient developmental issues", while Petersen and Spiga (1982) list a variety of "developmental challenges".

Mastering relevant developmental tasks may best be described as solving ill-defined and highly complex problems. When life changes are too rapid or extreme, occur simultaneously, or are unusually timed, individuals are subjected to varied and extreme challenges in coping with their situation. This might lead to conditions which prevent adolescents from continuously tackling and solving relevant developmental tasks (Coleman, 1978). According to Antonovsky (1981), individuals tend to become more vulnerable during periods of biological, social and psychological transition. A 14-year-old adolescent, for example, will be affected quite differently by the onset of a chronic illness, than a young adult who has already solved most of the developmental tasks of adolescence. Empirical studies of how adolescents cope with illness have shown that mastery of relevant developmental tasks is impeded or delayed (Hauser et al., 1984; Seiffge-Krenke & Brath, 1990). It has also been established that stressful life events during adolescence are related to emotional and behavioural problems (see for a review Compas, 1987). Compas distinguished between acute and chronic demands (such as acute or chronic diseases or enduring conflicts in the family), normative demands (e.g. school transition) and major events (e.g. parental divorce). These different types of events need not be mutually exclusive. Many of them are age-related and have a particularly high frequency during adolescence, e.g. physical growth/menarche, changes in social roles, family and school transition. It is also the case that the effects of general cultural events may differ dramatically across age-groups. The cohort which experienced adolescence during the economic depression of the 1930s has a very different event history from a present-day cohort.

Early studies of life events during adolescence generally made use of lists generated by adults and used for adult samples. In recent years, the development of the Adolescent Perceived Event Scale (Compas, Davis, Forsythe & Wagner, 1987) has offered better opportunities for the assessment of life events during adolescence. Open-ended lists of daily and major life events were obtained from a sample of over 600 adolescents aged between 12 and 20 years (Compas, Davis & Forsythe, 1985). This yielded a list of 213 non-redundant life events and daily stressors with three slightly different sets of items representing events of early, middle and late adolescence.

Although earlier research has provided a strong foundation for the study of stress and critical life events, it seems likely that considerable advantages can be derived from exploring the role of daily stressors in the lives of adolescents. Evidence has emerged which suggests that, as with adults, daily stress may play an important role in adolescent development (Baer, Garmezy, McLaughlin, Pokory & Wernick, 1987; Compas, Davis & Forsythe, 1985; Rowlinson & Felner, 1988).

To date, however and in contrast to research with adults, prospective studies of stress and emotional/behavioural problems in adolescents have been rare and have only recently begun to provide support for the role of stress as a risk factor (Cohen, Burt & Bjorck, 1987; Swearingen & Cohen, 1985; Compas & Phares, 1986). Cohen et al. (1987), for example, found that negative events accounted for a small (5%) but nonetheless significant proportion of variance in depression and anxiety.

Several authors have suggested that an integrative model of stress should include both types of events, since major events may lead to an increased number of daily stressors and these, in turn, may lead to symptoms (Felner, Farber & Primavera, 1983; Kanner et al., 1981). A recent retrospective analysis of stress and symptoms in older adolescents during the transition from high school to college lent support to this hypothesis (Wagner, Compas & Howell, 1988). Major events were related to daily stressors, which were associated, in turn, with psychological symptoms, but no independent relationship between major life events and symptoms was found.

Perceived Stress in Everyday Problems and Minor Events

The results obtained by Compas and his colleagues indicate that the relation between stress and maladjustment may not be linear. While such work has started to clarify the relationships between the two, it is still true that the cumulative effects of both major and minor stressful events and processes are not yet fully understood.

Our own research, which has used different methods to assess major and minor events, has confirmed the stressful character of everyday problems. Girls appear to be particularly vulnerable in this regard. Using a cross-sectional design, 1028 German adolescents aged 12 to 19 were asked to name the frequency and intensity of a series of 64 problems and the extent to which each problem had bothered them (Seiffge-Krenke, 1984). The problems stemmed from 7 developmentally relevant domains including: School (e.g. "I got a bad grade"); Future ("I'm afraid I might not get the job I want"); Parents ("I had an argument with my parents"); Peers ("My friend doesn't understand me"); Heterosexual relationships ("I am worried that my boy friend will leave me"); Leisure-time ("I feel isolated"); and Problems with the self ("I feel depressed").

The level of strain experienced by the subjects ranged from medium to low and the sequence of problems they described, corresponded to results found in earlier studies (e.g. Remmers & Radler, 1962; SHELL-study, 1981): future-related problems were followed by achievement and school problems and thereafter came interaction difficulties with parents and peers. Interestingly, fearful future anticipations occurred in totally different cohorts even though adolescents' life-conditions could be regarded as having changed considerably during the past 30 years. In our study, fearful future anticipations consisted of items representing personal fears ("I am afraid I might not get the job I want") and fears regarding social problems ("The increasing destruction of the environment frightens me").

Somewhat surprisingly, the level of perceived stress was fairly uniform across the genders. Males tended to refer more to problems with the opposite sex, while females reported more self-related problems concerning their body and behaviour. Early adolescence emerged as the only period which is perceived as quite stressful across all of the different domains. School-related problems, future-related problems, problems with peers and problems with the self peaked in early adolescence (see Figure 8.1).

Gender differences were analysed with the help of t-tests. Family-related problems were only rarely indicated. This was mainly true of adolescents whose parents had had an academic education (7% of our sample) and therefore had more space at home and greater financial resources. These parents might also have differed in parental style, e.g. been more tolerant. Adolescents from other socio-economic groups also expressed few fears and troubles concerning the family. As they grow older, both males and females report family troubles more frequently. Despite this, their orientation towards their parents remains generally positive.

School-related problems at age 12 were reported by male adolescents significantly more frequently than by female adolescents ($t = 3.0, p = < 0.05$). On the other hand, significantly more females than males reported problems with peers ($t = 3.2, p = < 0.02$) at age 14.

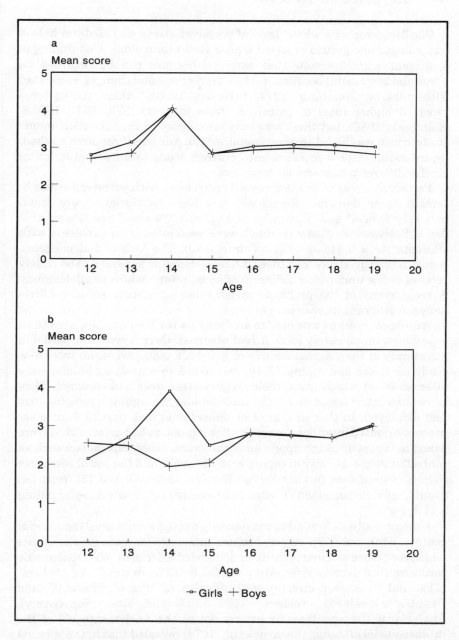

FIG. 8.1. Perception of problems in two domains by male (*n* = 479) and female adolescents (*n* = 549) in various age groups: a = future-related problems, b = problems with peers.

For the group as a whole, level of perceived stress was medium to low, but younger age-groups reported higher stress than older. This finding is consistent with the view that early adolescence can be regarded as particularly stressful because of school transitions and changes associated with puberty (Hamburg, 1974; Petersen, 1986). Other studies have reported higher rates of perceived stress for girls (Hill, 1987; Hill & Holmbeck, 1986), but there was only a tendency in this direction in our study, which was based on questionnaire data. A different research method, interviewing after a problem has occurred, leads to an accentuation of gender differences, as will be described.

Perceived stress in one domain was correlated with perceived stress in certain other domains. Significant and high correlations were found between "School" and "Future" ($r = 0.51$) and "Parents" and "Peers" ($r = 0.50$). Problems in "Leisure time" were associated with problems with "Parents" ($r = 0.41$) and "Peers" ($r = 0.40$). The lack of independence between perceived stress in these different domains appeared to be closely related to the underlying influence of social relationships in adolescence. A great many of the problems investigated, constitute social conflicts between different interaction partners.

A different method was used to analyse how the young people appraised a problem, immediately after it had occurred. Over a six-week period, a subsample of the original sample of $n = 1028$ took part in an interview study on stress and coping. They were asked to contact us immediately after an event which taxed their adaptive resources had occurred. They were then interviewed about the problem and the coping strategies they had employed. In this way, most of the subjects took part in four to six process-oriented interviews directly after a problem had arisen. They were asked to report upon the appraisal of the event, event parameters such as controllability, their way of coping with the event and the social resources they had used (see further Seiffge-Krenke, 1992). Of the 116 reported events, only 7% consisted of critical life events (e.g. "I saw a roofer falling and dying").

Unexpectedly, 74% of all spontaneously quoted events involved a social conflict, while only 19% referred to non-interactional conflicts, i.e. events which concerned self and identity or demanded a decision. With males, this social conflict usually referred to the fields "Leisure time" and "School" (41% and 31%, respectively), with females to "Peers", "Parents" and "Identity/self-related problems" (28%, 20% and 20%, respectively). Analysis of the spontaneous utterances of the adolescents using the process-model of coping (Lazarus et al., 1974) revealed that first appraisal of each of the events was by and large aversive in the sense that it was regarded as a loss or a threat. Interestingly, female adolescents reported four times more threat than males.

The process of secondary appraisal used by the adolescents, involved a more precise analysis of a specific situation and the personal resources which were available. Male adolescents tended to regard problems as new and simple, whereas females described them as familiar and complex. Nearly all adolescents (92%) described the situation as highly relevant for them and as having far-reaching consequences (60%). Subjects tended to perceive many barriers in solving the problem at hand. For girls, these barriers were both internal and external, while boys saw them as mainly external. Girls also reported higher expectations of failure to solve the problem than boys (42% vs. 21%, respectively). Females reported more network and relationship stressors than males, they felt more threatened by an event and were more pessimistic about solving the conflict involved. Analysis of tertiary appraisal (see Lazarus et al., 1974) after the coping process revealed that girls continued to report higher levels of ongoing stress than boys. For them, the level of underlying conflict arising from the event was still very high, though less stressful than at the stage of primary appraisal (Seiffge-Krenke, 1992).

These results concerning the stressfulness of minor events and gender differences in perceived stressfulness are in line with those of Compas (1987) and Compas and Phares (1986). Where gender differences are concerned, our findings indicate that female adolescents not only rate more events as threatening than do males, they also report a higher rate of ongoing stress after the coping process has taken place. This supports Lazarus' (1984) suggestion that certain hassles have major significance for further coping, i.e. they create a particular pattern of vulnerability which means that the individual experiences psychological stress in the ordinary transactions of life. This suggestion implies that it is not so much major events, but rather the ongoing series of irritating, frustrating, and distressing daily hassles which matters most in the experience of stress. Our findings show that minor events or everyday problems may remain psychologically salient over time and require continuing adaptive efforts which may ultimately be more taxing than efforts aimed at coping with major events. What then is the relationship between daily hassles, major events and psychological response? Wagner, Compas and Howell (1988) used a three wave panel design to test whether negative daily events mediate the relationship between major negative events and psychological symptomatology. Their results, derived from adolescents during the transition from high school to college, support the validity of an integrative model of stress. Both negative daily events and major life events contribute to psychological symptomatology.

COPING WITH EVERYDAY PROBLEMS

There are at least three issues related to adolescent coping which warrant further investigation: the type of coping strategies used by adolescents and the function they serve; age, sex, and cultural differences in coping behaviour; and finally, cross-situational consistency or variability in coping. The third of these areas has been only rarely investigated. This has arisen because of the absence of methods for assessing adolescent coping across situations. This problem appears to have been solved with the recent development of a promising instrument (Daniels and Moos, 1990) which allows the integrated assessment of life stressors and social resources in eight domains (e.g. health, parents, school, etc.). Ebata & Moos (1989) and Moos (1989) have also developed an instrument for assessing coping responses in the Coping Responses Inventory (Youth Form).

We chose two different methods for analysing coping behaviour. Young people's reaction to a problem was investigated by means of process-oriented interviews conducted immediately after the event had taken place (see previous section). Anticipatory coping was assessed by means of the Coping Across Situations-Questionnaire (CASQ). This consists of a two-dimensional matrix covering 20 coping strategies across 8 age-specific problem situations (Seiffge-Krenke, 1989b). The latter consisted of Studies, Teachers, Parents, Peers, Opposite Sex, Self, Future and Leisure-time. These eight domains were found to represent the issues usually considered by adolescents to be age-specific, salient and sources of conflict. The Questionnaire explores three factors which represent three different coping styles: Active Coping by means of Social Resources (e.g. "I discuss the problem with friends"); Internal Coping ("I analyse the problem and think of various possible solutions"); Withdrawal ("I withdraw, because I am unable to change the situation"). The third factor may be regarded as dysfunctional in that no immediate solution is reached. It includes intrapsychic defences such as denial, regression and withdrawal. The three factors together account for 53.2% of the variance and their Cronbach alphas were 0.80, 0.77 and 0.76 respectively. Cross-cultural studies on adolescents from Israel (Seiffge-Krenke & Shulman, 1990) and Finland (Seiffge-Krenke, 1991a) have revealed a similar three factorial structure, though the Israeli sample showed a slight change in sequence: Internal Coping emerged as the first factor and Active Coping as the second. In the study involving 1028 German adolescents aged 12 to 19, the subjects presented themselves as competent copers, well able to deal with problems arising in several developmental areas. Functional coping modes dominated; dysfunctional coping being employed very rarely and only for certain types of problem. The latter mode occurred particularly often with self-related problems (e.g. "discontented with oneself"), of which about one third of responses involved withdrawal (Seiffge-Krenke 1989a). A replication study with Finnish adolescents produced comparable results.

The ratio of functional to dysfunctional coping was highly stable over time (Seiffge-Krenke, 1984). We analysed the coping behaviour of unselected groups of adolescents who were tested three times over an eighteen month period. Stability coefficients ranged between 0.59 and 0.87 and were especially high for support-seeking behaviour. Cross-cultural comparisons produced comparable patterns of functional relative to dysfunctional coping, with a ratio of 4:1 (Seiffge-Krenke & Shulman, 1990; Seiffge-Krenke, 1991a). The percentage of Active Coping which emerged was 41% in the Finnish, 57% in the German and 40% in the Israeli sample. The percentage of Internal Coping was 39%, 22% and 44% respectively. Thus, across eight developmental fields the percentage of Internal Coping in the Israeli sample was twice as high as in the German sample. On the other hand, the highest percentage of Active Coping was shown by the German sample. The most important results to emerge from these different studies are the general dominance of functional coping strategies in all three countries, the emphasis of Internal Coping in the Israeli sample and the emphasis of Active Coping in the German sample. In the Finnish sample, Active Coping and Internal Coping were more evenly balanced.

The three samples differ with respect to emphasis on direct action and help-seeking behaviour as compared to internal reflection concerning possible solutions. Furthermore, the tendency to apply dysfunctional coping across all situations was generally low and roughly comparable across the Finnish, German and Israeli samples (20%, 21% and 16% respectively). If this response tendency is examined with regard to specific situations, some marked differences become apparent. In problem areas relating to Self and Leisure-time, the percentage of Withdrawal responses reported by the German sample is twice as high as in the Israeli sample, while in situations relating to Parents and Teachers, both cultures have about the same Withdrawal rates (see Figure 8.2). In the Scandinavian sample, problems with Teachers elicit the highest Withdrawal rates. In Future-related situations, the percentage of Internal Coping is very similar for Finnish and Israeli adolescents (50% and 49%) and considerably higher than for the German sample (31%). The most prominent developmental task, the pressure to find a job in a society with a high youth unemployment rate, evokes an increased withdrawal tendency in the German sample. The Finnish adolescents, on the other hand, are much more oriented towards Future. They show a picture of motivational loss in School-related problems, while their orientation towards Future is rather strong. In general, the results of these studies show that while there are culture-specific modes of coping for certain tasks or problems, the broad tendency is for adolescents in all three cultures to employ similar modes

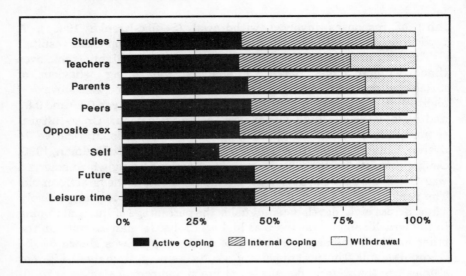

FIG. 8.2. Percentage of active coping, internal coping and withdrawal in eight developmental fields, *n* = 548 Finnish adolescents.

of coping. As Figure 8.3 shows, the use of internal forms of coping ("I analyse the problem and work out possible solutions") and the willingness to compromise increase with age.

Discussions with parents and adults become less important as the adolescents grow older; they are only referred to with regard to areas such as "School" or "Future". On the other hand, social support from Peers increases with age. Striking sex-differences emerge in the use of social resources, especially in domains such as "Parents", "School" and "Self-related problems". As they grow older, girls seek advice, help, comfort, or sympathy from others more often than boys, regardless of the nature of the problems. Girls discuss their problems with others more often and try to clarify their difficulties by talking about them openly. These trends are in line with research on adults, indicating a general tendency for females to rely more on social networks than do males (Haan, 1974; Belle, 1981). They are also more likely than males to seek help in extra-familial settings (Ilfield, 1980).

The picture changes if one moves from anticipatory coping to the situation following the occurrence of an event or problem relating to an area such as Parents, Peers, etc. As pointed out earlier, males and females differ in their appraisal of the same normative event. Girls assess the same events (bad marks at school, quarrel with the family, etc.) as four times more threatening than do boys of the same age (Seiffge-Krenke, 1992). The majority of all of the everyday events which were described involved a social

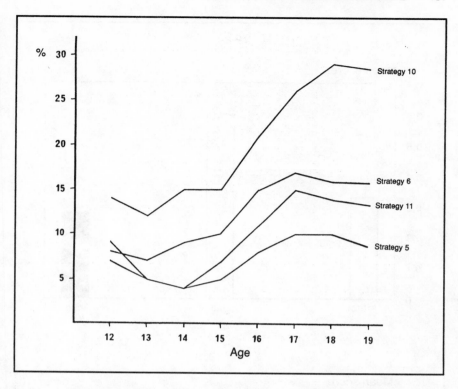

FIG. 8.3. Changes in coping with age, n = 1028 German adolescents. Strategy 10 = I think about problems and try to find different solutions. Strategy 6 = I try to talk about problems with the person concerned. Strategy 11 = I compromise. Strategy 5 = I accept my limits.

conflict. A content analysis of these conflicts revealed several main themes: Betrayal and Humiliation, for example, were frequent themes with peers; Autonomy, a frequent theme with parents.

Analysis of the coping processes actually used in responding to these events led to a division into three broad categories. This revealed that the adolescents referred much more frequently to affects (40%) and cognitions (40%) than to actions (20%). The most frequently employed cognitions were information seeking, cognitive control and analysis of the behaviour of others. On the affective side, negative emotions such as anger and anxiety prevailed. Actions included initiatives, opposition, submission and apathy. Two thirds of all of the items which were categorised as "action" included reported inhibitions of action. As can be seen in Figure 8.4, adolescents' reactions differed in amount of emotion, cognitions or actions reported, depending on the theme of the conflict and the interaction partners

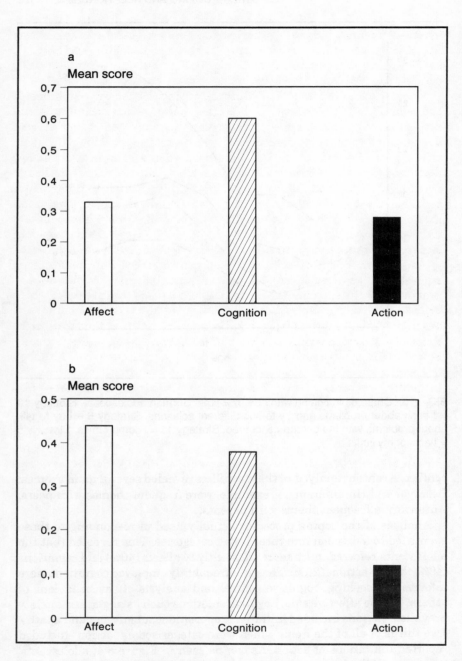

FIG. 8.4. Emotions, cognitions and actions reported as reaction to conflicts stemming from different areas: a = autonomy, b = betrayal.

involved. Events which were experienced as very stressful, e.g. losses ("My friend left me") or critical life events ("I saw a roofer falling and dying") evoked many affects and at the same time resulted in an inhibition of actions.

Conflict with parents (about "Autonomy") initiated many cognitions. If the adolescents fell in love, on the other hand, affects, cognitions and actions were balanced, i.e. the proportion of actions was higher. Events which were thematically similar produced concordance coefficients which were high and significant with respect to emotions and cognitions and low and nonsignificant with respect to actions. This indicates that even though adolescents think and feel in a similar way with respect to a particular problem, they differ in the ways in which they respond. The small concordance coefficients for activities may also express knowledge of different social norms. As Argyle et al. (1981) have shown, specific situations require their own rules for defining adequate social behaviour.

As is clear from this summary, empirical research on coping during adolescence has revealed a considerable degree of diversity within this age group. Generally speaking, adolescents adopt a functional approach which leads to a choice of coping strategies that are specific to the problem. When describing their likely response to anticipated events, they tend to describe themselves as successful copers. The situation changes dramatically, however, if they become directly involved with a concrete event. Although the events or problems which were described in the interviews correspond in quality to those referred to in the questionnaire (i.e. they were also events frequently experienced in fields such as Leisure time, Peer group, School, Parents and so on), process analysis revealed different patterns of response. Subjects more often reacted emotionally and rarely saw possibilities for applying action-oriented strategies. They focused mainly on situational cues which were relevant for planning their behavioural strategies (Nisbett & Wilson, 1977) and hesitated to take on a more active role. Girls expressed most stress in response to the events or problems. Where a social conflict was involved, they also saw it as being more permanent. Over time, this conflict tended to diminish as the young person learned to cope with it, but it continued to exist. One of the main functions of the coping strategies applied after a problem had taken place was to work through emotions aroused by the event or problem. Action blockage was most typical in events perceived as most stressful, e.g. critical life events which happened by chance during the course of the study.

PARENTS AS A SOURCE OF SUPPORT AND STRESS
Family Climate and Coping Behaviour

Two important points emerge from research which addresses individuation by focusing upon the family process (White et al., 1983; Hauser et al., 1984; Grotevant & Cooper, 1985): 1. adolescent development is viewed in terms of a transformation of the reciprocal patterning of the parent-child relationship; 2. the finding, which is of particular importance with regard to coping, that the quality of family relations is linked to measures of adolescent competence. In studies addressing the question of coping and family relations more directly, results confirm the saliency of certain family dimensions. Perception of family cohesion (Walker & Greene, 1987) and an index of family stress (Siddique & D'Arcy, 1984) can be more powerful predictors of adolescent well-being than specific negative life-events. Given these and similar findings (Rutter, 1983; Felner, Aber, Primavera & Cauce, 1985), some investigators have concluded that the quality and nature of the family climate is strongly associated with the style of coping adopted by the adolescent and that the latter subsequently affects the adolescent's level of adjustment.

Shulman, Seiffge-Krenke and Samet (1987) compared adolescent coping styles across differently perceived family climates. Family climate was measured with the Family Environment Scale (FES; Moos & Moos, 1976) and coping by means of the coping questionnaire (CASQ; Seiffge-Krenke, 1989b). One hundred and eighty seven Israeli adolescents aged 15 to 17 participated in the study. A cluster analysis revealed four distinctive types of family climate. Adolescents from Cluster 1 ('Unstructured Conflict-Oriented') perceived a high degree of conflictive interaction and lack of support within the family context. Apart from an emphasis on achievement, family members did little to support personal growth. Organisation and control within the family were perceived as low. In contrast to this, adolescents from Cluster 2 ('Control-Oriented') perceived their families as emphasising control and exerting pressure towards the structuring of family activities and explicitness of family rules. Ethical issues were of importance and achievement was stressed. Family members were described as supporting each other, but refraining from expression of emotions. Adolescents felt that they had a low level of independence. Adolescents from Cluster 3 ('Unstructured Expressive Oriented') perceived a substantial degree of cohesion and unity in their families, combined with encouragement of open expression of feelings. In addition, the family was described as supporting individual independence without pressure for achievement. Family rules and organisation appear to be approached in a laissez-faire atmosphere. Adolescents from Cluster 4

('Structured Expressive-Intellectual Oriented') described an emphasis on family relationships. Independence was encouraged, combined with an appropriate level of organisation and clear rules.

Comparison across the different clusters revealed a significant difference in coping styles, F (3, 183) = 3.35, p < 0.001). Table 8.1 shows that Active Coping was lowest in adolescents in Clusters 1 and 3. Where Withdrawal was concerned, adolescents from Cluster 1 exhibited the highest level of dysfunctional coping style. No difference was found between the four cluster groups with respect to Internal Coping.

No interaction was found between family type and age or gender of the adolescents making use of one or other of the three coping styles. When coping styles used by adolescents from the different family climates across the eight conflict domains were analysed, significant differences again emerged between the four family clusters on Active Coping, F (3, 183) = 3.28, p < 0.05) and Withdrawal, F (3, 183) = 5.26, p < 0.001). Where Active Coping was concerned, the domains of Studies, Parents and Self contributed to the differences. As to Withdrawal, perceived family climate predicted adolescents' dysfunctional coping, regardless of the domain in which the problem was encountered.

A replication of this study on two strictly controlled, parallel samples of German (n = 353) and Scandinavian (n = 521) adolescents produced similar results especially with respect to perceived family climate and

TABLE 8.1

Adolescent Coping Styles across Four Family Climate Clusters. Means, Standard Deviations and Results of Significance Testing are shown for 187 Israeli Adolescents

Coping Styles	Cluster 1 Unstructured Conflict Oriented	Cluster 2 Control Oriented	Cluster 3 Unstructured Expressive-Independence Oriented	Cluster 4 Structured Expressive-Intellectual Oriented	Test of Significance Overall F	Pair-Wise Scheffé
Internal Coping	M = 5.34 SD = 1.67	5.96 2.27	5.77 1.63	5.52 1.82	0.94[a]	—
Active Coping	M = 4.02 SD = 1.70	4.97 1.49	4.31 1.55	4.84 1.77	3.28*	1 ≠ 2, 4** 2 ≠ 3[b]
Withdrawal	M = 2.37 SD = 1.47	2.24 1.67	1.73 1.34	1.39 1.15	5.26**	1 ≠ 3* 1, 2 ≠ 4***

[a] = NS; [b] = p < 0.10; * = p < 0.05; ** p < 0.01; *** = p < 0.001

dysfunctional coping (Seiffge-Krenke, 1992). The cross-cultural comparison, including the German, Scandinavian and Israeli samples, showed that families whose offspring had the highest Withdrawal rates were uniformly characterised by poor cohesion, minimal expression of feelings and highly conflictual interactions (see Figure 8. 5). These families —especially in the Scandinavian and German samples—exerted high control over their adolescent members and neglected the individuality of their offspring.

The analysis indicated that adolescents with a higher level of functional coping saw their families as more cohesive and organised and as showing respect for individual development. Perception of a lack of family support or an over-controlling family climate was related to a higher level of dysfunctional coping. Adolescent perception of family climate was also found to be related to task or situation characteristics. Young people who saw their families as supportive and oriented towards individuality employed a higher degree of Active Coping via social resources in the domains of Studies, Parents and Self. In the domains Peers and Opposite Sex, coping behaviour was least related to family dimensions. The

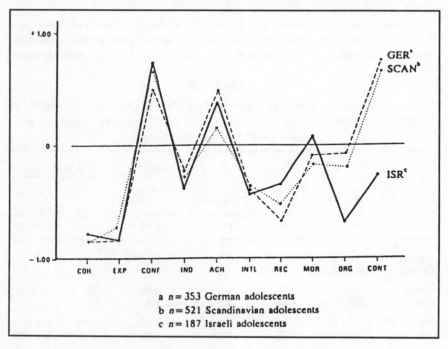

FIG. 8.5. Family climate (measured by Moos Family Climate Scale) and coping behaviour: unstructured conflict-oriented families.

association between dysfunctional coping style and family climate was found across most developmental domains and was validated in cross-cultural research. Thus, Withdrawal can be regarded as a deep-rooted type of coping behaviour. No difference in Internal Coping was found across the four family types. These studies were all conducted on non-clinical samples and this underlines the fact that adolescents, irrespective of family climate, appraise stressful situations in a similar fashion.

Stern and Zevon (1990) have recently extended this research by assessing adolescents' specific coping responses as a function of age, type of stressor and quality of family environment. Seventy-three adolescents aged 15 to 18 completed the Ways of Coping Scale (WCS; Folkman & Lazarus, 1985) and the Family Environment Scale (FES). The adolescents were asked to name recent events which they had experienced as stressful and then to consider these events when completing the WCS. Problem-focused coping and seeking social support were the most frequently used coping responses. Younger adolescents used emotion-based coping strategies to a greater extent than older adolescents. The relationships between adolescent coping and perceived family climate were similar to those found by Shulman, Seiffge-Krenke and Samet (1987). Negative perception of the family environment was associated with the use of more emotionally based coping strategies such as wishful thinking, denial and tension reduction.

The influence of family climate emerges clearly when adolescents are required to reflect about their preferred coping behaviours in anticipated stressful situations. In particular, what happens when an adolescent encounters a problem within the realm of family? Is coping behaviour similar to that employed in other types of anticipated situation? A typical occurrence which requires the adolescent's attention or response is when a conflict or disagreement emerges in the family. In recent years a growing body of research has been concerned with this topic.

Types of Conflict and Conflict Resolution

When conflicts at home occur, mundane issues predominate: family chores, time to come home or go to bed, dating, grades, personal appearance, and eating habits are the main matters of concern. As Hill and Holmbeck (1986, p. 158) stated ironically, conflicts, instead of being about basic values, are primarily about "hair, garbage, dishes, and galoshes." Smetana (1988) for example, found that doing chores, getting along with others, regulating activities and adolescent's personality were the most frequently cited conflicts. Respectively, they accounted for 18%, 17%, 12% and 12% of all conflicts. Apart from chores and achievement, the types of issues leading to conflict did not vary in frequency from pre-adolescence to late adolescence. Conflict over chores, especially cleaning one's own room, and achievement peaked in early adolescence, coinciding with changes in school and pubertal status (Hamburg, 1974; Hill & Holmbeck, 1986). Some studies indicate that adolescents have more conflicts with their mothers than with fathers (Montemayor, 1982); perhaps because mothers are more involved in regulating the everyday details of family life. When asked to identify the parent with whom they had conflicts, adolescents reported that 52% of their conflicts were with both parents, 35% with mother alone and only 14% with father alone. For girls, the results are more consistent with the prevailing notion that early adolescence is a period of particular disruption in parent-child relations (Hill, 1987; Hill & Holmbeck, 1986). A replication of the Middletown study of Lynd and Lynd (1929) by Caplow, Bahr, Chadwick, Hill and Williamson (1982) shows that the issues around which conflicts arise have not changed much in the past 60 years.

Analysis of specific coping strategies used when problems with the parents appeared, revealed an increasing readiness to compromise with age. In a sample of 1028 German adolescents aged 12 to 19, 19% of the 12-year-olds compared to 34% of the 19-year-olds were prepared to compromise. Furthermore, quarrelling with parents was increasingly discussed with friends (7% against 33%) and with the parents themselves (17% against 41%) as the adolescents get older (Seiffge-Krenke, 1984). This latter result underlines the age-related movement towards more symmetry and mutuality in the parent-adolescent relationship. Thus, when asking a youngster how he/she will cope with a problem with parents, the response reflects a tendency to cope in a functional way. In cross-cultural research on adolescents from Germany, Finland and Israel, we found that dysfunctional coping, e.g. Withdrawal, was not a frequent coping style when responding to problems involving parents. It was only reported by 15% of the German, 17% of the Israeli and 18% of the Finnish adolescents (Seiffge-Krenke & Shulman, 1990; Seiffge-Krenke, 1991a). In a telephone survey of 10th graders, Montemayor and Hanson (1985) found that 47% of conflicts with parents are solved by walking away and only 15% are marked by negotiation. Withdrawal as a coping strategy in parent-adolescent conflicts is apparently higher in their study than in ours.

Smetana's (1988) work on conflict resolution strategies is relevant in this context. She asked family members how conflicts were resolved and coded responses into two sets of categories: process of conflict resolution and type of conflict solution. Parents and children did not differ significantly in reporting that adolescents acceded to parental demands in 56% of all conflicts, whereas parents acceded to child demands in only 18% of conflicts. As with Montemayor and Hanson (1985), joint discussion accounted for only 13% of all conflict resolutions. Similar trends can be found in a study by Vunchinich (1987). Analysis of family dinner conflicts involving adolescents revealed that parents and adolescents reached a compromise in only 14% of cases. In other cases, one party either stands off, withdraws or submits. These "solutions" can hardly be described as active modes of coping.

Referring back to the interview study which focused on ways of coping with problems, immediately after they had occurred, it should be remarked that subjects tended not to report many activities, but did express many thoughts concerning quarrels with parents. In the light of the comparatively low level of reported emotions, we formed the impression that conflict with parents is an event with which adolescents are well acquainted, which involves much reflection, but which does not necessarily lead them to experience a need to act.

Between 15 and 25% of parents complain about conflicts with their adolescents (Montemayor, 1986). Estimates of the frequency of arguments between parents and adolescents averaged about two arguments per week with the parents (usually the mother) and about three arguments with siblings. In our interview study, the adolescents reported at least one quarrel per week with their parents. These findings indicate that conflict occurs in even the most positive, close relationship, but that extreme levels of conflict are not characteristic of "normal" families. Conflicts are solved before they escalate into serious difficulties.

In clinical samples, frequency and intensity of conflicts increase. This is often associated with changes in family context such as unemployment (Elder, 1974), insularity (Wahler, 1986) or adolescent abuse (Garbarino & Gilliam, 1980). Family structure may also be influential. More parent-adolescent conflicts are reported in divorced, single-parent, and step-parent families than in families in which both natural parents are present (Montemayor, 1984; Wallerstein, 1985; Garbarino, Sebes & Schellenbach, 1984). If these findings are considered with regard to the reported changes in the pattern of family structure (e.g. Hill, 1987), it appears that an increasing rate of parent/adolescent conflict can be anticipated.

While these findings indicate that adolescents and parents are in conflict from time to time, they show that neither parents nor adolescents tend to employ active modes of coping in a real situation. In the main, both parties simply disengage from each other. How can this pattern of interaction or disengagement contribute to the development of coping in adolescence, since in many cases, active coping is not employed?

SIGNIFICANT OTHERS AS MODELS
FOR COPING

Parents fulfil many different functions for the developing adolescent, one of which is that they act as models for coping behaviour. Role change is normally a major feature of adolescent development and it is evident that the models available to the young person at this stage of life are potentially of great significance (Coleman & Hendry, 1989). It may be that general attitudes towards active problem solving, sensitivity towards situation-specific characteristics and a flexible response in dealing with certain problem situations on the part of the parents are crucial for the development of adequate coping behaviour in the young person.

The research discussed in the two preceding sections leads to contradictory conclusions. On one hand, an optimal family atmosphere combining closeness and individual autonomy is related to active forms of adolescent coping. On the other hand, data concerning adolescents' behaviour in family conflicts show that withdrawal (standing off), i.e. inactive coping is the most frequent type of behaviour. This contradiction can be resolved by suggesting that adolescent "acquisition" of adaptive coping behaviour within the family is a two-step process. Individual coping involves autonomous behaviour and responsibility which are major developmental tasks in adolescence (Blos, 1964). In order to achieve individuality, a youngster has to differentiate him/herself from the family (Grotevant & Cooper, 1985). Family disagreements or conflict may serve to facilitate this process. Vunchinich (1987) has pointed out that in more than two-thirds of cases a family conflict is restricted to two turns. This suggests that its function is not to solve a problem (compromise is reached in only 14% of cases), but rather to emphasise the distinctive views and attitudes of the different family members, including the adolescent. Being allowed one's separateness, combined with closeness and support (Shulman, Seiffge-Krenke & Samet, 1987) allows the young person to explore ways of coping adaptively with common, stressful conditions. Optimal family paradigms have been described as facilitators and promoters of adolescent functioning (see Constantine, 1987). However, a supportive family atmosphere is not in itself sufficient for the adoption of adaptive coping. Adolescents generally employ more emotion-focused strategies when they actually have to cope with a problem (Blanchard-Fields & Irion, 1987). Before adulthood, youngsters are probably not fully capable of differentiating among stressful events and defining those which are controllable and require an active coping approach and those which are uncontrollable and require emotion-focused reactions.

In short, it appears that active coping in adolescence does not arise from a supportive family atmosphere alone. It is likely that the parental model of adaptive coping will directly influence the adolescent mode of coping. In a recently completed study (Shulman, Carlton-Ford, Levian & Hed, submitted) the relationship between parental coping and the adolescent (normal and learning disabled) mode of coping was examined. As Table 8.2 shows, parental mode of coping (as measured by F-COPES, McCubbin et al., 1981) contributes to adolescent coping. This result holds for both active and inactive coping.

Thus far, research on coping has failed to address intergenerational aspects of coping behaviour. Research related to this topic is found in identification research (e.g. Conger & Petersen, 1984) and deals with the extent to which the adolescent incorporates the attitudes and characteristics of another person. A further research area from which we may gain knowledge about the significance of parents as models for coping behaviour are studies which investigate the relationship between the family's level of functioning and the organisation and adaptation of the

TABLE 8.2

Learning Disabled and Non-Learning Disabled Adolescents' Levels of Coping and Parental Coping: Hierarchical Regressions, Fs and Betas

Variable/Step	LD			Non-LD		
	r^2	F	beta	r^2	F	beta
Internal Coping						
1. Reframing	0.00	0.04	−0.15	0.03	0.61	0.10
2. Passive appraisal	0.34	5.74**	−0.61	0.09	1.09	0.18
3. Acquiring social support	0.41	4.96**	0.27	0.13	1.04	0.21
Active Coping via Social Resources						
1. Acquiring social support	0.19	5.41*	0.43	0.17	4.64*	0.35
2. Reframing	0.19	2.59	−0.06	0.30	4.78	0.37
3. Passive appraisal	0.21	1.86	−0.14	0.30	3.05	0.03
Withdrawal						
1. Passive appraisal	0.05	0.10	−0.17	0.04	1.06	−0.23
2. Acquiring social support	0.11	1.41	−0.44	0.04	0.52	−0.05
3. Reframing	0.36	3.87*	−0.52	0.09	0.71	0.22

* $p < 0.05$, ** $p < 0.01$

offspring. Elder (1974) and Baumrind (1968) studied the type of parental model which is most adaptive for the adolescent and found parental control and perceived authority to be crucial. All of these studies provide much the same picture of the most appropriate model for parents to follow in interacting with their teenage children. Competent adolescents have parents who exercise reasonable control, but are also flexible and encourage independence.

Identification with the peer group is a further important factor which needs empirical examination (Turner, 1982). Sympathy and perceived similarity are relevant for social comparison and modelling in situations where the peer group provides a model for coping. It should be borne in mind, that early theories stress the emergence of adolescent subcultures (Coleman, 1974) and emphasise the negative influence of certain adolescent behaviour patterns such as drug and alcohol abuse, dangerous driving or pre-marital sexual behaviour. Labouvie (1986) investigated the relationship between alcohol and drug abuse in adolescence and coping. He points out that many cultures provide prescriptions for the use of alcohol or drugs in conjunction with desirable and emotionally uplifting occasions. It seems reasonable therefore, to expect that substance use in connection with active coping efforts is more normative than is its use in connection with reactive coping efforts. Labouvie also remarks that while substance use as an active or reactive coping action is in no way unique to the period of adolescence, it is important to consider its role in relation to the particular social network of the adolescent. His research provides answers to questions concerning the areas in which friends are more influential and those in which parental influence is greater. Kandel (1986) also examined the drug behaviour of adolescents as a function of both the parents' self-reported use of alcohol and the best friend's use of marijuana. She found strong evidence for the overall role of peer influence. While parents and best friends both have an independent effect on adolescents' marijuana use, the effect of peers is much larger than the effect of parents. This was best seen in triads in which the adolescent is exposed to conflicting role models because parents' and friends' behaviour diverge, the one using drugs and the other not. When faced with such a conflict, adolescents are much more responsive to peers than to parents. Kandel's results confirm those of Labouvie (op. cit.), by showing that parental influence can work synergetically and strengthen peer influence. Opposite patterns of influence appear in connection with the formation of educational aspirations in the same triads. The effect of parents on adolescents' aspirations is much stronger than the effect of the best friend (Kandel & Lesser, 1969).

If Kandel's results are related to conformity research, it is possible to draw the conclusion that susceptibility to peer groups is higher in early and mid-adolescence than in late adolescence. Thus, the tendency to use a "dangerous" model for coping may increase during the initial stages of adolescence. As Jessor (1986) has pointed out, however, much risky behaviour disappears as adolescence comes to a close. For example, the transition towards an adult role is accompanied by a lowering of level of drug use. About 50% of the males who were problem drinkers as adolescents, cease to be problem drinkers as young adults.

Palmonari, Pombeni and Kirchler (1990) have also investigated identification with the peer group (see also Chapter 7, this volume). In a huge study of nearly 4000 adolescents, they tried to differentiate between adolescent membership of various types of peer groups and coping with developmental tasks. Their results indicate that high identifiers (e.g. adolescents who identify highly with their peer group) felt more secure in their groups and were therefore less inclined to reject peers who joined another group. Moreover, highly identified adolescents reported fewer problems with developmental tasks and got more support from their peers in coping with these tasks.

CONCLUSIONS

The study of stress, coping and relationships has emerged as an interesting and important area in adolescent research. As with research with adults, investigations of stress have emphasised the role of discrete major life events. More recently, the role of minor events, i.e. hassles and every day problems, has also been investigated. Our own research shows that female adolescents report more negative events than males and are more fatalistic in solving the underlying problems. They also report a higher percentage of ongoing stress which continues even after the coping process has been completed. Surveys of adolescent problems or strains show, not only that early adolescence is perceived as particularly stressful, but that females experience higher stress than males. Although research on the role of gender and developmental level is at an early stage, the results of our studies suggest that the number, intensity and effects of stressful events may vary with age and gender.

Our research on coping has drawn extensively on the conceptual framework of Lazarus et al. (1974). It has also been influenced by Tyler's (1978) emphasis on the importance of examining coping in the context of naturally occurring stressors. This led us to use two different methods in assessing stress and coping: a survey approach measuring anticipatory coping with stressful events, and an interview procedure, immediately after a stressful event or problem has occurred. As a result, we regarded real-life stressors, even quite minor ones, as being of possible significance. Our findings concerning the process of coping with these everyday stressors illuminated Lazarus' model by showing that no reaction was a frequent coping mode among adolescents. Thus, in coping after an event has taken place, blockage of action or passivity were much more prominent than with anticipatory coping. This finding points to the knowledge of social norms on the part of the adolescent. It also illustrates that while adolescents are working through the emotions aroused by an event/problem no reaction can be effective—in the sense used by Lazarus et al. (1974)—as a coping mode. Cognitive and behavioural efforts to alter the source of stress as well as attempts at regulating the negative emotions associated with stressful circumstances are important in reducing the negative effects of a range of stressful events (Compas, 1987). Our results show that we not only need an integrated model of psycho-social stress (see Wagner, Compas & Howell, 1988), we also require an integrated model of the coping process which takes account of how the different stressors that occur in real-life conditions in adolescence are mastered.

Lazarus and Folkman's (1984) theoretical model of stress and coping places heavy emphasis on the role of cognitive processes in determining what is experienced as stressful and how one copes. In applying this model to adolescents, it is important to account for changes in cognitive functioning with development. Coping research has rarely investigated age-differences and where it has done so, it has usually used samples covering a broad age range (McCrae, 1983). Our research revealed substantial age-differences in the use of internal coping strategies, e.g. reflection about possible solutions. It also showed that compromising increases with age. In future research, we intend to go beyond chronological age and take account of the adolescent's level of cognitive functioning, since these two variables cannot be considered as equivalent.

In analysing adolescents' social support systems, we tried to focus upon more than one relationship. At present, however, the function of peers and friendship is just emerging as a new feature in coping research on adolescents. Many more results are available concerning family relations and coping behaviour and different measurement procedures have produced similar results in this area (Stern & Zevon, 1990; Shulman, Seiffge-Krenke & Samet, 1987). Cross-cultural studies have established a relationship between aspects of family climate and coping strategies, showing the extent to which parental behaviour can be helpful or detrimental to the development of coping behaviour in young people. Further integration of these findings may help to substantiate the notion that a sense of family support and organisation contributes to a functional, interpersonal style of coping. Parental emphasis on personal growth encourages the individual's sense of mastery and this is reflected in a low level of withdrawal. If this line of thought is pursued, it can be argued that the sense of family cohesion and support in asserting individuality are the precursors of adolescent adaptive coping. These ideas are consistent with theoretical and research formulations on the role of the family in adolescent development and adaptation (Blos, 1967; Grotevant & Cooper, 1985; Shulman & Klein, 1982).

How does this perspective square with parent-adolescent conflicts? As Montemayor (1983) has shown, sixty years of empirical research has failed to produce evidence of parent-adolescent turmoil. This does not mean that no conflict takes place, in fact we have tried to illustrate manifestations of parent-adolescent stress, certain areas of conflict and frequent ways of coping with these conflicts. However, we have to stress that methodological shortcomings are frequent in research on parent-adolescent relationships and too little attention is given to cohort differences.

During the past decade, there have been remarkable changes in the quantity and quality of research on family-adolescent relations. Current research is often guided by concepts and theories derived from the family process and developmental literature which stress the distinctive cognitive, social and biological features of adolescence. Unfortunately, the kind of families on which this literature is based bears little relation to the kind of families in which adolescents grow up nowadays. The "Dick and Jane families", as Hill (1987) ironically put it—i.e. a household with one working father, a housewife mother and two school-age children—was representative of 60% of American households in 1955 and had shrunk to 7% in 1985. Most of the studies reported in the literature were carried out in the USA. While there are certainly differences in divorce rate, migration and percentage of working mothers between some European countries and the United States, it must be confessed that little is known about adolescents reared in single-parent or reconstituted families and there is also a gap of knowledge concerning ethnic and structural variations in adolescent family life. Western societies have shifted from patriarchal and agricultural bases to domination by a large-scale market economy. Parents play a lesser role in placing their children occupationally and normative regulation of courtship and marriage has been largely removed from the purview of the family (Reiss, 1971). Despite this, as we have tried to show, parents continue to be more influential than is commonly believed. Recent research (Grotevant & Cooper, 1986; Youniss, 1980) shows that adolescence is not only a stage of development for the child, it is also so for the parents, who have to participate in the individuation process through transformation of their own roles and self-understanding. Family members are therefore forced to respond and adapt to changing roles and functions, while re-negotiating and re-structuring the specific nature of their interpersonal relationship. This comes back to coping in adolescence in that competent adolescents have parents who exercise reasonable control, but are flexible and encourage independence (Baumrind, 1968; Kandel & Lesser, 1972; Leahy, 1981).

A basic issue is the extent to which coping development proceeds in response to peer or to parental influences. Where the relation between peer relationships and coping is concerned, we have shown that this perspective has been largely neglected until very recently. Negative functions of peers as models for coping dominated (Kandel, 1986). The differential influence of parents or peers as models for coping is yet not fully understood. The influence of parents appears to derive from their role as definers of norms and standards and from provision of a family climate which fosters competence and autonomy. Peers, on the other hand, are attractive role models for some behaviour, which, due to its timing in adolescence, tends to be perceived as deviant.

It is not only necessary to conceptualise peer versus parental influence in terms of specific issues; peer influence and peer group must themselves be differentiated according to their prevailing orientation. We have discussed adolescent friendship and peer influence without any differentiation being made with regard to the adolescent's sex. Most of the general processes underlying the formation and dissolution of friendship are comparable across the sexes, but intimacy and closeness of relationship are of greater importance in female adolescents (Buhrmester & Furman, 1987; Buhrmester, 1990). Additional differences appear in the relative influence of parents and peers. Girls, in general, appear to be more receptive than boys to interpersonal influence, whether it emanates from parents or friends. This is consistent with the finding that female adolescents rely more on social resources in coping with stressful events (Belle, 1981; Ilfeld, 1980).

We also have to take into account that from mid-adolescence onwards, parents are replaced by peers as trustworthy addressees for personal problems (Rivenbark, 1971). Several writers stress the adolescent's perception of friendship as a supportive relationship and underline that the peer relationship provides a new perspective through which the young person discovers the power to co-construct ideas and to receive validation through exchange with co-equals (Berndt & Perry, 1986). This implies that adolescents use their friends as important sources of social support and assistance in coping. Because there has been a tendency to concentrate on the negative aspects of peer influence in coping research, the ways in which friends provide positive help in coping with problems remain largely unknown.

CHAPTER NINE

Loneliness, Attitude Towards Aloneness, and Solitude: Age Differences and Developmental Significance During Adolescence

Alfons Marcoen and Luc Goossens

LONELINESS IN ADOLESCENCE: A THEORETICAL MODEL

The results of any study on loneliness depend largely on the researchers' often implicit conceptualisation of the variables under investigation, the choice of measuring instruments and the age of the subjects. The first section of this chapter aims to describe the general design of an ongoing research programme against the background of the available literature on the subject. This will help to clarify the contributions made by the series of studies described in subsequent sections. The literature will be selectively reviewed with special emphasis on three topics: basic conceptual distinctions in the study of loneliness; theoretical and empirical issues in the measurement of loneliness; and finally, age trends and the developmental significance of adolescent loneliness.

Basic Conceptual Distinctions

In recent years, loneliness has been the focus of considerable attention among social psychologists and, to a lesser extent, among developmental psychologists (see Hartog, Audy & Cohen, 1980; Hojat & Crandall, 1987; Peplau & Perlman, 1982, for reviews). Three clear conceptual distinctions can be made within this research literature: loneliness; attitude to aloneness; and solitude.

Loneliness is typically defined as "the unpleasant experience that occurs when a person's network of social relationships is deficient in some important way, either qualitatively or quantitatively" (Perlman & Peplau, 1981, p. 31). Such a deficit occurs when a subject's interpersonal needs cannot be satisfied within his or her social network. As a result of these unmet needs, the subject experiences a variety of aversive affective states, of which feelings of abandonment and desertion are likely to be the most dominant. This entire complex of negative feelings is what is referred to when the term "loneliness" is used, by laymen and social scientists alike. Feelings of loneliness are often situationally determined and tend to be short-lived. The toddler who watches his mother leave the school on his very first day in pre-school, the primary school child whom other children exclude from a ball game on a free afternoon and the adult who goes through a marital break-up, all experience this type of loneliness in varying degree. Some people, however, feel loneliness in many different settings and it occurs so frequently that it comes to resemble an enduring personality trait.

The scientific approach to loneliness, which sees unmet social needs as underlying feelings of loneliness, differs somewhat from the lay viewpoint. In everyday contexts, close links are often made between loneliness and being alone, i.e. the absence of other people from the immediate surroundings. In non-academic conversations, loneliness is virtually defined as "being sad because one is alone". Social scientists, however, have increasingly come to emphasise that loneliness is a subjective experience and is not synonymous with objective social isolation. "People can be alone without being lonely, or lonely in a crowd" (Peplau & Perlman, 1982, p. 3). With this important distinction in mind, social psychologists have increasingly focused attention upon the subjective experience of being alone.

A second important construct in the study of loneliness is attitude to aloneness. This refers to a generalised reaction rather than to a particular experience of social isolation. Two different clusters of reactions to being alone can be distinguished. Some may be afraid of being alone, feel uneasy when they lack the company of others, and within a short period of time, they try to establish contact with others in order to put this unbearable situation to an end. Others, however, may be attracted to being alone and may experience positive feelings while alone, so that they try to prolong rather than to end the situation. These radically different experiences appear to be rooted in two different attitudes towards being alone, namely, "aversion to aloneness" and "affinity for aloneness".

The third concept discussed in the literature is solitude. This term refers to any active and constructive use which is made of time spent alone. It is sometimes referred to as "constructive solitude" (Rubenstein & Shaver,

1982). While the construct bears some resemblance to positive attitude to aloneness, a clear conceptual distinction can be made between the two constructs. A positive attitude to being alone simply means that one positively values the mere fact that no one else is around, even if it is only because one does not want to be disturbed by others. Solitude implies a desire to be alone in order to become engaged in an activity that has intrinsic appeal. Theorists differ on the precise definition of solitude (see Rook, 1988, p. 581 for further discussion of this distinction). Some authors seem to equate solitude with "keeping busy" (Rubenstein & Shaver, 1982), whereas others refer to periods of withdrawal which are necessary for self discovery, artistic accomplishment or other creative activity (Storr, 1990; Suedfeld, 1982). It is to the latter form of solitude that particular properties, such as promotion of mental health (Suedfeld, 1982), are ascribed.

It should be added that many theorists, particularly those in Europe, regard a person's ability constructively to spend time on his own as a sign of emotional maturity. Within the German phenomenological tradition, "Einsamkeit" (or being alone) is considered by both philosophers and psychologists (e.g. Kölbel, 1960) as a means of realising the strengths of one's character and psychological maturity as a result of spending periods of time on one's own (See also De Jong-Gierveld & Raadschelders, 1982, pp. 105-106). Psychoanalytic authors (e.g. Winnicott, 1958) have also referred to the capacity to be alone as one of the most important signs of maturity in emotional development. Underlying this capacity is the experience, as an infant or small child, of being alone with a particular supportive figure usually the mother, or a mother symbol. Gradually, this ego-supportive environment is introjected and becomes a part of the individual's personality. This process means that the capacity actually to be alone is typically acquired during childhood.

The three of concepts loneliness, attitude to aloneness and solitude together constitute the theoretical basis for scientific research on loneliness. The following section discusses how each of these different constructs can be measured.

Measurement Issues

Most empirical effort has been devoted to the measurement of loneliness while attitude towards aloneness has received more limited attention. Currently there is no measure whatsoever of the construct of solitude. The brief overview of the most popular instruments which follows, emphasises the problems associated with some of these measures. (See Marangoni & Ickes, 1989 and Russell, 1982, for more comprehensive reviews of problems in measuring loneliness). Thereafter, the position adopted in the present chapter towards these measurement issues will be discussed.

Loneliness is often measured by means of a single item ("How often do you feel lonely?"). In responding to this question, subjects are asked to tick one of a series of alternatives indicating different frequencies of being lonely (e.g. almost all of the time, much of the time, some of the time, occasionally, never). In addition to this measure, a number of multiple item measures exist in which loneliness is conceived of as a unitary phenomenon involving a common substrate of experiences of rejection, abandonment and the like. These measures simply probe the intensity of these feelings and completely disregard their origin or cause, their duration (i.e. their state- or trait-like quality), or possible means of alleviating the emotions involved. Well-known examples of this type of instrument include the Revised UCLA Loneliness Scale (Russell, Peplau & Cutrona, 1980) and the Children's Loneliness Scale (CLS; Asher, Hymel & Renshaw, 1984). The former is specifically designed for use with young adults and is very popular for research with that age group, while the latter is used in the upper grades of primary school. The scores obtained with these instruments are highly correlated with those derived from single-item measures of loneliness which have frequently been employed as measures of concurrent validity.

These traditional measures of loneliness have increasingly come under attack. The main objection levelled against them is that the precise nature of the social deficits experienced by the lonely person, is never determined. This is a serious objection indeed, if one follows many researchers, in believing that the general experience of loneliness can be differentiated on the basis of specific interpersonal deficits experienced in different relationships.

The major impetus for this kind of criticism has been derived from theoretical work which distinguishes between the "loneliness of emotional isolation" and the "loneliness of social isolation". According to this view, initially developed by Weiss (1973, pp. 18-19), the former type of loneliness occurs when a person suffers from "the absence of a close emotional attachment", e.g. when he or she lacks an intimate love partner. The latter type occurs when the person painfully experiences "the absence of an engaging social network", e.g. when no interaction with groups of relatives, friends, or neighbours is currently available to him or her. Weiss further believed that different relationships offer specific relational satisfactions, for which he coined the term "relational provisions".

Later work has expanded on these theoretical views and rightly pointed out that intense feelings of emotional and social loneliness can also be experienced by a person who has an intimate partner and has access to a social network, but who fails to obtain the social provisions he needs within these relationships. In line with these ideas, multidimensional measures of loneliness have been developed to assess current dissatisfaction within existing relationships. A well-known example of this approach is the Differential Loneliness Scale (DLS; Schmidt & Sermat, 1983). This instrument probes for loneliness occurring in romantic/sexual, family, friendship and community or group relationships.

Measuring attitudes to aloneness also presents a host of problems. Reliable and valid questionnaire measures of the construct have not yet been developed. However, some information on the topic can be derived from single items which form part of broader instruments, such as sentence completion tests which are designed to explore the entire social world of the subject. (These measures will be briefly discussed in the section on the developmental framework for adolescent loneliness). Measurement techniques have been developed to assess subjects' direct experience of being alone and these are readily available.

The most widely used measure is the Experience Sampling Method (ESM; Csikszentmihalyi & Larson, 1987; Larson, 1989). This method is designed to analyse subjects' use of time, or more precisely, the ecology of daily life. As such, it provides data on both the time that people spend alone and the time they spend in the company of others. Participants in ESM-studies are provided with electronic pagers which they carry throughout a one-week period. At randomly chosen times each day, subjects are signalled by the pagers and asked to report on what they are doing. Each subject provides 35 to 45 reports a week. When paged, subjects report on their objective situation and on their subjective states. They are asked to say where they are, whom they are with and what they are doing (objective data) and to describe their feelings and their motivational and cognitive state (subjective data). Taken together, the ESM-data provide a representative sample of a subject's daily experience, aggregated across an entire week.

One of the many ways to analyse the rich body of data assembled in this way is to contrast subjects' objective conditions at the different times when they are paged. Typical conditions, referred to as "contexts", include: alone, with family, with friends, or with classmates. Both the prevalence and the average experience of time spent alone can be determined empirically and compared with the time spent with others (aggregated across the three remaining categories: family, friends and classmates). The most striking advantage of this ingenious technique is that the subjective data on aloneness represent direct reports from subjects who were actually alone at the time of reporting. They do not represent some kind of general attitude towards being alone, assessed by means of a questionnaire completed at a single moment in time, when the subject might well have been in the company of others.

In the present chapter, the position adopted towards the measurement of loneliness and aloneness might be described as essentially eclectic and pragmatic. As many of the relevant theoretical distinctions as possible were incorporated into the instrument developed for the research programme. A convenient "one-time" assessment was adopted, instead of a more sophisticated, time-consuming and labour intensive measure such as the Experience Sampling Method. Finally, the instrument was constructed explicitly for use with pre-adolescents and adolescents, the target population for the research programme—a population for whom few measures were currently available .

Where the concept of loneliness was concerned, a need was felt to distinguish between different types of loneliness experienced in different relationships. It is widely believed that the most important relationships during childhood and adolescence are those with parents and peers. Furthermore, earlier efforts to develop a preliminary loneliness scale (Marcoen & Brumagne, 1985) had, as expected, already revealed that in the particular age range under study, loneliness was largely confined to these two relationships. With these considerations in mind, two different scales were developed. Each scale set out to probe for feelings of rejection, abandonment and desertion occurring within the relationships with parents and peers, respectively.

For attitudes to aloneness, two scales were constructed. The first assessed aversion to aloneness (including items such as "I do not like to be alone") and the second, affinity for aloneness (including items such as "I want to be alone" and "I enjoy being on my own"). This attitudinal type of measure was regarded as being complementary to direct assessment of subjects' experience when they are actually alone, such as is provided by time-sampling methods (ESM).

In summary, a multidimensional measure containing four subscales was developed. The subscales measure (a) loneliness in relationships with parents, (b) loneliness in relationships with peers, (c) negative attitude to aloneness and (d) positive attitude to aloneness. The questionnaire, which admittedly is fraught with all of the deficiencies of single occasion self-report assessments, covers both loneliness and attitude to aloneness, two of the central concepts in contemporary research on loneliness. At present, its principal limitation is that it is unable to provide a measure of a third concept—solitude, or active and constructive use of time spent alone.

The instrument was developed specifically for research with pre-adolescents and adolescents. The following section will discuss the developmental framework for adolescent loneliness developed in the ongoing research programme.

A DEVELOPMENTAL FRAMEWORK FOR ADOLESCENT LONELINESS

Building on earlier theoretical work and reviews of the literature, an attempt was made to (a) predict normative developmental trends in adolescent loneliness and aloneness and (b) to specify how each of these phenomena would be related to important developmental processes presumed to take place during adolescence.

Predicted Age Trends

Certain authors (Brennan, 1982; Perlman, 1988) have claimed that high levels of (uni-dimensional) loneliness are very common in adolescence and have enumerated a series of developmental factors which may contribute to this increased loneliness. Changes in the social, cognitive and biological domain all seem to play an important role in the process. The young adolescent is confronted with a whole set of novel social expectations. He or she should be popular with peers, have dates and experience success in different domains of social and academic life. New cognitive abilities and the biological changes of puberty foster emotional maturation and bring about strong interpersonal needs and a search for new ways of relating to others. At the same time, the adolescent has not yet acquired sufficient experience in the social world, nor the social skills to keep relationships going. As a result, it is not unlikely that loneliness will ensue. Finally, adolescence involves a complete re-organisation of the social world of the developing individual. Parents are relinquished as primary attachment figures and involvement with same-sex peers increases dramatically.

In the present project, the last of these developments was taken as a point of departure for formulating hypotheses about age differences. Despite the relative importance of parents and peers at different points in time during adolescence, a decrease in parent-related loneliness and an increase in peer-related loneliness were not predicted during this period. Rather it was believed that parents continue to be important and that adolescents seek to remain connected to both mother and father, even while they are progressing towards the establishment of their own individuality. However, this joint process of individuality-in-connectedness (Grotevant & Cooper, 1986) leads parents to change their relationship with their offspring in the direction of greater equality. A growing body of research indicates that this process takes some time and is typically accompanied by some disequilibrium, if not turmoil in parent-child relationships (Youniss & Smollar, 1985). Parent-related loneliness is not an inevitable consequence of this situation, of course and need not be experienced by every adolescent. On average, however, the ongoing re-negotiation of family roles is likely to lead to an increase of this type of loneliness.

During the same period, feelings of loneliness will decrease in relationships with peers. The emerging capacity for intimate same-sex friendships, one of the most systematic changes in social development in early adolescence, radically changes relations with peers in the direction of greater involvement and increased sharing of thoughts, fears and feelings (Petersen, 1988). As a result, it was anticipated that loneliness would be less likely to be a feature of this type of relationship as adolescents grow older.

It was predicted that affinity for aloneness would increase during the course of adolescence, with a concomitant decline in its counterpart, aversion to aloneness. This hypothesis was based on the idea, central to the present research project, that a person's capacity to engage in periods of solitude is a sign of emotional maturity and should therefore be more common as adolescents approach adulthood. An implicit assumption in this line of reasoning is that adolescents' positive attitude to aloneness, which is conceptually related yet distinct from solitude, fulfils the same developmental function as solitude itself.

It is worth remarking that results obtained with the Experience Sampling Method (ESM) do not fully support the developmental predictions outlined here. They indicate that some adolescents come to value periods of social isolation in a positive way, while others continue to react in purely negative terms to being alone (Larson, 1990; Larson & Csikszentmihalyi, 1978; Larson, Csikszentmihalyi & Graef, 1982).

Despite this work, the predicted age trends in adolescents' attitudes towards aloneness are in line with results emerging from earlier research on adolescents in which the London Sentence Completion Test was used. This instrument includes stems like "When there is no-one else around ..." and "If a person is alone ...". Research with British (Coleman, 1974), United States and New Zealand adolescents (Kroger, 1985) has shown that the percentage of negative themes elicited by these stems peaks at age 12, while the percentage of positive endings is highest among 17-year-olds.

No gender differences were expected in either parent- or peer-related loneliness. Earlier reviews on research using uni-dimensional measures such as the UCLA Loneliness Scale have revealed few significant gender differences (e.g. Borys & Perlman, 1985). It was expected that this finding would also apply to the use of other measures of loneliness. Likewise, no gender differences were expected in aversion to or affinity for aloneness. Some researchers have hypothesised that girls, because of their higher level of affiliation motivation, would be more likely to respond negatively to being alone than boys. However, this contention is not supported by recent research (Wong & Csikszentmihalyi, 1991).

In summary, it was predicted that loneliness in the relationship with parents will increase from pre- through late adolescence, whereas peer-related loneliness will decrease over the same period. It was also predicted that aversion to aloneness will gradually decline throughout adolescence and that there will be a concomitant increase in affinity for aloneness.

Associations with Core Developmental Phenomena

In earlier work, both heightened feelings of loneliness and increased prevalence of time spent alone during adolescence have been related to the struggle to achieve identity formation which typically takes place during this period in the life-span (Larson, 1990; Perlman, 1988). The present research programme expands on these earlier theoretical efforts by formulating specific hypotheses regarding associations between adolescents' feelings of loneliness and their resolution of different developmental tasks.

Following Erikson (1968), the acquisition of a sense of identity and the establishment of intimate relationships with others were considered to be the most important developmental tasks of late adolescence. Generally speaking, lower levels of loneliness may be expected in subjects who have successfully achieved both of these tasks. Marcia (1980), building on Erikson's dichotomy of identity versus role confusion, has distinguished four different resolutions of the identity crisis. Within his theoretical framework, one might hypothesise that adolescents who have achieved a more advanced resolution of the task of identity formation will score significantly lower on both the parent- and peer-related loneliness scales than is the case with adolescents who have resolved this task less successfully.

These tasks might be regarded as typical of the adolescent period of development. However, during adolescence, developmental issues which seemed to have been resolved during the childhood years, tend to re-emerge and call for continuous, age-specific adjustments, if not for complete re-working. Attachment to parental figures (Bowlby, 1969; 1973; 1980) seems to be an example of such a task, in that it requires continuous attention from the developing person. Attachment, defined as the behavioural system which tends to maintain or re-establish the proximity of a caregiver, has been studied predominantly in infancy. However, it is increasingly recognised that major shifts in the attachment system may take place during later phases in development and during adolescence in particular (Ainsworth, 1989). This raises the possibility that different levels of loneliness may reflect adolescents' different approaches to attachment to parents. One might hypothesise, for example, that adolescents who are securely attached to their parents will experience lower levels of parent-related loneliness than do their insecurely attached age-mates.

In short, it can be expected that, during adolescence, both loneliness and attitudes to aloneness will be related to subjects' resolution of the identity and intimacy crises and to their particular style in dealing with attachment issues arising during this period. A set of more detailed hypotheses for each of these core developmental phenomena will be advanced in later sections of this chapter. First, however, consideration will be given to the development of the multidimensional instrument used to test these hypotheses.

MEASURING LONELINESS: THE DEVELOPMENT OF A MULTIDIMENSIONAL INSTRUMENT

Nine different groups of subjects were used in the development of the research instrument. The groups fall into two categories. Four groups were used to carry out empirical checks on predicted developmental trends in loneliness and aloneness and on the psychometric soundness of the scales employed. In this chapter, these groups of subjects will be described as the main samples. All four groups contained large numbers of subjects and covered a wide age range. Samples 1 (Marcoen, Goossens & Caes, 1987) and 2 (Peeters, 1986) comprised 444 and 338 subjects, respectively. Subjects in these samples were at the 5th, 7th, 9th and 11th grade levels. The subjects in Samples 3 (Goossens, Marcoen & De Smedt, 1989) and 4 (Van Hees, 1990) comprised 412 and 200 pupils, respectively, from Grades 7, 9 and 11.

In referring to different grade levels in these samples, the American grade system has been taken as a general frame of reference. All of the students in Samples 1 to 4 actually attended schools in Belgium. Belgian grade levels are typically designated as "Primary Grade 1 to 6" and "Secondary Grade 1 to 6". Taken together, these correspond to American Grades 1 to 12. Mean ages at each of these grade levels are roughly similar to the average age of students in the corresponding grade in the American educational system. On average, then, subjects in the 5th, 7th, 9th and 11th grade are 11, 13, 15 and 17 years of age, respectively.

Additional samples were recruited in order to examine the psychometric properties of the self-report instrument and to explore developmental antecedents and correlates of both loneliness and attitude to aloneness. A total of 430 subjects at the 10th and 12th grade level were included in Sample 5 (De Saeger, 1991). Sample 6 (Grietens, 1988; Marcoen & Goossens, 1989) comprised 169 subjects at the 9th and 12th grade levels. Finally, Sample 7 (Terrell-Deutsch, 1990) included 494 pre-adolescents (Grades 4 to 6) from the Toronto area (Canada). The final sample provides a cross-cultural check on the usefulness of the newly developed loneliness measure. All of the other samples comprised subjects from the Dutch-speaking part of Belgium. All samples contained roughly equal numbers of boys and girls.

The research instrument, the Louvain Loneliness Scale for Children and Adolescents (LLCA) is made up of four subscales: loneliness in the relationships with parents (L-PART); loneliness in the relationships with peers (L-PEER); aversion to aloneness (A-NEG); and affinity for aloneness (A-POS). The instrument was originally developed for use with Dutch-speaking subjects. An English translation of the scale (which is identical to the version used by Terrell-Deutsch, 1990, except for slight changes in wording), with items listed according to a priori scale assignment, is provided in the appendix to this chapter. Each of the subscales comprises 12 items which are answered on a 4-point scale: "often", "sometimes", "seldom" and "never". For most items, these response alternatives are scored 4, 3, 2 and 1, respectively. Some of the items of the parent-related loneliness (L-PART) subscale are scored in the reverse direction. Scores on all four subscales range between 12 and 48.

The LLCA and, where appropriate, other instruments were group-administered during normal school hours by Master's students in Psychology. Total testing time never exceeded 50 minutes, i.e. the normal duration of a classroom period in Belgian schools.

Psychometric Properties

Initial inquiries into the psychometric qualities of the new loneliness instrument followed a three-pronged approach. This involved setting out to determine whether each of the four subscales could (a) make a differential contribution to the measurement of loneliness and attitude to aloneness, (b) exhibit adequate levels of internal consistency and (c) evince a substantial degree of factorial validity.

Intercorrelations among the four subscales of the Louvain Loneliness Scale for Children and Adolescents were assessed with each of the four main samples. Median correlations are presented in Table 9.1. As can be seen, some subscale overlap is found between the different subscales and between the peer-related loneliness (L-PEER) and affinity for aloneness (A-POS) scales, in particular. The maximum amount of shared common variance, however, is rather low (up to 12%). The L-PART and L-PEER scales, although significantly inter-related in some samples, clearly tap different aspects of adolescents' experience of loneliness (only 4% of shared variance). Finally, affinity for and aversion to aloneness should not be considered as opposites; each of these scales probes largely independent aspects of subjects' evaluation of being alone.

TABLE 9.1

Median Intercorrelations Among the Subscales of the Louvain Loneliness
Scale for Children and Adolescents (LLCA) in the Four Main Samples

	Subscale		
Subscale [a]	L-PEER	A-NEG	A-POS
L-PART	0.20	0.08	0.18
L-PEER		0.19	0.35
A-NEG			−0.04

[a] L-PART = Parent-related loneliness; L-PEER = Peer-related loneliness; A-NEG =
Aversion to aloneness (Aloneness negative); A-POS = Affinity for aloneness (Aloneness
positive).

Internal consistency (Cronbach alpha) and congruence with a priori
scale assignment (Tucker coefficient of congruence) were examined in
seven of the samples and are shown in Table 9.2. As can be seen, the
reliability estimates obtained for all subscales are uniformly high in the
Belgian (Dutch-speaking) samples. The English version of the scale, as
used with a sample of Canadian subjects (Sample 7), also exhibits high
levels of internal consistency. Congruence with a priori scale assignment
is quite satisfactory, as can be inferred from the findings on subscale
inter-correlations. It should be added here that the four-factor structure of
the instrument was also replicated in the Canadian sample (Terrell-Deutsch,
1990), using varimax rather than congruence rotation. On the basis of the
results, we may conclude that the newly developed loneliness measure exhibits
low subscale overlap, excellent reliability and high factorial validity.

Construct Validity

The validity of the multidimensional loneliness measure was assessed by
calculating correlations with conceptually related measures. In view of the
specific content of the different subscales of the instrument, a two-step
procedure was adopted. First, an attempt was made to demonstrate that
two of the scales measure loneliness, whereas the other two probe for
subjects' attitude to being alone. Secondly, the L-PART and L-PEER scales
were shown to measure important aspects of adolescents' relationships
with parents and peers, respectively.

With regard to the first objective, both the Louvain Loneliness Scale for
Children and Adolescents (LLCA) and the Children's Loneliness Scale
(CLS; Asher et al., 1984) were administered to two different samples. These

TABLE 9.2

Internal Consistency (Cronbach Alpha) and Congruence with
Hypothesised Four-Factor Structure (Tucker Coefficient) for the
Subscales of the Louvain Loneliness Scale for Children and Adolescents
(LLCA) in Different Samples

Sample	Subscale [a]			
	L-PART	L-PEER	A-NEG	A-POS
	Cronbach Alpha			
1	0.88	0.87	0.81	0.80
2	0.86	0.87	0.80	0.80
3	0.86	0.88	0.81	0.82
4	0.85	0.87	0.84	0.80
5	0.92	0.86	0.86	0.84
6	0.88	0.87	0.81	0.80
7	0.88	0.86	0.76	0.76
	Tucker Coefficient			
1	0.87	0.97	0.92	0.94
2	0.97	0.87	0.92	0.90
3	0.97	0.90	0.94	0.92
4	0.95	0.88	0.93	0.93
5	0.98	0.92	0.94	0.95
6	0.96	0.87	0.94	0.88

[a] L-PART = Parent-related loneliness; L-PEER = Peer-related loneliness; A-NEG = Aversion to aloneness (Aloneness negative); A-POS = Affinity for aloneness (Aloneness positive).

were the Canadian sample (Terrell-Deutsch, 1990) and Sample 8 which included 136 pre-adolescents (Grades 5 and 6) from the Dutch-speaking part of Belgium (Bijttebier, 1991). Another sample (Sample 5) was given the LLCA and Dutch versions of the Privacy Preference Scale (PPS; Marshall, 1974) and the Privacy Questionnaire (PQ; Pedersen, 1979). Each of the latter two instruments contains a scale labelled "Solitude" which is very similar in content to the affinity for aloneness (A-POS) subscale found in the LLCA. The relevant correlations between these measures are presented in Table 9.3.

TABLE 9.3

Construct Validity of the Louvain Loneliness Scale
for Children and Adolescents (LLCA):
Correlations with Other Measures of Loneliness and Aloneness

		Subscale [a]			
Sample	Measure	L-PART	L-PEER	A-NEG	A-POS
		Loneliness [b]			
7	CLS	0.36	0.75	0.06	0.22
8	CLS	0.39	0.79	0.26	0.43
		Aloneness [c]			
5	PPS-Solitude	0.19	0.11	−0.17	0.59
5	PQ-Solitude	0.11	0.16	−0.26	0.69

[a] L-PART = Parent-related loneliness, L-PEER = Peer-related loneliness, A-NEG = Aversion to aloneness (Aloneness negative), A-POS = Affinity for aloneness (Aloneness positive); [b] CLS = Children's Loneliness Scale; [c] PPS = Privacy Preference Scale; PQ = Privacy questionnaire.

It was expected that the Children's Loneliness Scale (CLS) would show high correlations with either the L-PART or the L-PEER scale, or most probably with both of them. It was also hypothesised that the CLS would produce low correlations with the two scales which tap subjects' attitude to aloneness. Conversely, both solitude scales were expected to correlate strongly with the A-POS scale and much less with the other three scales. A quick glance at Table 9.3 indicates that these expectations are completely borne out by the data. However, one slight qualification should be made. It appears that the Children's Loneliness Scale measures peer-related rather than parent-related loneliness.

It may be noted here that the correlations between the CLS and L-PEER scales and between the solitude scales and the A-POS scale should not be compared directly, because the solitude scales are somewhat less reliable than the Children's Loneliness Scale. As a result, the correlations between the solitude scales and the A-POS scale may have been somewhat under-estimated. In order to circumvent this problem, estimates of the "true" correlations between the constructs under study were made. The correlations between the L-PEER scale and the Children's Loneliness Scale were increased to 0.85 and 0.89, respectively, in Samples 7 and 8 when the correction for attenuation was applied. A similar correction yielded equally high correlations between the A-POS scale and the solitude scales in the Privacy Preference Scale and the Privacy Questionnaire ($r = 0.83$ and 0.85, respectively). One may conclude, therefore, that the L-PEER and A-POS scales share between 69% and 79% of "true" common variance with existing measures of loneliness and aloneness, respectively.

The second step of the validation procedure shows that the L-PEER scale measures important dimensions of adolescents' relationships with friends, while the L-PART scale is a valid measure of relational dissatisfaction with parents. A sample of 175 Belgian adolescents from Grades 9 and 12 (Sample 9; Segers, 1985) was asked to complete the LLCA and to rate their relationships with mother, father and friends on four basic dimensions of interpersonal relations defined by Wish, Deutsch and Kaplan (1976). These dimensions were: competitive or hostile versus cooperative; unequal versus equal; superficial versus intense; and formal versus informal. Correlations between the loneliness scores and the relationship ratings are shown in Table 9.4.

As can be seen, significant positive correlations were obtained between the scores on the parent-related loneliness scale and the ratings for both mother and father on all four relational dimensions. Likewise, significant

TABLE 9.4

Correlations between the Parents and Peers Subscales of the LLCA and Relationships with Significant Others Rated on Four Basic Interpersonal Dimensions

| | Interpersonal Dimension | | | |
Subscale	Competitive-hostile	Unequal	Superficial	Formal
	Mother			
Parents (L-PART)	0.66**	0.47**	0.69**	0.31**
Peers (L-PEER)	0.19*	0.12	0.20*	−0.07
	Father			
Parents (L-PART)	0.63**	0.52**	0.57**	0.41**
Peers (L-PEER)	0.25**	0.16*	0.21*	−0.06
	Friends			
Parents (L-PART)	0.03	−0.03	−0.01	0.03
Peers (L-PEER)	0.33**	0.32**	0.25**	0.26**

* $p < 0.05$,   ** $p < 0.01$

positive correlations emerged between subjects' scores on the peer-related loneliness scale and their ratings of their relationships with friends on all four dimensions. As high scores reflect negative evaluations, these findings indicate that subjects scoring high on the parent or peer scale tend to see their relationships with their parents or with peers, respectively, as more hostile, more unequal, more superficial and more formal. The aversion to and affinity for aloneness scales were essentially unrelated to subjects' ratings of their relationships with significant others (mother, father and friends).

The construct validity of the two loneliness subscales of the LLCA was further supported by significant associations in the predicted direction with Hayden Thomson's (1989) Relational Provision Loneliness Questionnaire (see Terrell-Deutsch, 1990), with a measure of self-consciousness (Goossens et al., 1989), known as the Situation Scale for Adolescents (SISA; Goossens, 1984) and with a biographical data sheet which tapped adolescents' social, psychological and ecological conditions (Marcoen et al., 1987).

In summary, the results strongly support the construct validity of the L-PART and L-PEER loneliness scales. Promising findings have also been gathered on the validity of the A-POS scale. The validity of the A-NEG scale is somewhat more problematic. It is clear that much additional research is needed on the construct validity of this particular subscale.

DEVELOPMENTAL FINDINGS

Two different types of results will be presented in this section. First, attention will be given to age and gender differences in adolescents' feelings of loneliness and attitude to aloneness. Thereafter, relationships with other important developmental phenomena during adolescence will be examined.

Age and Gender Differences

Subjects' scores on the four subscales of the Louvain Loneliness Scale for Children and Adolescents (LLCA) in the four main samples were analysed by means of Grade × Gender ANOVAs. Mean scores on the L-PART scale as a function of grade level are presented in Figure 9.1. A significant grade effect was obtained for this subscale in all four samples, $F(3, 436) = 4.08$, $p < 0.01$, $F(3, 328) = 9.65$, $p < 0.001$, $F(2, 406) = 4.39$, $p < 0.05$ and $F(2, 194) = 5.97$, $p < 0.01$, for Samples 1 through 4, respectively. Tukey-Kramer a posteriori tests (alpha set at 0.05) revealed a clear developmental trend. Seventh graders ($M = 17.73$) scored significantly lower than 11th graders ($M = 20.17$) in Sample 1. Subjects at Grade 9 ($M = 22.27$) were found to score higher than both 5th and 7th graders ($M = 18.62$ and 17.36) in Sample

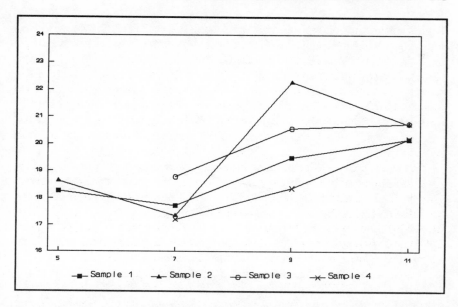

FIG. 9.1. Mean scores on the parent-related loneliness scale (L-PART) as a function of grade level in four different samples.

2. In addition, 11th graders (M = 20.72) obtained a higher score than did 7th graders. Seventh graders in Sample 3 (M = 18.78) again scored significantly lower than both 9th and 11th graders (in order M = 20.56 and 20.75), who did not differ significantly from each other. Finally, 11th graders (M = 20.19) obtained significantly higher scores than 7th graders (M = 17.21) in Sample 4 with scores for 9th graders (M = 18.37) falling in between.

It is clear that, as expected, subjects' mean score on the L-PART scale gradually increases from pre- through late adolescence. This result is consistent with the contemporary idea (Youniss & Smollar, 1985) that overall satisfaction with the relationship with parents tends to decline during adolescence because of the re-negotiation of family roles and family functioning which takes place during this period. We have to add, however, that the age (or grade) trend is not a truly linear one. Subjects' score on the L-PART scale is lowest at Grade 7 and increases in higher grades.

Adolescents' mean scores on the L-PEER scale as a function of grade level are shown in Figure 9.2. A significant grade effect emerged in Samples 1 and 2 only, $F(3, 436)$ = 12.59 and $F(3, 328)$ = 11.88, respectively, for both $p < 0.001$. In both cases, a posteriori tests revealed that 5th graders (M = 24.04 and 26.35, respectively) scored significantly higher than 7th, 9th and 11th graders (means range between 19.23 and 21.83). In short, as had been

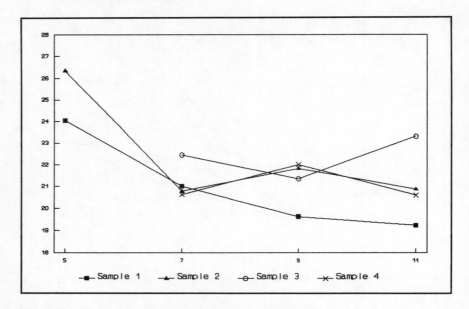

FIG. 9.2. Mean scores on the peer-related loneliness scale (L-PEER) as a function of grade level in four different samples.

anticipated, subjects' score on the L-PEER scale decreased from pre-through late adolescence. However, the decrease is not linear. A sudden drop in peer-related loneliness occurs between pre- and early adolescence. Some between-group variability is also observed. For example, the results for Sample 3 suggest an increase from Grade 9 to Grade 11, though the observed age difference is non-significant.

Subjects' scores on the A-NEG scale as a function of grade are presented in Figure 9.3. Significant grade-effects were again found in Samples 1 and 2 only, $F(3, 436) = 7.87, p < 0.001$ and $F(3, 328) = 4.01, p < 0.01$, respectively. In Sample 1, 5th graders ($M = 33.29$) were found to score significantly higher than 7th, 9th and 11th graders (means between 29.32 and 30.86). Fifth and 7th graders in Sample 2, who were not found to differ from one another ($M = 34.24$ and 34.33, respectively), obtained significantly higher scores than 9th ($M = 31.62$) and $M = 11$th graders ($M = 32.41$). In adolescence proper (Grades 7 to 11) no age-differences whatsoever are observed (Sample 3) or a (non-significant) curvilinear trend (Sample 4) is found to emerge. In the light of these results, a linear decreasing trend may be cautiously inferred. This result is again in line with the initial hypotheses.

Age- (or grade-) trends in A-POS may be found in Figure 9.4. A significant grade-effect emerged in Samples 3 and 4, $F(2, 406) = 9.44, p < 0.001$ and $F(2, 194) = 3.90, p < 0.05$, respectively. Eleventh graders ($M = 33.43$) scored

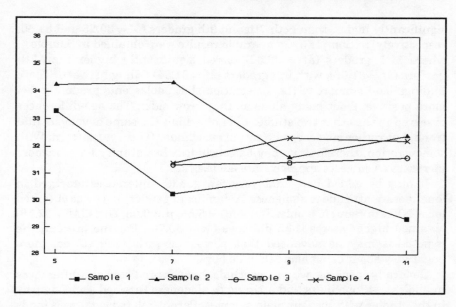

FIG. 9.3. Mean scores on the aversion to aloneness scale (A-NEG) as a function of grade level in four different samples.

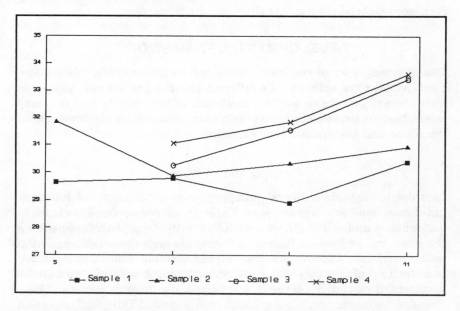

FIG. 9.4. Mean scores on the affinity for aloneness scale (A-POS) as a function of grade level in four different samples.

significantly higher than both 7th and 9th graders (M = 30.25 and 31.55, respectively) in Sample 3. Comparable results were obtained in Sample 4, where 11th graders (M = 33.62) scored significantly higher than 7th graders (M = 31.06), with 9th graders (M = 31.84) falling between. These findings lend support to the expectation that adolescents gradually feel more positive about being alone as they grow older. The age-differences observed in the other two studies did not exhibit the same developmental trend, but rather suggest some sort of curvilinear (U-curve) pattern. With some caution, therefore, it may be concluded that affinity for aloneness increases as subjects approach late adolescence.

It may be added here that very few gender differences emerged in loneliness or attitude to aloneness. A significant gender effect was observed for A-NEG in Sample 3 only, $F(1, 406)$ = 5.55, $p < 0.05$. Girls (M = 32.18) obtained higher scores than did boys (M = 30.70). For the present, the hypothesis may be advanced that adolescent girls tend to feel more negatively about being alone than do boys.

Generally speaking, we may conclude that the predicted age-differences in adolescent loneliness and attitude to aloneness received some support in the studies with the four main samples. Parent-related loneliness tends to increase and peer-related loneliness to decrease as adolescents grow older. Aversion to aloneness decreases with advancing age, whereas affinity for aloneness tends to increase throughout adolescence.

DEVELOPMENTAL FRAMEWORK

Two different types of empirical efforts will be presented in this section. First, adolescents' scores on the different subscales of the new loneliness measure will be related to their resolution of the identity and intimacy crises. Second, the role of adolescents' attachment style as predictor of both loneliness and aloneness will be examined.

Identity and Intimacy

In order to measure subjects' emerging sense of identity and intimacy, uni-dimensional scales were used. These scales assess the experience of self-reliance and self-worth in association with identity achievement, on the one hand and validation and affection through the establishment of intimate relationships, on the other. An additional measure was employed in order to compare subjects' identity development with Marcia's (1980) prototypical resolutions of the identity crisis, the identity statuses. These statuses, "Achievement, Moratorium, Foreclosure and Diffusion", represent specific combinations of two basic dimensions, identity commitments and exploration of identity alternatives, each of which may be present or absent.

The term "commitment" refers to an important life-choice made by an adolescent which involves social self-definition and represents a matter he or she cares about or values (an educational or vocational goal, an ethical value, etc.). "Exploration" refers to a period of decision-making in which the adolescent either investigates a number of identity options involving possible commitments (breadth of exploration) or explores one option by means of different approaches (depth of exploration).

Adolescents in the Achievement status have strong commitments after a period of exploration. Moratorium subjects are still in a period of exploration and have vague commitments at best. Adolescents in the Foreclosure status have strong commitments, but have not experienced a period of exploration or crisis. Finally, Diffusion subjects do not have strong commitments and are not currently in a state of crisis. In fact, they may never have gone through such a period.

For initial exploration of the developmental context of adolescent loneliness, subjects in Sample 6 (Grietens, 1988; Marcoen & Goossens, 1989) were administered the Louvain Loneliness Scale for Children and Adolescents and a series of identity and intimacy scales. The latter comprised Dutch translations of the Identity and Intimacy subscales of the Erikson Psychosocial Stage Inventory (EPSI; Rosenthal, Gurney & Moore, 1981) and the Extended Objective Measure of Ego-Identity Status (EOM-EIS; Grotevant & Adams, 1984). The Objective Measure yields four quantitative scores which correspond to Marcia's four identity statuses: Identity Achievement, Moratorium, Foreclosure and Diffusion. Each of these four scores is a summation of subjects' scores related to the ideological and interpersonal domains of identity formation (so-called Total Identity scores).

The general hypothesis was that positive resolution of the identity and intimacy crises of late adolescence would be associated with lower levels of parent-related loneliness, peer-related loneliness and aversion to aloneness, but with higher levels of affinity for aloneness. The latter prediction was again based on the assumption that a positive attitude to aloneness bears some resemblance to solitude (or constructively spending time on one's own) which is considered to be a sign of psychological maturity.

More specifically, both uni-dimensional identity and intimacy (Rosenthal's EPSI) were expected to reveal significant negative correlations with parent- and peer-related loneliness and aversion to aloneness. Predictions regarding the multidimensional identity measure (Adams' EOM-EIS) were somewhat more complex. Scores on the non-commitment status scales (Moratorium and Diffusion) were expected to show positive associations with the first three loneliness scales (i.e. L-PART, L-PEER and A-NEG). On the other hand, scores on the identity scales which reflect strong commitments (Achievement and Foreclosure) were expected to exhibit negative correlations with these three scales.

Expectations for the A-POS scale were exactly the opposite of those for the other three scales. Higher scores for identity, intimacy and commitment identity statuses (Achievement and Foreclosure) were expected to be associated with greater affinity for aloneness. Finally, higher scores on the non-commitment identity status scales (Moratorium and Diffusion) were expected to parallel lower scores on affinity for aloneness.

In order to test these hypotheses, the scores on the four loneliness and aloneness scales obtained in Sample 6 were regressed on the six identity and intimacy scales. Significant regression weights (betas) are presented in Table 9.5. The set of identity and intimacy measures accounts for 15 to 32% of the variance in the loneliness and affinity for aloneness scores (adjusted squared multiple correlation). As the Table shows, the score on the aversion to aloneness scale is difficult to predict from these variables.

More importantly, most of the significant betas were in the predicted direction, at least in the case of the two loneliness scales. Higher levels of parent-related loneliness were found among subjects who obtained high scores on the Diffusion scale. The reverse held for Foreclosure where a negative correlation was observed. Four variables proved effective predictors of peer-related loneliness. As expected, lower levels of loneliness

TABLE 9.5

Significant Standardised Weights (Betas) in the Regression of Loneliness Scores on Identity and Intimacy Variables

| Predictor | Loneliness subscale [a] | | | |
	L-PART	L-PEER	A-NEG	A-POS
Identity		−0.36**		−0.21*
Intimacy		−0.25**	0.25**	
Achievement		0.23**		0.21**
Moratorium				0.24**
Diffusion	0.26**	0.16*		−0.19*
Foreclosure	−0.29***			
Adjusted R^2	0.15	0.32	0.04	0.17

[a] L-PART = Parent-related loneliness; L-PEER = Peer-related loneliness; A-NEG = Aversion to aloneness (Aloneness negative); A-POS = Affinity for aloneness (Aloneness positive).
* $p < 0.05$,   ** $p < 0.01$,   *** $p < 0.001$

in peer relations were found in adolescents who scored higher on the unidimensional identity and intimacy scales. Further, again confirming expectations, subjects high on Diffusion showed higher levels of peer-related loneliness. The positive association between subjects' score on the L-PEER scale and the Identity Achievement scale was an unexpected finding.

Only one variable was related to aversion to aloneness. Contrary to expectations, adolescents who scored higher on intimacy tended to have more negative views on being alone. A confused pattern of results emerged for the A-POS scale. The negative relation with Diffusion and the positive association with Achievement had been anticipated. However, lower levels of affinity for aloneness were found in adolescents who scored higher on the uni-dimensional identity scale and subjects high on Moratorium held more positive views on being alone. Both of these results were unexpected findings.

In conclusion, most of the hypotheses on the associations between subjects' feelings of parent- and peer-related loneliness and their emerging sense of identity and intimacy received some empirical support. The findings for affinity for aloneness were somewhat discouraging.

The results indicate that much additional research seems to be needed on the association between loneliness and identity development, particularly for affinity for aloneness. However, the fact that a sizeable portion of the variance in both peer- and parent-related loneliness could be accounted for by a set of short and crude measures of identity and intimacy is a particularly promising result.

Attachment Style

Identifying patterns of attachment in adolescence calls for a different approach to that used with young children. In infancy a child's attachment style is determined through direct observation of his or her behaviour in a strictly controlled situation, known as the Strange Situation (Ainsworth, Blehar, Waters & Wall, 1978). In this situation, the child's behaviour is objectively assessed during brief episodes of separation from and reunion with the primary caretaker and when reacting to an unknown adult. After infancy, however, the fact that children have moved to the level of internal representation means that the actual presence of the caregiver may no longer be needed to infer a person's attachment style (Main, Kaplan & Cassidy, 1985). Through their day-to-day interactions with their caregivers, children develop internal working models of attachment which represent generalised expectations regarding interpersonal relations.

One promising model of attachment in adolescence has been introduced by De Wuffel (1986). In line with Bowlby's (1973; 1980) theoretical ideas,

De Wuffel identified two basic dimensions in caregiver-child relationships, namely, predictable support from attachment figures and freedom to explore. These two dimensions are expected to generalise to a capacity for interpersonal trust and a sense of self-reliance or independence, respectively. More importantly, De Wuffel (1986) went on to develop a series of self-report measures for reliably assessing the basic dimensions in his conceptual model.

Adolescents' position on the basic dimensions of support and exploration can be inferred from their appraisals of everyday events with their primary caregivers, i.e. with their parents, as revealed in the Family Episodes Rating Task (FERT). Another measure, the Adolescent Interpersonal Orientation Questionnaire (AIOQ) yields total scores for both interpersonal trust and independence as experienced in relationships with peers. Following the logic of De Wuffel's model, adolescents' interpersonal orientation (AIOQ) has to match their attachment style (FERT). The former is considered to be an expansion or generalisation of the latter.

Using these two instruments, four basic groups can be distinguished, each with its own particular style of attachment. Subjects who score high on both experienced support and exploration are described as Securely attached. Adolescents low on support and low on exploration are labelled Anxious-ambivalent. Subjects who score low on support but high on exploration are referred to as Avoidantly attached. Finally, adolescents high on support but low on exploration are labelled Dependently attached.

Because of the model's intuitive appeal, it was decided to conduct an exploratory study on loneliness and attachment style using the conceptual model and assessment methodology developed by De Wuffel (1986). Subjects in Sample 4 (Van Hees, 1990) were administered the Family Episodes Rating Task (FERT), the Adolescent Interpersonal Orientation Questionnaire (AIOQ) and the Louvain Loneliness Scale for Children and Adolescents (LLCA). Following the procedures outlined by De Wuffel (1986)—basically a median-split on both the support and exploration dimensions derived from the FERT, with appropriate checks on concurrent validity using the scores obtained on the AIOQ—each of the 200 adolescents in the sample was classified into one of the four attachment groups. Roughly equal numbers of subjects fell into each of these groups: Securely attached, 47; Dependently attached, 50; Avoidant attachment, 40; Anxious-ambivalent, 63.

A series of four one-way ANOVAs was then performed with attachment group as the independent variable and subjects' score on each of the four LLCA scales as the dependent variable. Mean scores on the loneliness and attitude to aloneness scales as a function of subjects' attachment style are shown in Table 9.6. The four groups were not found to differ from one another on the A-POS scale. However, significant effects were obtained for

TABLE 9.6

Mean Scores on the Louvain Loneliness Scale for Children and
Adolescents (LLCA) in Four Attachment Style Groups

| LLCA Subscale [a] | Attachment Style | | | |
	Secure	Dependent	Avoidant	Anxious Ambivalent
L-PART	16.77	16.57	22.15	19.04
L-PEER	17.72	20.88	21.28	23.57
A-NEG	30.11	34.30	31.50	31.76
A-POS	30.85	32.07	33.66	32.09

[a] L-PART = Parent-related loneliness; L-PEER = Peer-related loneliness; A-NEG = Aversion to aloneness (Aloneness negative); A-POS = Affinity for aloneness (Aloneness positive).

the L-PART and L-PEER scales and for the A-NEG scale, $F(3, 196) = 13.26$, 9.28 and 4.46, respectively, with all values significant at $p < 0.01$ or beyond. Pairwise a posteriori tests (Tukey, alpha set at 0.05) revealed that each of these three scales differentiated the four attachment groups in a distinctive way.

Avoidant subjects scored significantly higher than all the other attachment groups on the L-PART scale. In addition, Anxious-ambivalent subjects obtained a significantly higher score on this scale than adolescents in the Dependently attached group with Securely attached subjects falling between. The latter group of subjects (Securely attached) scored significantly lower on the L-PEER scale than did all the other groups. Subjects who tend to be Dependently attached scored significantly higher on the A-NEG scale than Securely attached subjects; the other two attachment groups fell between the former groups.

Taken together, the loneliness and attitude to aloneness scales highlight the specific characteristics of the four attachment groups, each of which has its own weaknesses and strengths in the interpersonal domain. Subjects in the Avoidant and Anxious ambivalent groups, who experience a lack of support in their relationships with their primary attachment figures, feel more lonely in their relationships with their parents than do the other two groups. The Securely attached group is distinguished from the group of Dependently attached subjects by its low level of peer-related loneliness. Finally, the latter group of subjects, who fail to engage in adequate levels of exploratory behaviour, are characterised by their inability to be alone. All of these results seem to make sense within the explanatory framework of attachment theory. The only unexpected finding is that the A-POS scale failed to differentiate between the four attachment groups and, in particular, between the Securely attached individuals and the other groups.

It is fair to say that current evidence for the association between adolescent loneliness, on the one hand and subjects' sense of identity, intimacy or attachment style on the other hand, is at best, mildly positive. However, the preliminary results reported in this chapter do provide the first steps towards the establishment of a developmental framework for adolescent loneliness and aloneness which is certain to be expanded further by future research.

RETROSPECTS AND PROSPECTS

Looking back on the present chapter, it can be concluded that a more fully worked out conceptualisation of adolescent loneliness has led to the development of a four-scale instrument which measures loneliness in relationships with parents and peers, and aversion to and affinity for aloneness. The research reported in the chapter shows clearly that four basic objectives have been achieved: (1) Each of the four aspects of loneliness and aloneness can be measured reliably by means of a separate subscale, with limited subscale overlap and high factorial validity; (2) All four subscales exhibit a reasonable level of construct validity; (3) Each of the different aspects of loneliness and aloneness evidences a normative developmental trend during adolescence; and (4) all are related, in specific ways, to important developmental phenomena during adolescence.

Some of the results, however, were clearly divergent from the initial hypotheses. The non-linear trends for both parent- and peer-related loneliness (L-PART and L-PEER) were initially something of a surprise. The finding that the L-PART scores are lowest in Grade 7 has some intuitive appeal, because this grade level marks the transition from primary to secondary school in the Belgian educational system. One may venture that parents pay more attention to their children's academic progress and school adaptation in this transitional period and, while doing so, meet their offspring's relational demands.

This particular interpretation in terms of school transition, however, makes the fact that the L-PEER score is significantly lower in Grade 7 than in Grade 5 all the more striking. The transition to secondary school involves a move into a different school context and may be seen as increasing rather than decreasing feelings of peer-related loneliness as adjustment to a new group takes place.

Several explanations may be advanced for the results obtained. First, 7th graders already have adequate social interaction skills, because of the rapid increase in the capacity for intimacy during pre-adolescence (Petersen, 1988), which enables them to find new friends within the new school context or to find compensation through other relationships in their social networks. A second possibility is that the transition to secondary school does bring about feelings of peer-related loneliness, but these feelings are short-lived and subside after a few weeks or months, as is the case in other transitional periods of a person's academic career, such as the transition to college (Cutrona, 1982). In this context, it is noteworthy that all questionnaire sessions with the LLCA were conducted several months after the start of the school year, because, for understandable reasons, school principals typically refuse any testing during the hectic start of the school year. Whichever explanation is appropriate, it is clear that short-term longitudinal research, in which a group of subjects is followed through the transition to secondary school and into the first year in the new context, is necessary to answer all of the questions arising around the Grade 7 results.

Some unexpected findings were also observed with regard to the correlations between loneliness and attitude to aloneness, on the one hand and identity, intimacy and attachment style, on the other. Although it is difficult to provide a clear explanation for some of these findings, some reasons can be offered for the unexpected results with the A-POS scale. These explanations centre on two aspects, the conceptualisation of the crucial variables in the process of identity development and the content of the A-POS scale.

Higher scores on the A-POS scale were associated with higher scores on the Moratorium scale. This finding is at odds with the initial hypothesis which stated that making strong commitments is the crucial variable in identity development and hence should be associated with greater affinity for aloneness. The defining feature of subjects in the Moratorium status is precisely that they have not yet found strong commitments and are still in the process of exploring several alternative paths to identity. An alternative conceptualisation, of course, is that exploration rather than commitment is the crucial variable in identity formation. Adolescents in the Moratorium status, who suffer from a temporary stagnation in development and explore several alternatives while being unable to arrive at strong identity commitments, may tend to retreat into aloneness and hence obtain high scores on the A-POS scale. It is particularly difficult to put this alternative hypothesis to an empirical test by means of the traditional identity status measures, because subjects' exploration and commitment are necessarily mingled in these instruments. The development of more differentiated identity measures, in which levels of exploration and commitment are assessed separately, may help clarify this issue.

There is an alternative way to account for the unexpected association between the Moratorium score and A-POS, and for the fact that the latter scale failed to differentiate between the four attachment groups. This involves accepting that, strictly speaking, affinity for aloneness cannot be described as a sign of psychological maturity—as has been done in the present research programme. Instead, one has to assert that solitude is a concept of a more limited nature which refers to active and constructive use of aloneness. In view of this, it should be associated with more advanced forms of identity and with secure attachment.

The A-POS scale, in its present form, contains many items which tap a reactive rather than an active desire to be alone, i.e. the items test whether one wants to get away from others rather than wanting to engage all by oneself in an activity which is intrinsically rewarding. A reliable and valid measure of the experience of solitude would permit an adequate test of the hypothesised associations with psychological maturity. Current field efforts within the ongoing research programme are devoted to the development of such an instrument. In all, it seems fair to conclude that the concept of solitude, which has acted as an important source of inspiration for the research efforts and has not yet been adequately distinguished from a positive attitude to aloneness, is bound to come to the fore in later phases of the research programme.

It is also appropriate to speculate on ways in which the developmental framework introduced in this chapter might be extended in order to clarify further the meaning and significance of loneliness in the developing social world of the adolescent. By and large, loneliness has been thought to be confined to relationships with parents and same-sex partners during both childhood and adolescence. From mid-adolescence onwards, however, relationships with opposite-sex partners are increasingly important. An additional scale measuring feelings of loneliness in heterosexual relationships could easily be developed along the lines which guided the construction of the L-PART and L-PEER scales. This would allow empirical testing of the hypothesis that loneliness with regard to opposite-sex relationships increases towards the end of adolescence.

Three further developments would be necessary in order to achieve this. First, important additional distinctions would have to be made with regard to the core constructs in the developmental framework. Second, hypotheses regarding associations between these constructs and both loneliness and attitude to aloneness would have to be modified. Finally, the measurement of the core developmental variables would have to be improved, particularly with regard to intimacy. A distinction would also have to be made between adolescents' ideological identity and their interpersonal identity. Such developments could lead to testing of the hypothesis that late adolescents who have achieved a strong sense of identity in the interpersonal domain, i.e. who know what they want from their relationships with opposite-sex partners, will suffer less from heterosexual loneliness. Where intimacy is concerned, an alternative would have to be developed to the scale used in the present research programme. This instrument primarily measures adolescents' capacity to relate meaningfully to same-sex partners and to feel at ease in social contacts with others (Rosenthal et al., 1981). A measure which captures adolescents' ability to relate to members of the opposite sex in mutually satisfying ways seems to be much more appropriate.

These suggestions for theoretical extensions and for improvements in measurement devices illustrate the potential value of the proposed developmental framework of adolescent loneliness. It is evident, however, that complete insight into the role of heterosexual relations for the developing person and into the significance of loneliness as it emerges in this type of relationship will necessitate research on young adulthood (ages 18 to 25), the prime time of heterosexual relationship formation. The research described here provides many guidelines as to how such further investigations might best be approached.

ACKNOWLEDGMENTS

The authors gratefully acknowledge the assistance of Patricia Bijttebier, Paul Caes, Ilse De Saeger, Christiane De Smedt, Hans Grietens, Annick Peeters, Edwin Segers and Sofie Van Hees in data collection. Special thanks go to Rob Stroobants, who skilfully handled all statistical analyses. All correspondence should be directed to the first author at the following address: Catholic University of Louvain, Center for Developmental Psychology, Tiensestraat 102, B-3000 Leuven, Belgium.

APPENDIX

Numbers refer to actual order of appearance in the questionnaire. Items keyed in reverse direction are preceded by a minus sign.

The Louvain Loneliness Scale for Children and Adolescents (LLCA)

Parent-related Loneliness (L-PART)

-1. I feel I have very strong ties with my parents.
-3. My parents make time to pay attention to me.
11. I feel left out by my parents.
-16. I find consolation with my parents.
18. I find it hard to talk to my parents.
-25. I can get along with my parents very well.
-30. My parents are ready to listen to me or to help me.
-37. I have the feeling that my parents and I belong together.
-38. My parents share my interests.
-43. My parents show real interest in me.
45. I doubt whether my parents really love me.
-48. At home I feel at ease.

Peer-related Loneliness (L-PEER)

4. I think I have fewer friends than others.
5. I feel isolated from other people.
7. I feel excluded by my classmates.
9. I want to be better integrated in the class group.
15. Making friends is hard for me.
17. I am afraid the others won't let me join in.
23. I feel alone at school.
27. I think there is not a single friend to whom I can tell everything.
33. I feel abandoned by my friends.
35. I feel left out by my friends.
41. I feel sad because nobody wants to join in with me.
47. I feel sad because I have no friends.

Aversion to Aloneness (A-NEG)

8. When I am lonely, I feel bored.
10. When I am alone, I feel bad.
12. When I feel lonesome, I've got to see some friends.
14. When I feel bored, I am unhappy.

20. When I am lonely, I don't know what to do.
22. To really have a good time, I have to be with my friends.
24. When I am lonely, time lasts long and no single activity seems attractive.
29. When I am alone, I would like to have other people around.
32. When I am bored, I go to see a friend.
34. I feel unhappy when I have to do things on my own.
39. When I am lonely, I go to see other people myself.
42. When I am bored, I feel lonesome.

Affinity for Aloneness (A-POS)

2. I withdraw from others to do things that can hardly be done with a large number of people.
6. I want to be alone.
13. I am looking for a moment to be on my own.
19. When I am lonely, I want to be alone to think it over.
21. When I have an argument with someone, I want to be alone to think it over.
26. When I am alone, I quieten down.
28. To think something over without disturbance, I want to be alone.
31. I am happy when for once I am the only one at home, because then I can do some quiet thinking.
36. I want to be alone to do some things.
40. I keep away from others because they disturb me with their noise.
44. Being alone makes me take up my courage again.
46. At home I look for moments to be alone, so that I can do things on my own.

CHAPTER TEN

The Young Person's Relationship to the Institutional Order

Nick Emler

Social theorists are generally agreed that a qualitative change occurred in European societies sometime around the end of the eighteenth century. It was a change that transformed the character of social relationships and with them the entire moral fabric of society. One analysis of this transformation locates its origins in the progressive rationalisation of productive labour and so labels it the Industrial Revolution. Whatever the origins, this period in European social history was characterised by several roughly concurrent trends which included industrialisation, urbanisation, mass literacy and secularisation. Furthermore it saw the emergence in recognisably modern form of what is now the dominant kind of political unit, the nation state.

The Industrial Revolution was also seen to create two rather different spheres of social life, two contrasting types of social relation (Cooley, 1909). On the one hand was the private sphere of the family and friendship relations, the sphere of the primary group. This was taken to be a society of small-scale, informal, face-to-face and relatively long-term personal relationships. Solidarity was based on personal and emotional ties of kinship and affection. On the other hand was the public sphere of institutional relationships, the sphere of the secondary group. This was taken to be a society of more anonymous, formal, impersonal and transitory relationships in which commitments were contractual and rationally calculated.

There is now some doubt as to whether the transformation in social relationships wrought by the industrialisation of Western societies was either so discontinuous with the past or precisely of the kind envisaged by social theorists in the nineteenth and early twentieth centuries. Wellman (1979), for example, has questioned the conclusion that the community disappears in the mass society, that a clear division really does emerge between a relatively limited private domain and a much larger segment dominated by emotionally superficial and largely formal role relationships. However, the analyses provided by the earlier social theorists did have the merit of drawing attention to a pervasive feature of contemporary life; the prevalence of formal, large-scale institutions and organisations, or what Weber (1947) called "bureaucracies".

There are two things to notice here. The first is that much of the public, and indeed private, business of our lives is conducted within frameworks provided by bureaucracies. In adult life we are likely to be employed in formal organisations, our education will have been provided by such organisations and organisations of this kind will also deliver health care and security. A range of public services will be coordinated through large-scale bureaucratic organisations and behind everything will lie the administrative machinery of the state. Even relations between private individuals and the conditions of family life will be regulated by state bureaucracies.

Weber applied his thesis about the rationalisation of social relationships primarily to productive labour. He foresaw that economic enterprises organised around wage-labour relations would be progressively bureaucratised. But he saw that this process also applied to the apparatus of government. The nation state in its contemporary form only becomes possible with the development of means for the effective administration of mass populations, and bureaucracy provides these means.

The second thing to notice is the special character of bureaucratic relations. Weber argued that the bureaucracy differs from other kinds of social organisation, notably those based on ties of personal loyalty and those based on respect for custom and tradition, in a number of crucial respects. It rationalises the relation between the individual and the system: individuals are formally clients, customers or members, with formally defined rights, entitlements and obligations which depend on status. It also rationalises membership status, awarding positions on the basis of technical qualifications rather than, for example, on the basis of personal preferences or family connections. Finally, it rationalises norms and authority relations. What Weber called the "legal-rational" orientation of bureaucracy is perhaps its most distinctive feature.

Weber distinguished formal or legal-rational authority from other varieties in a number of ways, but four are central. The first is that all positions of formal authority exist within a rationally organised hierarchy "an institution or organisation" and have no legitimacy except in terms of their positions in this system. The second is that each position always has specific, explicit, formally defined and limited spheres of jurisdiction; authority is rationally partitioned. The third is that holders of such authority can only legitimately exercise it in accordance with formally defined, impersonal and impartial criteria and not in the service of personal interests. And the fourth is that office holders have formally defined duties and obligations which are likewise distinct from their personal inclinations.

If the social revolution which accompanied the industrial revolution hastened the spread of bureaucracy it did not so much create distinct spheres of social relations as introduce new principles into the regulation of all social relationships. It created what Mitchell (1969) has called a structural order for social relationships. The state seeks to rationalise all relationships by formally defining the rights and obligations of all citizens, rights which are backed up by formal guarantees of protection and obligations which are to be enforced by formally defined sanctions. This pattern is then reproduced in the various institutions within the state so that individuals will also have formal rights, entitlements and obligations in their institutional roles as patients and doctors, employees and employers, pupils and teachers and even as parents and children.

INSTITUTIONS IN THE SOCIAL WORLDS OF ADOLESCENTS

The purpose of this long preamble, of course, is to make a point about the social worlds of adolescents, a point that will provide the theme for the remainder of this chapter: relations with the institutional order assume a particular significance in adolescence. The reasons for this are various. At the beginning of adolescence the typical child's life will revolve around the family, friends and school. The institutional or structural order will impinge on life, with one very important exception, in only a relatively limited way. There is also an argument that at the beginning of adolescence children have difficulty in construing relationships except in personal terms or in terms of broad social categories such as male and female.

By the end of adolescence, most of the formal entitlements and obligations of the adult citizen will have been acquired. A majority of individuals will have entered the labour market, if they are not undergoing more intensive and advanced preparation in higher education for a particular segment of this market. And the labour market in the contemporary nation state is dominated by highly bureaucratised employment relations. Over the course of adolescence individuals will have made various transitions towards adult status and towards placements within the social order which will owe much to the kinds of accommodations they have made to the requirements of the institutional order.

Let us consider first of all the kinds of experience adolescents will have of formal organisations and formally ordered relationships. These will include experience of commercial organisations, encountered through the purchase of goods and services. Certainly over the course of childhood there will have been extensive if episodic and vicarious experience of relatively impersonal commercial transactions. Consequently by age ten or eleven children already have a well-developed understanding of the institutions of buying and selling (cf. Berti & Bombi, 1988). But much of their experience will have been as onlookers, making sense of the activities of their parents and other adults. In adolescence they will increasingly make these transactions themselves and increasingly on their own behalf. Thus adolescence sees a change in the individual's role as commercial customer and consumer.

Both children and adolescents will also have some direct experience of health care organisations but this will be in most cases even more occasional and may remain strongly personalised, as a relationship with the family doctor for example.

For most individuals adolescence brings more extensive recognition of the degree to which activities are subject to legal regulation. In this period of life there are typically increasing opportunities to be in public places and to participate in activities beyond the direct supervision of parents or other adults. Young people are increasingly expected to exercise control over their own behaviour and are increasingly held legally responsible for their actions. Whereas earlier in childhood parents stood between the child and the law, in adolescence this relationship becomes more direct. And indeed many young people will have direct personal contact with the law-enforcing agencies and agents of the state over the course of their adolescence.

This may partly be a function of the greater capacity of adolescents to do things that are legally proscribed. Increases during adolescence in size, strength and skill open up new behavioural possibilities. Adolescence also brings with it a range of physical capacities in advance of the formal entitlement to exercise them. These include capacities for physical labour, alcohol consumption, driving motor vehicles and sexual relations.

Finally, all adolescents will have one institutional experience in common; they will all have had several years direct experience of formally ordered relations in the shape of their schooling. In this respect, there is continuity between childhood and adolescent experience. There may be some differences associated with adolescence; the schools may be larger units than those of the childhood years and they may be associated with greater formality. Also beyond some point, the precise timing of which varies across countries, continued participation in full-time formal education becomes voluntary. The decision made at this time "whether or not to leave full-time education" is fundamental for its repercussions upon almost every detail of the individual's subsequent life course (e.g. Banks et al, 1991). How young people adapt to formal education is central to their relations with the institutional order of society generally and we shall need to return to this later in the chapter.

At this point we may note that adolescence represents a significant new phase in the individual's relations with the institutional order. To begin with this is not so much because of changes in educational experiences but because of a combination of physical changes and increased independence. In a sense a crisis or decision point arises early in adolescence, but perhaps not of the kind described Erikson's (1968) writings on youth. Rather it is a crisis in relations with the wider community in which the choice is: "Will I allow the state to mediate in and stipulate the terms of my relations with others or will I seek to conduct these relations directly?".

The thesis of this chapter is as follows. At the heart of young people's relation to the institutional order is their orientation to formal authority. The most important context for the development of their relationships with the institutional order and the formal authority it embodies is probably formal state education. Finally, the kind of accommodation young people make to formal authority is reflected in the degree to which they engage in delinquent activities.

The remainder of this chapter will develop this thesis and its implications and will set out the empirical and theoretical basis for these various claims and the ways in which they are related to one another. In particular it will be necessary to justify the link between involvement in delinquency and orientation to formal authority. It therefore begins with the interpretation of delinquency entailed in this thesis.

ACCEPTING VERSUS REJECTING THE INSTITUTIONAL REGULATION OF CONDUCT

Why should delinquency be regarded as an expression of young people's orientation to formal authority or of their relations with the institutional order? After all, criminologists, sociologists and psychologists have offered many other interpretations of juvenile crime. According to strain theorists (e.g. Merton, 1969) delinquency is the use of unofficial and illegitimate means for pursuing legitimate and culturally valued ends, namely the acquisition of wealth. Strain theory assumes that all individuals have internalised and accepted the value of these ends in childhood. In adolescence, a section of the population, those from working class backgrounds, discover that legitimate means for achieving these ends, namely well-paid jobs, are likely to be unavailable to them.

Cultural diversity theory (cf. Sutherland & Cressey, 1970) assumes that a single society contains a variety of subcultures each with different values.

The values of some sub-cultures support forms of behaviour which other more dominant sub-cultures define as crime.

Social control theorists such as Hirschi (1969) have argued that everyone is susceptible to criminal behaviour in so far as this is perceived to be rewarding. They will only be restrained to the extent that they have attachments to significant others, to the extent that they have commitments to the conventional order (for example, investments in careers that would be put at risk by criminal behaviour) and to the extent that they have beliefs that punishment is the likely consequence of crime. Thus control theorists attach no special significance to the institutional order except insofar as institutions can be sources of commitments and of rewards and punishments.

The same is true of at least two influential psychological theories. Behaviourists have argued that children acquire behavioural habits, whether through observational learning or through systematic punishment and reward, or some combination of the two. The habits themselves may be good or bad; the learning mechanism involved is indifferent to their content. Delinquency simply reflects a surfeit of anti-social habits. Biogenetic theories are based on the assumption that patterns of behaviour are influenced by inherited characteristics. Generally, theorists writing within this framework have assumed that crime reflects some genetically transmitted feature which creates a deficit in the capacity to become socialised. Eysenck (1977) has provided one of the most thoroughly developed theories of this kind. According to Eysenck the basis for behavioural control is conditioned anxiety and the capacity to acquire such stimulus-reponse connections strongly and rapidly is genetically determined. Other theorists have stressed an incapacity to experience remorse or to form emotional attachments as being at the root of criminal behaviour.

Interestingly, one of the few theories which suggests a strong link between involvement in crime and orientation to authority is psychoanalysis. In psycho-analytic theory the Oedipal crisis is resolved when the young child internalises the image of the father as an authority for its conduct. This internalised representation of authority then directs the child's conduct when the father is physically absent. It also mandates deference to the father's wishes and instructions and, by generalisation, to the demands of all authority. In the hands of other writers, however, submission to authority becomes pathological (e.g. Adorno et al, 1950) and the childhood superego a threat to civilised society rather than one of its foundations. What most psychology has taken from Freud is not a lesson about the sources of respect for authority but the idea that the truly socialised individual is directed by internalised moral standards alone and not by susceptibility to any form of external control. Thus Eysenck's theory of criminality gives no significant role to social control; crime occurs to the extent that internalised controls are weak. Those theories of moral development that have in other respects remained closer to Freud nonetheless also assume that the process of socialisation is largely one of acquiring moral autonomy based on internalised standards and controls (e.g. Hoffman, 1977). Thus crime, including juvenile crime, is interpreted in most contemporary moral psychology not as a failure to respond to the social control that institutions and organisations seek to exercise but more simply as a failure of self-control.

Interestingly this interpretation has its roots in analyses of the same social changes that Weber had described in terms of the rationalisation of human relations and the rise of bureaucracy. The important difference is that moral psychology has been much more strongly influenced by Adam Smith, Ferdinand Tonnies and others who saw these social changes in terms of the increasing anonymity of industrial and urbanised society. Under these conditions, it was assumed, social control is not practical. Society must therefore depend more extensively on individual self-control. For theories based on this analysis, adolescence assumes significance as the first important test of the success of moral socialisation. If their childhoods have equipped them with a properly functioning conscience adolescents will continue to observe the standards of civilised conduct as they move increasingly beyond the direct supervision of adults. If not, the same lack of parental control will allow them to be increasingly delinquent.

The flaws in this analysis and in the assumptions about society on which it rests have been spelled out in detail elsewhere (e.g. Emler & Hogan, 1991; Emler & Reicher, in press). Here it will only be noted that such evidence as is available suggests that most behaviour of any signficance is available for social control. The issue must therefore be why social control and particularly organisational control, does not always work and in particular works less well in adolescence.

There are two popular interpretations of juvenile criminality which imply a link to relations with authority, though both attribute delinquency to forms of personal psychological deficit. One links delinquency to deficits in social skills (e.g. Spence, 1981). It suggests that young people who are delinquent mishandle encounters with authority. They lack the social skills to respond "appropriately" when confronted by people in authority (Freedman et al, 1978).

There are some attractions to this interpretation. It allows that all young people may misbehave to some extent but when confronted by officials, policemen or others in positions of responsibility, some of them fail to do the appropriate things, to show respect and deference or regret for their misdeeds. Instead they are hostile, abusive, brazen and confrontational. This elicits a punitive reaction from authority (Piliavin & Briar, 1964) and sets up a positive feedback loop of escalating mutual hostility. One specific attraction of this analysis is that it offers a plausible interpretation of the link between primary and secondary deviance.

Its principal weakness lies in the lack of clear evidence either that juvenile offenders are deficient in social skills or that their reactions to authority, which indeed are more likely to be hostile and confrontational, should be interpreted as skill deficits (Renwick & Emler, 1991). Its merits are that it does draw our attention to the importance of encounters with authority in the lives of adolescents and the ways in which these encounters are handled.

The second interpretation has a more cerebral emphasis. That is, it directs attention to processes in the head of the individual actor rather than to the dynamics of relations between social actors. This is the cognitive-developmental analysis of delinquency following Kohlberg (cf. Jurkovic, 1980; Jennings, Kilkenny & Kohlberg, 1983) and it assumes that delinquents differ from non-delinquents in the quality of their moral judgment and decision-making processes. Kohlberg (1976) argued that these processes undergo a series of improvements which can be described as stages in the development of moral reasoning. At each successive stage the individual makes a more adequate analysis of the moral obligations which exist among individuals and between individuals and their communities. Each stage sees a reinterpretation of the relationship between individuals and authority. A critical transformation in the interpretation of this relationship occurs between the second and third of the stages described by Kohlberg. This also marks the transition between what Kohlberg called respectively preconventional and conventional moral reasoning.

At Kohlberg's stages 1 and 2, actions are judged in terms of the wants, interests or fears of the individual. There is no recognition that society entails shared standards of conduct. Rules and expectations are perceived as external to the self and relations with all authority are interpreted in individual and personal terms. The significant shift between stages 2 and 3 involves reference to shared standards of what is right or desirable in deciding what are one's obligations. Thus the individual who reasons about moral obligations at the third stage assumes that there are standards of virtue which he or she shares with others, including others in positions of authority. Nonetheless, there is still no explicit recognition of the formal character of institutional authority in Weber's sense. This only emerges clearly at stage 4 where it is recognised that the social system has a superordinate legitimate authority and the obligation to comply with legal authority is distinguished from the obligation to comply with standards of decent, considerate interpersonal behaviour. At the same time, the impersonal requirements upon office-holders to discharge specified duties is distinguished from less formal expectations about acting considerately or with good intentions.

The crucial claim made by Kohlberg and his colleagues is that at each successive stage delinquency becomes less likely. It makes sense both theoretically and in terms of the observed patterns of delinquency and moral reasoning that reasoning at the first and second stage leads to delinquent conduct more frequently than does reasoning at the third and fourth stage. On the one hand it seems plausible that a stage 3 and particularly a stage 4 analysis of the individual's obligations towards authority and the law would more consistently lead to the conclusion that certain forms of conduct are morally wrong. On the other, it is well documented that involvement in delinquency first increases and then decreases over the course of adolescence (cf. Hirschi & Gottfredson, 1983). During this same period conventional moral reasoning is likely to emerge for the first time (Colby & Kohlberg, 1987).

Thus one might speculate that as individuals enter adolescence and their conduct becomes increasingly dependent upon internal control, then they will become progressively more delinquent. But this trend will be checked and ultimately reversed as this internal control becomes increasingly based upon conventional moral reasoning. The most delinquent adolescents will be those slowest to develop moral reasoning at the conventional level. Again the principal weakness of this interpretation is the lack of evidence directly linking moral reasoning level and delinquency. It also provides no explanation for the marked sex differences in delinquency; there are no parallel sex differences in moral reasoning. Its merit lies in directing our attention to the fact that institutional authority is a phenomenon which individuals must comprehend and interpret in some way and to the possibility that this comprehension undergoes further significant changes in adolescence.

A point not to be forgotten about Kohlberg's theory is its assumption, shared with other moral psychologies, that behavioural control is properly vested in the individual and not in the system. Individuals may, at stage 4, recognise that they have obligations to the social system but they are assumed to be properly free to make this determination themselves. But even this seems to shift the balance too far in favour of the system and Kohlberg concludes that stage 4 is ultimately unsatisfactory as an analysis of moral obligations. He postulates a further level of moral development, the principled level at which obligations to more abstract principles of justice, equality and respect for human life take precedence over any obligations to a local social system or officials acting on its authority. In this respect, Kohlberg's moral position converges with that of crowd psychology and its descendants.

The basic thesis of crowd psychology is that the behaviour of individuals becomes less civilised and more criminal when individuals are gathered together in crowds. This idea was first popularised by Le Bon (1896) but later developed by McDougall, Freud and Floyd Allport among others. Freud for instance suggested that the crowd exercises a form of hypnosis on its members and this has the effect of undermining the superego. The idea later appeared in experimental social psychology, for example in the work of Asch (1951) on conformity; of Latane and Darley (1970) on bystander intervention in emergencies; of Wallach, Kogan and Bem (1962) on the risky shift; and of Zimbardo (1970) on de-individuation. These research programmes seemed to indicate that individuals would abandon standards of truth and honesty, ignore their moral responsibilities and behave recklessly if not quite unpleasantly in the presence of a group. One implication appeared to be that groups have these immoralising effects on individuals because they increase the individual members' sense of personal anonymity.

This immediately suggests another interpretation of adolescent crime: adolescence provides more opportunities for peer association and to the extent that young people associate in groups they will therefore be inclined to criminal behaviour. It is true that adolescent crime is overwhelmingly a collective activity (Emler, Reicher & Ross, 1987), but there is no evidence that delinquent adolescents are any more likely than non-delinquents to associate in groups (Morash, 1983).

Arguably the more significant consequence of crowd psychology has been to render all group influence morally suspect. This may become clearer if we consider an offshoot of crowd psychology, what might be called "holocaust psychology". This variant suggests that moral dangers lie not just in groups but in the leadership of groups. In the version of holocaust psychology developed by Adorno and his colleagues (Adorno et al, 1950) the dangers arise to the extent that some individuals are unduly deferrential to the authority of the in-group. Milgram (1974) extended this thesis by suggesting that almost any individual and not just those with authoritarian personalities, is inclined to defer to authority. Thus the threat to civilisation is posed not by the criminal propensities of individuals but by the power of state bureaucracies. This analysis converges with that of Kohlberg in the conclusion that only persons with sufficiently robust moral autonomy will resist pressures to obey institutional authorities. In the 1960s and 1970s adolescence was examined by psychology for signs of the emergence of such autonomy (e.g. Haan, Smith & Block, 1968) and rather less in terms of other kinds of accommodation with authority.

To conclude this section two points can be made. Delinquency has become somewhat marginalised in mainstream psychology as "crime". By this is meant that there has on the one hand been a tendency to regard crime as a pathology of behaviour, as outside the range of normal human conduct and on the other a tendency to assume that it is confined to a small minority of the population: most people are law-abiding and their conformity is unproblematic; in just a few cases the process of socialisation goes awry and criminal behaviour is the result.

It is argued here that, on the contrary, crime or at least delinquency must be regarded as normal and commonplace. Almost everyone breaks some laws or regulations some of the time and the only difference between those people conventionally described as criminal and the rest is one of degree. Very few adolescents engage in robbery involving the use or threat of violence, but a high proportion will commit less serious transgressions such as spraying slogans on walls in public places, other forms of vandalism, minor theft, carrying weapons or getting into fights. If we recognise that rule-breaking is a continuum defined in terms of range, frequency and seriousness and that there is considerable variation along that continuum within the population as a whole then new questions about the relationship between individuals and the institutional order are opened up.

The second point is that the proper scope of the institutional order is a central issue in political debate. The traditional division between left and right in political philosophy is based in part on judgments about the organisation of authority in society. Adolescence is certainly a period in which there is increasing engagement with political issues and one might expect this to include issues relating to the proper scope of state authority. Thus to the extent that individuals form attachments to political parties in adolescence they might be seen as developing preferences for one set of views about authority over another. However, very few adolescents take such an interest in the philosophical bases of political divisions and it is probably rare that young people in their teens envisage formal authority or the institutional order as political issues (cf. Banks et al, 1991). On the other hand these do loom large as personal issues for adolescents and the next section endeavours to show how.

ALTERNATIVE STRATEGIES FOR MANAGING SOCIAL RELATIONS

The link being proposed between juvenile delinquency and orientation to institutional authority can be understood by first considering again the nature of institutional authority. This, as has been argued, may be regarded as a system for managing relations between individuals. It provides means for co-ordinating activities, allocating duties and resources, resolving conflicts of interest and settling grievances. Consequently each individual stands in two kinds of relation to this system. One of these is a relation of constraint; the individual is required to abide by regulations, to observe formally defined proscriptions and prescriptions and to obey the instructions and directives of those who are formally authorised to issue them. The other relation is one of protection; the system offers individuals protection of their rights, their person and their property and provides them with means of redress when those rights are violated.

But if the institutional order is, among other things, a system for managing relations between people, is there an alternative? The answer is 'yes' and what Mitchell (1969) has called the 'personal order' provides such an alternative. This is the ordering of social relations in terms of the networks of personal ties, loyalties, obligations and antagonisms existing between specific individuals. It represents a range of informal means for achieving the same objectives as the structural or institutional order. People can coordinate and organise informally, making informal arrangements and deals. They can also cope with the hazards of social living by informal action. They can seek the protection of their friends, defend themselves directly and rely on retaliatory action when attacked or offended.

It is suggested, therefore, that these are two broad ways of managing relations with others, two kinds of strategy which individuals and communities can adopt to cope with the problems and requirements of social life. To some extent these approaches are in conflict, to some extent complementary. Young people will embrace a mixture of both. Delinquency reflects a greater commitment to the informal solution, non-deliquency to the institutional solution.

Is there any evidence to support this interpretation? Three kinds of evidence will be discusssed, relating respectively to the content of delinquency, to the relation between delinquency and beliefs about formal authority and to the relation of both to educational career.

Delinquent Action as the Conduct of Social Relations by Extra-legal Means

If delinquency is indeed part of an informal solution to the management of social relations then its content should reflect this. One prototypical form of adolescent delinquency is theft. But the fact that some adolescents fail to observe formal legal requirements regarding property is by itself not particularly revealing about their attitudes to the law as such. Most people would probably agree that theft is morally wrong quite apart from being legally proscribed and that its immorality is as strong a reason for desisting from theft as is its illegality.

What is more interesting is that adolescents who regularly steal also typically do other things which reflect the kind of informal solution outlined earlier (Emler, 1984; Emler, Reicher & Ross, 1987). They are more likely than their peers to break institutional rules and regulations, often in pursuit of friendship obligations (for example, providing friends with help on school tests, holding parties without permission, etc.). They are more likely to commit status offences (under-age smoking and drinking, truanting from school). They are more likely to accept stolen goods (reflecting a willingness to participate in an informal and extra-legal economy). And they are more likely to carry weapons and to attack enemies. Routine preparedness for and involvement in aggression can be seen as preference for informal solutions to grievances and the risk of victimisation, though of course these habits are open to other interpretations. However, Black (1983) has also argued that many crimes can be seen as forms of self-help justice; that is, they are motivated by a desire to rectify perceived injuries to the self. Black instances cases of theft arising from disputes over ownership, cases of vandalism directed against the property of someone who had offended the culprit and cases of assaults arising from provocation.

None of this should be taken to suggest that adolescent crime can be attributed entirely to any burning sense of injustice. Nor should it be taken to exclude the role of other factors in adolescent crime such as opportunity, intoxication, a lack of empathy with its victims, impulsiveness, a desire for fun and excitement, or a desire for material gain. The point is that many of these factors can tell us something about when delinquency occurs but they do not provide the whole story and certainly little about what links diverse delinquent activities into an overall pattern. We need also to recognise what general problems of social relations delinquent activity might be directed at solving.

Adolescent delinquency may represent an informal strategy in another respect. It provides a public demonstration that one is both willing and able to defend one's interests by direct retaliation (cf. Felson, 1978; 1981). Lest it be supposed that the concealed and covert nature of crime would ensure that it could not serve to convey such messages, it needs to be stressed that adolescent crime is in practice a relatively public activity. Young people who are regularly delinquent commit their misdeeds in ways that ensure their visibility (cf. Emler, Reicher & Ross, 1987). Consequently, young frequent offenders have a reputation for being tough, unemotional, brave and brutal, in other words a reputation as people disposed to violent retaliation against anyone who might offend them. Moreover, they are also themselves likely to know that delinquent behaviour gives rise to such reputations (Emler, Reicher & Ronson, 1987).

Finally, however, delinquency can be regarded not just as direct informal action to pursue and defend personal interests. It can also be seen as expressing an explicit repudiation of the alternative official system. Adolescent delinquency typically includes actions directed against the institutional order and its representatives, such as vandalising public property and attacking police officers. The confrontational style of relating to officials noted earlier is, it is argued, not just a by-product of misbehaviour but an intrinsic feature of the delinquent pattern. Interestingly, police records reveal fewer attacks on police officers by juveniles than adolescents themselves claim to make. This particular form of behaviour may therefore be exaggerated in self-reports. But the point of interest is that young offenders should wish to claim involvement in such action at all.

Attitudes and Beliefs about Authority

Is there any indication that young people hold beliefs about formal authority or about appropriate responses to victimisation which are consistent with the interpretation proposed here? If delinquent behaviour reflects a preference for informal solutions to the problems of social living and a rejection of formal solutions then one might expect to find that such behaviour will also be reflected in attitudes and beliefs about authority. Thus, adolescents who are particularly delinquent should also express attitudes which favour direct retaliation, which endorse aggression as a legitimate way of protecting one's rights and interests, which reject the idea that rules and authority are desirable and which reject the demands of institutional authority.

Clear links have been reported between attitudes to law and authority on the one hand and degree of involvement in delinquency on the other (Brown, 1974; Clark & Wenninger, 1964). In these two studies, however, attitude-behaviour relations were confounded with age effects; the samples spanned an age range from 11 to 18 years. It is known from other research that attitudes of the kind sampled change over this period; crime comes to be regarded less seriously and attitudes to the law and legal authoritites become less positive (Turiel, 1976; Mussen et al, 1977; Tuma & Livson, 1960). During the same period, general levels of involvement in delinquency increase, at least up to age 14-15 (Farrington et al, 1982). Studies by Reicher and Emler (1985) and Emler and Reicher (1987), in which age was controlled, revealed a strong relationship between delinquency and attitudes to authority.

These latter studies also confirmed that attitudes to institutional authority as such, do constitute a coherent and distinctive domain. Young people do not just hold beliefs about policemen, about the law, about the courts, about the authority of school teachers, or about the legitimacy of school rules, each as separate issues and relatively unrelated in their thinking. Their attitudes to all these matters are consistently related to one another. Data published by Rump, Rigby and Walters (1985; see also Rigby & Rump, 1979) point to similar conclusions about the generality of attitudes to institutional authority.

Can behaviour be explained in terms of attitudes? Do delinquents break the law because they have negative attitudes towards formal authority and do other adolescents abide by the law because their attitudes are positive? The correlation between attitudes and behaviour reported by Reicher and Emler (1985) is so high it is more reasonable to conclude that attitudes and behaviour are in fact two facets of the same orientation. In other words, young people develop an orientation to formal authority that is more or less positive and this orientation is expressed both behaviourally, in terms of degree of compliance with laws, regulations and the instructions of people in authority, and verbally in terms of attitudes and opinions about rules and authority. Attitudes show the same patterns as behaviour. Between 11 and 16 they become less positive, directly paralleling increasing levels of delinquent activity. And they are less positive amongst males than amongst females.

The content of young people's attitudes to authority provides further clues about preference for informal solutions that are consistent with this argument. As might be expected, prototypical attitudes are those which endorse rule-breaking and defiance of authority. But another significant theme concerns the impartiality of authority. Young people differ markedly in beliefs about the extent to which police officers are honest, are not unnecessarily brutal, are impartial in the protection they provide and so on. Thus, if an adolescent believes that the police and other legal authorities are unlikely to provide protection for his interests or redress for his grievances then direct action might seem like a more realistic personal solution. Of course it is difficult to decide what is cause and what effect here; adolescents may be reporting perceptions that their own actions have helped to confirm.

This problem of cause and effect is even more evident with respect to another strong theme in adolescent attitudes to authority. Adolescent opinions are sharply divided as to whether the authorities are themselves sources of victimisation. If some young people feel that they or the social categories to which they belong are unduly persecuted by the institutional system, then it might seem reasonable to them not only to reject the institutional solution but retaliate against the institutional order as well, to attack policemen or vandalise public property, for example. Nonetheless, the treatment they experience and report at the hands of institutional authorities may itself be a response to their own criminal habits.

Whether the institutional system somehow alienates a particular section of the adolescent population and so pushes it towards both informal solutions and retaliation, or whether some young people are unwilling or unable to accept the demands and requirements of the institutional system in the first place is the fundamental theoretical question. Some answers to this question will be examined later. Before that, let us briefly consider other aspects of young people's orientations to informal solutions.

There is rather less research which can answer questions about the attitudes of young people towards direct retaliation and other informal solutions to the risk or experience of victimisation. The small body of published research on this question has mostly been undertaken within the cognitive developmental framework. Piaget (1932) found that boys were more likely than girls to favour direct retaliation. Durkin (1959) suggested on the contrary that belief in the legitimacy of retaliation would give way with increasing age to attitudes favouring other solutions such as forgiveness or attempts at reconciliation. The implication is that by adolescence only a small minority of immature individuals will still cling to the view that retaliation is a legitimate strategy in the conduct of interpersonal relations.

Some more recent research (Emler & Ohana, 1992) reveals a different picture. First, there was no evidence of any developmental trend in opinions about appropriate responses to victimisation. Children's views fell into three broad categories, unrelated to age. One category involved suggestions that adults should be persuaded to intervene. This might be regarded as the childhood equivalent of the institutional solution: look to the appropriate authorities for protection and redress. A second category involved suggestions about persuading the culprit to recompense the victim. The third category included recommendations for various forms of direct action, such as taking back stolen property, by force if necessary and physically attacking the culprit. Though the categories of response were unrelated to either age or sex, they were related to the child's social class background; working class children were more likely to favour direct action.

It still remains to be determined whether these various preferences can also be found amongst adolescents and whether a preference for direct action is associated with delinquency. However, another study has revealed that delinquent and non-delinquent adolescents disagree about whether delinquents and non-delinquents respectively are people inclined to stand up for their rights. Those who are themselves more delinquent believe that delinquents are more likely to stand up for their rights, whereas those who are themselves less delinquent believe that it is the non-delinquents who are more likely to do so (Emler, Reicher & Ronson, 1987). This is at least consistent with the suggestion that delinquency and non-delinquency reflect alternative strategies of self-protection. However, in a follow-up study (Haswell, 1991) delinquents were seen, by more and less delinquent 14-16 year olds alike, as more likely to be people who stood up for themselves.

Finally, if a pattern of informal solutions to social organisation involves informal deals, alliances, agreements and obligations, as well as informal retribution, this also implies a certain quality of participation in a network of informal social relationships. Some writers have argued that juvenile delinquents are typically young people who have rather impoverished social relationships. Hartup (1983) has written that "delinquency among adolescents and young adults can be predicted mainly from one dimension of early peer relations ... not getting on with others" (p.165). However, there is little evidence that clearly supports this conclusion and much which indicates that adolescent delinquents have extensive and stable networks of personal relationships. Giordano, Cernovich and Pugh (1986) find that in some respects the strength and significance of personal ties may be even greater for delinquent adolescents than for their more law abiding peers. This is more consistent with what would be expected if the informal and institutional solutions in some degree operate as alternatives.

Education and Orientations to the Institutional Order

Formal education provides most children with their first direct and extended experience of a formal organisation and institutional authority. It seems likely, therefore, that this experience will be the basis on which children construct a preliminary understanding of formal authority and the principles according to which it operates. And it appears that by 10-12 years children do have quite a well developed understanding of many of those features that are definitive of formal or legal-rational authority as defined by Weber (Emler, Ohana & Moscovici, 1987; Emler, Ohana & Dickinson, 1990). Certainly, within the context of the school their insight into formal authority is more advanced than the research of Adelson (1971), Furth (1978) and Kohlberg (1976) had previously seemed to suggest.

Does experience of formal education also shape attitudes to institutional authority? Given the prominence of school in the lives of young people, one would expect that their attitudes to authority generally would be related to their attitudes to formal authority as encountered in the school. In fact, adolescents' attitudes to school rules and regulations and to the authority of teachers are closely related to their attitudes to the law and to other forms of institutional authority (Reicher & Emler, 1985; Rigby & Rump, 1979).

The next question is whether these attitudes and the associated patterns of behaviour are related to particular patterns of experience in education. Again the answer is in the affirmative. The connection between delinquency and educational career is well documented. Adolescents who are more delinquent than their peers are increasingly more likely to be in lower streams or curriculum tracks across the course of their secondary schooling (Hargreaves, 1967; Kelly, 1975), less likely to enter public examinations (West & Farrington, 1977), more likely to drop out of school (Hathaway, Reynolds & Monachesi, 1969), more likely to have records of low academic attainment and more likely to leave school with poor academic records and examination results (Hargreaves, 1967; Hindelang et al, 1981; Kelly, 1975; Jensen, 1976; Rhodes & Reiss, 1970).

Academic career shows the same pattern of association with attitudes. Thus, for example, attitudes to formal authority are strongly related both to level of academic attainment and to school leaving age in the United Kingdom (Emler & St. James, 1990).

What is to be made of these associations? One interpretation is that the course taken by young people's educational careers shapes their orientation to authority. Young people who experience failure at school then begin to reject formal education and the system of authority with which, for them, it is so strongly associated.

Something of this kind has been argued by control theorists. Hirschi (1969) for example suggested that people will continue to obey the law so long as they also continue to maintain investments or commitments which would be put at risk by criminal behaviour. Investment in educational attainment and, through this, career aspirations would constitute a particularly important commitment for adolescents. But if this investment had irrevocably and obviously failed then they would be free to engage in delinquency; there would be nothing to lose. In Hirschi's interpretation, however, there is no active rejection of the institutional system, only a turning away from an institution which no longer has any hold over the individuals concerned.

There is an alternative analysis which reverses the direction of causality. According to this analysis the school acts as an extended test of the child's capacity and inclination to accommodate to the requirements of a bureaucratic system (e.g. Danziger, 1971; Jencks, 1972). Jencks (1972) has argued that employers consider educational credentials not so much because of the particular technical or cognitive skills to which they attest but because they are reliable markers of an individual's success in accepting bureaucratic requirements. In so far as educational credentials signal a positive orientation to formal authority then they suggest the holder of these credentials will also adapt well to bureaucratic authority and control in the work-place. Thus educational attainment is not an influence on orientation to institutional authority so much as a product of this orientation.

This analysis also has its intuitive appeal. Success in school is certainly a function of ability but differences in ability do not explain all of the variance in attainment. One can see that doing well at school could also be a function of the child's adjustment to the peculiar requirements of the bureaucratic regime which he or she encounters there, accommodation to the routine and discipline of a formal timetable and to the authority of teachers.

Liska and Reed (1985) have used panel data to examine the competing claims of control theory and this alternative interpretation and conclude that the direction of causality implied in the latter has more support. It is also consistent with the empirical links between delinquency on the one hand and intelligence on the other. If educational failure produced delinquency then because educational failure is related to low intelligence delinquency should also be related to low intelligence. In fact there is no convincing evidence for any relation between delinquency and intelligence (e.g. Menard & Morse, 1984). This is what would be expected if the orientation to institutional authority that lies behind delinquency also influences educational career.

For the present, the evidence does appear to be more consistent with this interpretation but before reaching any final conclusions it would be preferable to see a direct test of the hypothesis.

There is, however, one respect in which experiences mediated by the organisation of schooling may contribute to delinquency. There are several indications that preferences for informal and delinquent versus institutional solutions are consolidated at a collective level. That is, these are not preferences which individual adolescents pursue by themselves. Rather they pursue one kind of solution rather than the other to the extent that they have consistent social support for this preference. Large city high schools tend to sort pupils into streams or curriculum tracks according to attainment. If the foregoing analysis is correct, this selection will be sensitive to their orientations to institutional authority. Hence those with the least positive orientations will regularly find themselves placed by the school in the company of others with similar orientations. This then provides a necessary condition, namely like-minded associates, for the more consistent pursuit of the delinquent solution.

CONCLUSIONS

It has been argued in this chapter that the orientations adolescents take towards the institutional system of society are reflected in their willingness to comply with laws and regulations and in their views about formal authority. It has been proposed that the institutional order is a system for regulating social relationships and that in so far as young people reject this system, they are opting for an alternative and more informal system of social regulation.

It would be wrong to conclude that adolescents are completely polarised on this issue. In practice, attitudes range from highly positive to ambivalent (Emler & Reicher, in press). And the conduct of most adolescents is somewhere between consistent compliance with law and authority and consistent serious violation of laws. In other words, the common pattern would seem to be a mixture of solutions. There are two issues that need to be distinguished here. One concerns the differentiation of preferences: what causes an individual to tend more towards one end of the continuum than the other? This is a question about individual differences. The other is a question about age changes: why are adolescents as a whole more negative about the institutional order than either children or adults? Let us take them in order.

Considered from the point of view of societies as a whole, the institutional system has many apparent advantages over the informal alternative. Its capacity to rationalise productive labour has generated considerable economic wealth. It has permitted the development and effective administration of large scale organised provision for welfare and security. And, in principle at least, it offers rational procedures for delivering justice.

So why are some individuals averse to this system to the point of preferring informal alternatives? It cannot be claimed that the informal solution, represented by delinquency, is a clearly more successful alternative for those adolescents who adopt it. First, they are actually more likely to be victims of crime than any other group in society so it cannot be said that their own delinquency has offered them reliable protection. Second, they are more likely to be among the economic and social losers in society to the extent that their poorer educational qualifications and earlier departure from full-time education exclude them from good jobs, good marriages and political influence. At the extreme they may face loss of liberty.

Nonetheless, there are several factors which could favour unofficial, informal and delinquent solutions to some degree. First, the institutional solution is inherently imperfect; it cannot, for example, deal with every little slight and injury that a person may suffer, yet even when the injury is small the sense of grievance is real. For such matters, informal reparations in the form of apologies and expressions of regret are common. The problems arise when culprits are unrepentant. We can only expect the police or the courts to intervene when some threshold of seriousness is passed and for some matters, for example family violence, that threshold might be rather high. And the threshold may be perceived, rightly or wrongly, as much higher by particular groups of individuals because of the categories to which they belong, for example, male, working class, adolescent members of ethnic minorities. This then provides a second factor increasing the relative attractiveness of unofficial solutions.

A third factor is personality or temperament. Willingness to abide by institutional rules and procedures is a relatively stable characteristic. Those individuals who are most delinquent in their adolescence will have been conspicuously poor at adjusting to school bureaucracy in their childhood (West & Farrington, 1973) and will likewise accommodate less well than others to the requirements of employment relations in adulthood. This suggests that the requirements of the bureacratic system are simply more congenial to certain personalities (cf. Hogan, 1983).

A fourth and related factor is the availability of personal resources for adapting successfully to different systems. Despite the inconclusive evidence the possibility cannot be dismissed that adolescents differ in the extent to which they are equipped to relate to formal authority. Upbringing, social background and sub-cultural definitions of masculinity, for example, could all lead to encounters with authority that are abrasive and confrontational rather than polite and cooperative. At the same time, middle class children may have more personal resources and social capital which they can exploit to secure the support and protection of the official system, combined perhaps with less practice in the arts of physical intimidation.

A fifth factor is social support, as argued earlier. Teenagers who are themselves delinquently inclined and find that they are surrounded by others who share their inclinations will pursue the delinquent solution more consistently than those whose inclinations represent a minority preference amongst their peers.

The second question is why teenagers as a whole should be less positive about authority than other age groups. There is in effect a cycle from the idealisation of authority in childhood, through disillusionment and increasing cynicism in adolescence, to realism in adulthood. But this is only to describe the movement of attitudes with age. A definitive explanation for this cycle is beyond the capacity of existing research evidence. If one is allowed to speculate, however, then one source of these attitude changes may be cognitive changes. Once children have worked out how formal authority is supposed to operate, at around 10 to 12 years, they may then become increasingly disenchanted by the way it appears to operate in practice. Late adolescence and adulthood may then see the emergence of further insight, perhaps on the basis of accumulated experience, into the practicalities of organisational functioning. Adolescents are only occasionally called upon to exercise authority themselves. If this role becomes a more common experience in adulthood then it may contribute to increasingly positive views about authority.

A second source of change may be patterns of social relationships. Departure from full-time secondary education is also departure from a pattern of informal association dominated by age equals and thus liable to impose an "in-group versus out-group" framework (cf. Levine & Campbell 1973) upon young people's relations with adult-dominated institutional authority. Interestingly the end of formal schooling also marks the beginnings of a decline in delinquent activity.

This chapter has had a lot to say about delinquency but it has been the intention to say something about problems common to all adolescents and the ways in which these problems are handled. All adolescents face the hazard of victimisation by others. All adolescents in contemporary industrialised societies are faced with highly bureaucratised social structures and must make some accommodation to the demands and requirements of those structures. This chapter has suggested that their responses to these various issues in the conduct of social relations are related.

It has not been possible to deal here with every facet of young people's relations with authority and it is as well to acknowledge this. There are many other dimensions to adolescent social relationships and to the identities they negotiate, construct and express within these relationships. Thus, identities pursued and expressed through deviant styles of dress, drug use, life-styles and sexual preferences all potentially introduce conflicts with institutional authority in its attempts to regulate conduct. To what extent such conflict is incidental or central to these identities is one possible avenue for future inquiry. Another is the extent to which institutional systems are sensitive to individual differences in orientation to authority and the different ways in which these systems may be organised to exact compliance. The social relations of adolescents can only fully be understood by also considering the other parties to these relationships and these include adults and the institutions they represent.

CHAPTER ELEVEN

Adolescence in a Changing World

John Coleman

The adolescent stage of human development is as much of a puzzle today as it was 20, 40, 60 years ago. True, research has provided answers to some of the key questions of the 1950s and 1960s. Many of these answers are reflected in the present volume. Today we no longer need to ask "Is there a generation gap?", or "Are parents or peers more influential during the adolescent years?". We can say something about these questions and about many others, as a result of empirical endeavour. Yet adolescence, perhaps more than most life stages, is as much a product of social and economic circumstances, as it is of biology and physiology. Adolescence in the 1990s can only be understood with reference to historical time and the confusion and uncertainty among both the young and their parents about the nature of the teenage years must be taken as a key element in the overall picture.

When faced with such confusion, it is not uncommon to turn to theory for some answers. Yet within developmental psychology there is an absence of appropriate theory pertaining to the adolescent stage. Throughout this volume there have been some passing references to theoretical notions, primarily to psychoanalytic theory. In most cases, though, this has simply been used as a jumping off point for the exploration of an empirical question—for example Zani's chapter (5) "Dating and Interpersonal Relationships in Adolescence". Havighurst (1953) is another theorist mentioned by authors in previous chapters, who refer specifically to his proposition that during adolescence there are a number of age specific tasks to be accomplished. These tasks are seen as socio-psychological markers of movement towards maturity and concern changes in family relationships, the assumption of occupational roles and so on. In many respects Havighurst's theory is similar to that of Erikson (1953) whose notion of developmental dilemmas or "normative crises" is now extremely well known.

The problem, however, is not simply the absence of theory. Two other difficulties arise. First, as Steinberg (1990) indicates, theories stemming originally from the beginning of this century have left unfortunate legacies which have hindered understanding. Second, the theories which are used, have not kept pace with changing circumstances and therefore we have only a sadly inadequate conceptual framework with which to make sense of adolescence in the 1990s. In this chapter I shall start by exploring the legacies of theory. I shall then turn to the changes in social and historical circumstances which have altered the adolescent experience over the last decade or so. This will then make it possible to consider critically the contributions of the chapters in this volume. I shall conclude by suggesting that a new approach is needed which will help produce a more coherent view of adolescence and which will serve as an aid not just to social scientists but to parents and professionals as well.

THE LEGACIES OF THEORY

Different theories have had varying degrees of impact upon our notions of adolescence. Without doubt, however, it is psychoanalytic theory which has had the most profound influence, as Steinberg (1990) so cogently argues. The three "legacies" to which I shall draw attention all stem from early themes within psychoanalysis and all have been enduring in their effect upon the research agenda. The three are the idea of discontinuity, the concept of storm and stress and the belief that separation or detachment are integral to adolescent development.

Discontinuity

The upsurge of instincts which is believed to occur at or around puberty is taken by psychoanalytic theorists to represent the starting point of the psycho-sexual developmental stage of adolescence. Prior to this the "latency" stage is believed to occur, during which psycho-sexual maturation remains in abeyance. Co-existent with this view is the idea that during the teenage years, regression and the use of primitive defence mechanisms reflect the struggle of the ego to cope with the powerful instinctual forces which come into play. The previously well-behaved and biddable child becomes a rebellious, ill-mannered adolescent. This view has led to the sense of discontinuity between the two stages. As Collins (1990, p. 85) puts it:

Since the mid 1970s, a major shift has occurred in the premises of research in this area and with it the nature of the family context of development during the second decade of life has come to be viewed in a new way. For much of its history, research on adolescents has emphasised the disruptive, disjunctive effect of the developmental changes of adolescence on attachment to parents. Influenced both by popular impressions and by psychological theories, particularly those influenced by psycho-analytic formulations, researchers focused primarily on the extent of generational disparity in values, decline in parental influence and debilitating conflicts. Research findings, however, have generally indicated a more multi-faceted view of changes experienced by families during the transition to adolescence.

The implications of this traditional view were considerable. The emphasis on the manifestation of new types of behaviour during adolescence steered researchers away from looking at the pre-cursors of such behaviour. Adjustment and relationships during the teenage years were conceptualised as occurring *de novo*, with very little thought being given to the glaringly obvious proposition that the groundwork for transition in adolescence must have been laid in childhood. Take as an example the development of personal autonomy and independence. As we now know, the negotiations which take place between parents and young people over this issue play a central part in aiding or hindering the adolescent adjustment process. Yet such negotiations have in fact been taking place for many years beforehand. The 8-year-old won't brush his teeth because "they're my teeth". The 9-year-old girl will wear a blue skirt but not a red one because "I want to choose how I look". The 10-year-old may already be engaged in a struggle over which friends are suitable and which are not. Thus the development of autonomy has its roots in earlier years. If we are to fully understand adolescence a new research agenda is needed which takes this into account.

Storm and Stress

"Storm and stress is now dead". Thus have numerous authors throughout the 1980s commenced their obituaries of this most enduring notion. No one now seriously believes that all young people experience major dysfunction, or that phrases such as "normative crisis" or "the psychopathology of everyday adolescence" bear much relation to adolescence as it is generally experienced. Nonetheless the "disturbance model" as Olbrich (1990) calls it, is not yet fully laid to rest and indeed is continuing to have an impact on the research questions posed today.

This impact is manifested in a number of ways. First, if we look at the body of research on adolescence in the family, it is clear that far more is known about parent/adolescent conflict than about harmony, and significantly more evidence is available on differences in values and attitudes, than on intergenerational similarities. As Steinberg (1990) points out, this is especially ironic since empirical evidence stemming back to the 1960s has emphasised the fact that positive family relationships are much more common during adolescence than disruptive ones.

Another effect to which attention needs to be drawn is the continuing negative image of young people in western society. Although the reasons for the creation and perpetuation of this image are undoubtedly complex and are not only to do with theory, few doubt its existence. Such a negative stereotype has far-reaching implications, most particularly in its effects on parents and policy-makers. As far as parents are concerned those whose children are nearing puberty experience what can only be called "anticipatory socialisation". Friends, neighbours and the media all conspire to raise anxieties and encourage the drawing up of contingency battle plans. Emphasis is placed on the problems that are likely to occur and the chances of harmonious relationships and parental competence being maintained are inevitably reduced. As far as policy makers are concerned, Furstenberg (1990) among others makes reference to the shift of economic resources in western countries from the young to the aged over the last decade. Is it too much to speculate that this may have something to do with the endurance of the negative stereotype?

Finally, it should perhaps be noted that the weight of empirical evidence which has accumulated in contradiction to the storm and stress viewpoint has led researchers into a new area of growing importance—that of coping—represented in this volume by the chapter "Stress, coping and relationships in adolescence" by Seiffke-Krenke and Shulman (8). As a direct result of the changed empirical perspective, these researchers have begun to ask the central question "What is it that differentiates those young people who adjust to the adolescent transition from those who do not?". A subsidiary and related question is "What are the skills and capabilities necessary for young people to assist them in the adolescent adjustment process?". I shall return to these questions at the end of the chapter.

Separation and Attachment

Since the appearance of Grotevant and Cooper's (1985) article there has been a growing recognition that the psychoanalytic notion of disengagement—the severing of the early emotional ties during adolescence—is in need of major revision. The word "attachment" has come increasingly to be applied as a core construct when describing the young person's relationship to his or her parents and a new and exciting field of research and speculation has opened up in this area.

Nonetheless it has to be recognised that the psychoanalysts made a powerful case. There are subtle and important changes which take place during adolescence, which lead to a greater distance between parent and teenager. At an overt level much of what the parent stands for may be challenged, even at times rejected. The young person does turn for emotional support to others outside the family, particularly his or her peer group. Perhaps most important of all this is the time when new loving relationships are formed with boy or girlfriend, inevitably altering the parents' role and diminishing the centrality of the mother and father in the relationship network. What has been lacking, however, in the single-minded focus on disengagement is, first, a recognition of the fact that while relationships with parents may alter they do not cease; second, an awareness that there are major gender differences and that in the mother-daughter relationship in particular, strong ties may continue to exist well past adolescence; third, a viewpoint which accepts that attachment and detachment are not mutually exclusive.

Rice (1990, p. 512), in his important review of attachment in adolescence, outlines the significance of the changing climate of opinion:

Recent life-span views of development have extended the definition of attachment beyond the mother-child dyad and beyond infancy and early childhood. Attachments are not necessarily restricted to just one individual; they can occur at all ages and with other specific people in addition to mother. In recent years, for example, there has been an attempt to establish a link between adolescent attachment relations and adolescent development and adjustment. Indeed, there is now considerable consensus that many important developmental tasks of adolescence find their resolution in a context of attachment and family relationships.

The legacy of theory in this area has been similar to that in the area of discontinuity. The research agenda has been focused on processes of separation, of achieving independence, of leaving home. We have a long way to go in exploring the ways in which both adolescents and young adults continue to derive support from and remain closely tied to one or both of their parents. Some of the methodological issues associated with this endeavour are outlined in the chapter by Honess and Robinson (3) entitled "Assessing parent-adolescent relationships". I see this as a key element in future research and I shall return to the issue of attachment later in this chapter.

HISTORICAL CHANGE

As I noted earlier, the last decade has brought with it such major changes in social, political and economic circumstances that inevitably the lives of adolescents have been altered in a variety of ways. Yet remarkably little attention seems to be directed to these changes when we delineate our research questions. Feldman and Elliott (1990, p. 494) put it well when they note:

> Even casual reflection suggests that the results of some previous research must be applied with caution if at all, to today's youth. For example, studies of minorities that were conducted in the United States before the mid 1960s may not be relevant to youth born after the civil rights movement and the black power movement. Similarly, conclusions drawn from research on the politically active youth of the 1960s may not apply to the more quiescent youth of subsequent decades. Likewise, old correlational data linking pre-marital sexual intercourse with problem outcomes may have little relevance for an era in which the majority have had sexual intercourse by age 16. These and many other examples emphasise that old findings need continuing reassessment and revalidation when they may be affected by changes in the larger social context.

Let me outline some of the new circumstances which are having an impact on young people in the 1990s and which cannot be ignored if we wish to develop a realistic understanding of adolescence. Consider the family. The nature of the family as it affects children and youth has altered in a quite dramatic way (Furstenberg, 1990; Hill, 1993). In the USA one in three teenagers will have experienced their parents' divorce by the age of 16. In the UK this figure is now one in four. What this means is that in many populations, every single young person experiences family breakdown, every child has a friend whose family consists of one parent only, every teenager accepts divorce as a part of life. If it has not happened to them it will have happened to a significant proportion of their class or peer group. To cope with the variety of family relationships an adolescent language is rapidly developing—involving "steps" and "ex-es"—and the facility with which this has happened is a mark of the adaptational process.

Alongside the increase in family breakdown and the growing number of single parents, is also the widening impact of step-families, a phenomenon that research has barely begun to take into account. Step-parent relationships and step-family circumstances pose particular strains and difficulties for teenagers (Coleman, 1991) and yet these have only just begun to enter the social science literature. The entry of a step-parent into the family affects young people in a variety of ways. Envy and jealousy, conflicts over discipline and boundaries, issues of sexuality, indeed the whole question of the role of a step-parent with adolescents—all these raise new questions about family functioning. The fact is that divorce and the change in family composition which results from it and from re-marriage, have altered young people's experiences in quite fundamental ways and raised key questions about parenting.

Looking at the change in family structure reminds us of the more general issues surrounding the parenting of adolescents. It is remarkable how little attention has been paid to this process and how limited the research has been. As Feldman and Elliott (1990, p. 495) say:

> Researchers also must consider the contexts themselves in greater detail than has been customary. For example, parents are not a monolithic entity. They, too, are subject to developmental pressures that may alter their interactions with their adolescent children in significant ways. A number of researchers have suggested that certain interactive patterns between teenagers and their parents arise from their being at developmental stages that mirror each other: young people are exploring what they can do with their lives even as parents are reviewing what they have done with their own.

What is clear from the evidence available so far (e.g. Raviv et al, 1992) is that parents of adolescents report this stage to be the most problematic and anxiety-provoking of all the stages of parenthood. Further it appears that there is uncertainty about where to seek help or information and an unwillingness to discuss such issues with friends or relations (Small and Eastman, 1991). If parents of teenagers suffer loss of confidence and a lowering of a sense of competence, what effect does this have on young people themselves? This too is a question we need to be addressing.

A second area which has had a significant impact on youth has been that of economic change. I have already referred to the possibility that economic resources have, during the 1980s, shifted from the young to the aged. In almost all western countries more teenagers have experienced poverty, inadequate housing and unemployment than in previous decades. We do not as yet know what long-term effect such disadvantage will have, but we can guess at it. Unemployment, in particular, demands more attention. The notion of gainful employment and the assumption of an occupational identity, lies at the heart of the adolescent story, which has been current throughout this century. We educate our young people and prolong their dependence, in order to enable them to enter the market place better qualified and better equipped. Yet youth unemployment is a direct negation of such a story and has implications for young people which extend far beyond the group that is directly affected (Coffield et al, 1986).

Winefield (1992), in a longitudinal study of youth unemployment, argues that for an adolescent to be without a job is a quite different experience to that of the adult unemployed. While unemployment for anyone may have an effect on the self-concept, unemployment for young people has significance for all aspects of social functioning. Of course such effects will be mediated, as Winefield indicates, by family, by parental employment experience and by the particular geographical setting of the individual concerned. Nonetheless unemployment is a major factor in determining the adolescent's outlook on life. The failure to recognise this within the research community is reflected, ironically, in the fact that *At the Threshold* (Feldman and Elliott, 1990) which is probably the most important book on adolescence to have appeared within the last ten years, deals only briefly with unemployment in a single chapter entitled "Leisure, work and the mass media".

The third social change to which reference needs to be made is that connected with culture and race. To a degree unprecedented in previous decades adolescents are sharing their lives with and being both directly and indirectly affected by those from other cultures. Again, this is a fact that is only just beginning to surface in the research literature, as for example in *When East meets West* (Feldman et al, 1992). Take a moment to reflect on this phenomenon. In Europe, boundaries between countries are disappearing. Germany is now one country. In certain parts of France there are large minorities of North African peoples. In Britain both Asian and Afro-Caribbean populations are growing and making an increasing impact on our culture. Other European countries have increasing numbers of Turks, Serbs, Poles, Croats. In the USA the numbers of Asians and Hispanics have in the last few years quite altered the ethnic composition of significant parts of the continent.

These facts reflect subtle changes which gradually alter the consciousness of the adult world. They have, however, a greater and more immediate impact upon young people, both through schools—the most visible environment where races are brought together—and through culture. Black music, Asian films, African literature—things like this are absorbed into a culture, often through young people.

Equally significant for adolescents are the experiences of those from ethnic minority groups who are attempting to integrate and find a place in the majority culture. The devastating impact of prejudice and racial hatred and the sensitive or insensitive manner in which a country deals with its minorities, are for young people significant elements of their world view. After all many adolescents themselves feel outsiders. Neither child nor adult, their status is ambiguous, their role in society ill-defined. The way other "outsiders" are treated is significant for them in a manner which is not readily acknowledged by adults. The changing cultural and racial composition of all western countries can only be an accelerating trend, one which is of high salience to the great majority of young people. It is time it was recognised as such by the research community.

THE PRESENT VOLUME

It is encouraging to be able to acknowledge that in this volume a number of chapters address issues raised within the framework of the concerns outlined here. Three chapters have direct application to theory and arise out of theoretical developments. Kirchler, Palmonari and Pombeni's work (Chapter 7) originates from an interest in Havighurst's conceptual framework and uses the notion of developmental tasks as a starting point for a series of investigations looking at the role of the family and the peer group. Studies reported show that young people who are able to establish a close relationship with peers have significant advantages in coping with developmental tasks. Furthermore, identification with peers was found to be related to identification with the family, indicating a significant overlap in the ability to maintain close contact with important others. This chapter refers directly to the issue of attachment mentioned earlier, arguing with Steinberg (1990), Hill (1993) and others that the development of autonomy can proceed hand in hand with the maintenance of strong family ties. Indeed the authors of this chapter argue that attachment is a major factor ensuring a positive transition to adulthood.

This theme is explored further in Honess and Robinson's outline (Chapter 3) of some up-to-date approaches to parent-adolescent relationships. The authors review the work of Grotevant and Cooper, Hauser and Powers and Adams and associates. All the approaches selected have been involved in exploring over the last few years the paradox of what Grotevant and Cooper have referred to as the individuality-connectedness continuum. There is no dispute among this group of researchers that a warm supportive family context has a facilitative impact on the growing adolescent. What still has to be explored is the proper balance between the granting of freedom and privacy for the young person to behave in ways that he or she sees as appropriate and the continuity of a parental bond that will inevitably involve some restriction. In the final part of their chapter, Honess and Robinson offer a valuable review of methodologies currently available for the study of family relationships.

Seiffge-Krenke and Shulman's Chapter 8 also falls into the group originating with theoretical concerns. The demise of the notion of storm and stress as an explanatory concept has led to a growing interest in coping, and these two authors have been in the forefront of this research endeavour. In their chapter they review the research findings which are currently available and cover, in particular, young people's perceptions of stress, the coping strategies of everyday life, and the role of the family as the source of both support and stress. It is clear from this chapter that much work still remains to be done on the coping process. While we are beginning to learn something about the basic strategies used, we still know very little about the longer term adaptational capabilities of adolescents. Understanding how young people cope with a concrete event—a stressor—is one thing; understanding how they cope with the transition from childhood to adulthood is quite another. Notions of vulnerability and resilience have yet to make a serious connection with the literature reviewed here by Seiffke-Krenke and Shulman.

Three other chapters are pertinent to questions of social change. First, Tyszkowa's contribution (Chapter 6) on the role of grandparents is particularly timely. In my earlier description of changes in the family I referred to divorce, single parents and step-families. One consequence of single parenting has been the reversal of a trend seen since the early part of this century—the marginalising of grandparents. Increased mobility led to less contact between extended family members and an inevitable decrease in the role played by grandparents in relation to their grandchildren. Today grandparents are becoming rapidly more central again, as single parents turn to their own parents for support and assistance. In Tyszkowa's chapter she examines the position of grandparents vis-à-vis their adolescent grandchildren and compares this with the situation pertaining in childhood. Results show a high degree of idealisation in both childhood and adolescence, but these results also highlight the need for further research in this area of growing importance.

Emler's Chapter 10 is another that addresses a question inextricably connected with the social and economic conditions in which young people grow up. The adolescent's relation to the institutional order is a complex and far too rarely addressed problem and here Emler courageously tackles a variety of concerns to do with the nature of authority, conformity, concepts of justice and injustice and the characteristics of adolescent crime. Emler argues that the young person's willingness to comply with laws and regulations is a reflection of his or her attitude to the institutional system of society. If this system is rejected, the adolescent opts for an alternative and more informal system of social regulation, one feature of which may well be delinquency. Of particular interest in this chapter—in the light of earlier comments on race and culture—is Emler's section on victimisation and teenagers' attitudes to authority—whether it is seen as even-handed or not. As Emler points out, if young people feel that they, or indeed others like them, are unduly persecuted by the institutional system, this is likely to increase their sense of injustice and encourage a rejection of institutional solutions. It may well be that for some the development of such attitudes are the pre-cursors of alienation, not just for minority cultures, but for those who identify with them.

The last chapter which I see as being related directly to issues of social change, is that by Zani "Dating and Interpersonal Relationships in Adolescence" (Chapter 5). The changing nature of sexual behaviour, most especially in the light of the AIDS/HIV phenomenon, is not something to which I referred specifically earlier in this chapter. Nonetheless, our need to understand the way in which early sexual relationships develop is more urgent today than at any period in this century and the contribution made by this chapter is highly significant for precisely that reason. Zani concentrates on three areas of concern: the nature of parental and peer influence on dating behaviour, the sequencing of the establishment of a dating relationship and the development of intimacy with a partner during adolescence. All three topics should be of major interest, for such issues are at the heart of the adolescent's experiences. Here too is an example of a range of behaviours which are continuously influenced by changing social circumstances and what little research there is must be outdated precisely because of rapid social change. In Britain, for example, there has been no substantive study of adolescents' sexual behaviour since the publication of Christine Farrell's book *My Mother Said* in 1978. The work of Zani and her colleagues in Italy shows only too clearly what needs to be done.

There remain three further chapters in this volume, each of which has a unique contribution to make. No doubt there are many schema within which these chapters could be placed. Here I intend to concentrate on the manner in which they address methodological issues and on the insights each provides in assisting us to clarify the problems and obstacles in research design. Before I do so it is worth recalling the words of Feldman and Elliott in their conclusion to *At the Threshold* (Feldman and Elliott, 1990, p. 500):

> As investigators expand the complexity of their questions about adolescent development, so too must their methods become increasingly complex. ... Although available methods are helpful, more innovations are needed to enhance the ability of investigators to observe and record the adolescent condition.

Let me first consider Jackson's Chapter 2 "Social Behaviour in Adolescence". This contribution provides a valuable and fresh perspective on an old problem—how can the complexity of social relationships be adequately described, especially during periods of major change such as adolescence? Jackson argues that there has been too little attention paid to the processes underlying social activity and social development and that as a result appropriate methodologies have been slow to appear. Jackson goes on to propose a model for the analysis of social interaction sequences in adolescence. Such a model makes possible a clear distinction between processing and action, a distinction which is especially significant during the teenage years. This is because at this time immaturity, either in cognition or social skills, may lead to discrepancies between processing and action, such discrepancies providing explanations for adolescent social difficulties.

A second important consequence of the model proposed is an opportunity to look at the information processing system utilised by both parties in social interaction. Such an opportunity highlights possible mis-communication, a critical but virtually unexplored area of adolescent social behaviour. The model has implications for a variety of other elements in social activity. Enough has been said however, to show that it is precisely in the development of such theoretical models that advances can be made in our conceptualisation of adolescence.

Chapter 4 by Silbereisen and Kracke "Variation in Maturational Timing and Adjustment in Adolescence" tackles another developmental issue which is similarly beset by methodological problems. Pubertal change, however, has been the subject of major research initiatives, especially during the 1980s and the work reported by Silbereisen and Kracke builds on such initiatives. The authors show how maturational timing affects relationships with both parents and peers. They also show how social factors may be viewed as influencing maturational timing and this leads them to develop a socio-biological perspective, which in turn raises methodological issues. Of especial importance, in the context of the present chapter, are two further arguments put forward by Silbereisen and Kracke. First, they believe that cultural influences, as for example in the setting of German re-unification, may play a part in determining a wide range of behaviours associated with puberty. Second, they argue that, since the pace of maturation results in part from processes which occur in childhood, no complete picture of maturation can be drawn without prospective longitudinal research. Such a view relates closely, of course, to the comments earlier in this chapter on the continuing impact of a notion of discontinuity in our construction of adolescence.

Finally, let me turn to Chapter 9 on loneliness by Marcoen and Goossens. The only chapter in this volume to outline a new research instrument, the article is of importance for a number of reasons. All too often social scientists are seen to concentrate their research efforts on subjects for which there is already a well developed scale or measure. Here, in contrast, the authors have tackled a topic which they believe to be of significance and have demonstrated how a new test can be devised. The subject of loneliness and its salience for young people, all too frequently goes unrecognised. In my own early work (Coleman, 1974) it became clear that to be alone has significant negative impact, especially for younger adolescents. Furthermore, in recent years, there has been a growing interest in social competence. The lonely, the bullied, those without friends, the unpopular ones—these young people suffer significant disadvantage. The instrument described in Marcoen and Goossen's chapter, and the results derived from its use, make a key contribution to our understanding of an especially vulnerable group.

THEORIES OF ADOLESCENCE

On this theme, Feldman and Elliott have stated (1990, p. 501):

Many earlier hypotheses that seemed to describe universal processes in adolescent development have not been as robust as they were once believed to be. The resulting move towards empiricism has had beneficial effects, but it also has had its costs. The field now is handicapped by a lack of theories to guide its questions. Some theories usefully can be imported from related areas of study and efforts to foster such cross-fertilisation would be worthwhile. But continued support of innovative attempts to identify and elaborate upon key underlying processes also is needed and few mechanisms exist to encourage such efforts.

The lack of a conceptual framework which takes into account both the empirical advances of the last 20 years as well as the changing social circumstances for young people in the developed world, is something to which I referred at the beginning of this chapter. Here in this final section I intend to outline briefly one theoretical framework—the life-span developmental approach—and one model of adolescent development—the focal model. Both, in my view, have a part to play in the construction of a more adequate conceptual framework relating to adolescence.

Life-span developmental psychology has emerged as a powerful theoretical position over the last 10 to 15 years. Its basic tenets have been stated in a variety of books and articles and useful sources are Belsky et al (1984) and Sugarman (1986). At its simplest level this approach to human development carries with it a number of fundamental assumptions. These can be summarised as follows:

1. There is a human ecology or context in human development. The intention here is to underline the importance of the environment in its widest sense and to point out that, for children and young people, the context of development is not just the family, but the geographical, historical, social and political setting in which that family is living. This is, of course, a point I have been making throughout this chapter. It is a viewpoint which owes much to Bronfenbrenner (1979) and his colleagues, but it is one which undoubtedly still requires greater emphasis if concepts of adolescence are to keep pace with history.

2. Individuals and their families reciprocally influence each other. This principle underlies the fact that neither a child nor a family is a static entity. Each grows, develops and changes and, most important, each influences the other at all times. The young person's maturation produces changes in the family, but at the same time alterations in family functioning and structure have effects upon the young person's development. Such a principle has also been referred to throughout this chapter. Its implications for the development of, for example, a fuller understanding of the parenting of adolescents cannot be underestimated.

3. Individuals are producers of their own development. Attention is being drawn here to the part that all individuals, of whatever age, play in shaping their own development. This is probably the most innovative of the four principles, having very wide implications for social science research. While it may be generally accepted that child and adolescent development results from an interplay of a variety of causes, the idea that the individual young person might be an "active agent" in shaping or determining his or her own development has not generally been part of the thinking of researchers in this field. The principle is integral to the focal model, to which we shall turn later in the chapter.

4. A multi-disciplinary approach must be taken for studying human development. This may seem like a statement of the obvious, but the fact that life-span developmental psychologists have laid particular stress on this principle has had surprising results and has brought together biologists, paediatricians, sociologists, ecologists and so on in co-operative projects on human development. Such co-operative work is undoubtedly paying substantial dividends.

Life-span Developmental Theory

The principles of life-span developmental theory can be seen to have become gradually recognised as essential in well-designed research programmes. The quality that distinguishes this theoretical model from other approaches is its interactive stance. It stresses reciprocal influences, it brings together different professional disciplines, it underlines the interaction between individual and family and the outside world. Life-span developmental psychology is not specifically concerned with adolescence, yet it is critical to the studies of adolescence because it provides an all important perspective. A striking example of this is to be found in Lerner (1985). In this paper the author considers three ways in which the adolescent interacts with the environment and thereby affects his or her own development. Lerner draws attention to the adolescent as stimulus, eliciting different reactions from the environment; as processor, making sense of the behaviour of others and as agent, shaper and selector doing things, making choices and influencing events.

Lerner's viewpoint provides a refreshing perspective on adolescence, one which takes into account some of the complexity with which we are all familiar in every day life. What this perspective lacks is any reference to the developmental or maturational process. For this dimension, we may turn to the focal model.

The Focal Model

The focal model grew out of the results of a study of normal adolescent development (Coleman, 1974). Briefly, large groups of boys and girls at the ages of 11, 13, 15 and 17 were given a set of identical tests which elicited from them attitudes and opinions about a wide range of relationships. Material was included on self-image, being alone, heterosexual relationships, parental relationships, friendships and large group situations. The material was analysed in terms of the positive and negative elements present in these relationship situations and in terms of the common themes expressed by the young people involved in the study. Findings showed that attitudes to all relationships changed as a function of age, but more importantly the results also indicated that concerns about different issues reached a peak at different stages in the adolescent process.

It was this finding that led to the formulation of a focal model. The model suggests that at different ages, particular sorts of relationship patterns come into focus, in the sense of being most prominent, but that no pattern is specific to one age only. Thus the patterns overlap, different issues come into focus at different times, but simply because an issue is not the most prominent feature of a specific age, does not mean that it may not be critical for some individuals of that age.

In many ways such a notion is not dissimilar from any traditional stage theory. However it carries with it a very much more flexible view of development and therefore differs from stage theory in three important respects. In the first place, the resolution of one issue is not seen as essential for tackling the next. In fact it is clearly envisaged that a minority of individuals will find themselves facing more than one issue at the same time. Second, the model does not assume the existence of fixed boundaries between stages and, therefore, issues are not necessarily linked with a particular age or developmental level. Finally there is nothing immutable about the sequence involved. In the culture in which the research was originally carried out, it appeared that individuals were more likely to face certain issues in the early stages of adolescence and different issues at other stages, but the focal model is not centred on a fixed sequence and it would be of very great interest to examine a variety of cultures in the light of this theory of development.

It is proposed that the focal model of adolescent development may provide a clue to the resolution of the apparent contradiction between the amount of adjustment required during adolescence on the one hand and the relatively successful adaptation among the general population on the other (Coleman and Hendry, 1990). If adolescents have to adjust to so much potentially stressful change and at the same time pass through this stage of their life with the relative stability which emerges from research studies, how do they do it? The answer which is suggested by the focal model is that they cope by dealing with one issue at a time. They spread the process of adaptation over a span of years, attempting to resolve first one issue and then the next. Different problems, different relationship issues come into focus and are tackled at different stages, so that the stresses resulting from the need to adapt to new modes of behaviour are rarely concentrated all at one time.

It follows from this that it is precisely with those who, for whatever reason, do have more than one issue to cope with at a time, that problems are most likely to occur. Thus, as an example, where puberty and the growth spurt occur at the normal time individuals are able to adjust to these changes before other pressures, such as those from parents and teachers, are brought to bear. For the late-maturers, however, pressures are more likely to occur simultaneously, inevitably requiring adjustments over a much wider area. Feldman and Elliott expressed their view as follows (1990, p. 485):

> More generally, adolescents face changes in essentially all aspects of their lives; their ability to cope with those changes depends not only on intrinsic strength and external support but also on the timing of the stresses. If disruptions are too numerous or require too much change in too little time, they may be hazardous. Concurrent major changes—for instance, going through puberty while entering a new school and losing an established circle of peer relationships—may be more than many adolescents can handle. Some of the problems associated with poverty may arise from the degree to which it promulgates changes over which neither adolescents nor their family can exert control.

The focal model is only one of a number of ways of conceptualising adolescent development, but it has two particular advantages. First, it is based directly on empirical evidence and, second, it goes at least some way towards reconciling the apparent contradiction between the amount of adaptation required during the transitional process and the ability of most young people to cope successfully with the pressures inherent in this process. Such a model evidently needs further testing, but since it was first proposed it has received substantial empirical support (Kroger, 1985; Simmons and Blyth, 1987; Hendry et al, 1992).

One major criticism of the model is that it is nothing more or less than the theory of life events (Dohrenwend & Dohrenwend, 1974) applied to adolescence. At one level this is correct. The focal model does argue that the more "issues" the young person has to cope with, the more indications of stress there are likely to be. The research of Simmons and Blyth (1987) provides excellent validation of this view. However, the focal model goes further—for it is in one highly significant respect quite different from life-events theory. While life-events theory implies simply that the more events that occur in an individual's life, the more stress there will be, the focal model suggests that the young person is an agent in his or her own development, managing the adolescent transition—where possible—by dealing with one issue at a time.

It will be recalled that in discussing the life-span developmental approach I mentioned Lerner's seminal paper published in 1985. In this paper the author outlines some of the ways in which the adolescent is active in shaping his or her own maturation. I see this concept as being central to the focal model—not only does the model imply that the young person copes better when facing one issue at a time, the model implies that in most circumstances the young person may actually be determining his or her own rate of development.

Such an idea may seem at first to be rather far-fetched. Yet a little thought will indicate that the concept is not so extraordinary after all. Consider for a moment the range of choices available to an individual in their current relationships. In any one day a teenager may choose to confront a parent over the breakfast table, to argue with a sibling, to accept the suggestion of a best friend, to stand up to an authoritarian teacher, to conform to peer group pressure, to resist the persuasion of a boyfriend or girlfriend and so on. Every one of these situations offers the young person a choice and all may well have a bearing on the interpersonal issues with which the focal model is concerned. I believe that most young people pace themselves through the adolescent transition. Most of them hold back on one issue, while they are grappling with another. Most sense what they can and cannot cope with and will, in the real sense of the term, be an active agent in their own development.

In outlining their agenda for future research endeavours Feldman and Elliott (1990, p. 495) have no doubt that the active role played by the young person in his or her own development should be central to our concerns:

Future research will need to examine in detail the role of the individual in shaping particular contexts. Lack of homogeneity within contexts gives individuals considerable latitude in shaping their own situations, at least within certain constraints. Too often adolescents are portrayed as passive recipients of circumstances and resources that others make available to them. In reality they play an active role in choosing and shaping the context in which they operate—their friends, their activities and their lifestyles. The desires of parents and society to provide environments that promote healthy development might be simplified if researchers could gain a clearer understanding of why and how teenagers either resist or cooperate with such efforts.

To conclude, both life-span developmental theory and the focal model have contributions to make to a more realistic conceptual structure. As chapters in this volume attest, the research endeavour is alive and well, but it urgently needs what Feldman and Elliott call an "organising framework" if it is to be seen as informing those who require it most—parents, professionals and policy makers. Young people are growing up today in a world of uncertainty, where values are unclear, where cultures are on the move, where the nature of the family is altering. Such circumstances inevitably affect the adolescent transition to adulthood. Research must be seen to be tackling the real life experiences of young people, rather than addressing academic preoccupations. Research must demonstrate that it can keep pace with social and political change and, in order to do so, it requires a coherent theory of adolescence. It is in this direction that our major challenge lies.

As I have indicated, chapters in this book together contribute to the painting of a rich picture of the social worlds of adolescents. Taken together, the various chapters represent many of the important elements of the changing social setting in which young people grow up today. Authors have tackled issues of sexuality, of authority, of family relationships, of grandparenthood. A framework has been outlined in which social relationships can be conceptualised and problems of peer-group influence, solitude and puberty have been explored. Such studies reflect clearly the enormous strides that been taken in ensuring that investigators pay attention, not only to the social nature of adolescence, but to the need for up-to-date and relevant information for all who live and work with young people.

References

Adams, J. F. (1981). Earlier menarche, greater height and weight: A stimulation-stress factor hypothesis. *Genetic Psychological Monographs, 104*, 3-22.

Adams, G.R. (1985). Family correlates of female adolescents ego-identity development. *Journal of Adolescence, 8*(1), 69-82.

Adams, G. R., Bennion, B. S. & Huh, K. (1987). *Objective measure of ego identity status: A reference manual*. Utah State University.

Adams, G. R. & Fitch, S. A. (1982). Ego state and identity development: A cross-sequential analysis. *Journal of Personality and Social Psychology, 43*, 574-583.

Adams, G. R. & Jones, R. M. (1983). Female adolescents identity development: Age comparisons and perceived childrearing experiences. *Developmental Psychology, 19*, 249-256.

Adams, G.R., Montemayor, R., Dyk, P. & Lee, T.R. (1991). *Adolescent Ego-Identity Development and Family Contributions*. Monograph in preparation.

Adelson, J. (1971). The political imagination of the young adolescent. *Daedalus, 100*, 1013-1050.

Adorno, T.W., Frenkel-Brunswik, E., Levinson, D.J. & Sanford, R.M. (1950). *The authoritarian personality*. New York: Harper.

Ainsworth, M.D.S. (1989). Attachments beyond infancy. *American Psychologist, 44*, 709-716.

Ainsworth, M.D.S., Blehar, M.C., Waters, E. & Wall, S. (1978). *Patterns of attachment: A psychological study of the strange situation*. Hillsdale, NJ: Lawrence Erlbaum Associates Inc.

Alexander, C.N. & Wiley, M.G. (1981). Situated activity and identity formation. In: M. Rosenberg & R. Turner (Eds.), *Social Psychology: psychological perspectives*. New York: Basic Books.

Allen, I. (1987). *Education in sex and personal relationship*. London: PSI Research Report, N. 665.

Alsaker, F.D. (1990). *Global negative self-evaluations in early adolescence*. Doctoral dissertation, University of Bergen, Norway.

Amerio, P., Boggi Cavallo, P., Palmonari, A. & Pombeni, M. L. (1990). *Gruppi di Adolescenti e Processi di Socializzazione*. Bologna: Il Mulino.

Anderson, S.A. & Fleming, W.M. (1986). Late adolescents' identity formation: Individuation from the family of origin. *Adolescence, 21*(84), 785–796.

Andersson, T.A. & Magnusson, D. (1990). Biological maturation in adolescence and the development of drinking habits and alcohol abuse among young males: A prospective longitudinal study. *Journal of Youth and Adolescence, 19*, 33-41.

Antonovsky, A. (1981). *Health, Stress and Coping*. San Francisco: Jossey-Bass.

Apter, A., Galatzer, A., Beth-Halachmi, N. & Laron, Z. (1981). Self-image in adolescents with delayed puberty and growth retardation. *Journal of Youth and Adolescence, 10*, 501-505.

Arcana, J. (1981). *Our mothers' daughters*. London: The Women's Press.

Argyle, M., Furnham, A. & Graham, J. A. (1981). *Social situations*. Cambridge: Cambridge University Press.

Arkowitz, H., Hinton, R., Perl, J. & Himadi, W. (1978). Treatment strategies for dating anxiety in college men based on real-life practice. *Counselling Psychologist, 7*, 41-46.

Aro, H. & Taipale, V. (1987). The impact of timing of puberty on psychosomatic symptoms among fourteen- to sixteen-year-old Finnish girls. *Child Development, 58*, 261-268.

Asch, S. E. (1951). Effects of group pressure on the modification and distortion of judgments. In: H. Guetzkow (Ed.), *Groups, leadership and men*. Pittsburg: Carnegie Press.

Asher, S. R., Hymel, S. & Renshaw, P. D. (1984). Loneliness in children. *Child Development, 55*, 1456-1464.

Baer, P. E., Garmezy, L. B., McLaughlin, R. J., Pokory, A. D. & Wernick, M. J. (1987). Stress, coping, family conflict and adolescent alcohol use. *Journal of Behavioural Medicine, 10*, 449-466.

Bandura, A. (1981). Self-referent thought: A developmental analysis of self-efficacy. In: J.H. Flavell & L. Ross (Eds.), *Social Cognitive Development*. Cambridge: Cambridge University Press.

Banks, M., Bates, I., Breakwell, G., Bynner, J., Emler, N., Jamieson,L. & Roberts, K. (1991). *Careers and identities*. Milton Keynes, UK: Open University Press.

Barenboim, C. (1981). The development of person perception in childhood and adolescence. *Child Development, 52*, 129-44.

Barkow, J.H. (1984). The distance between genes and culture. *Journal of Anthropological Research, 40*, 367-379.

Barratt, B. B. (1977). The development of peer perception systems in childhood and early adolescence. *Social Behaviour and Personality, Vol. 2*, 351-360.

Barrera, M. (1981). Social support in the adjustment of pregnant adolescents: Assessment issues. In: B.H. Gottlieb (Ed.), *Social networks and social support* (pp. 69-96). Beverly Hills, CA: Sage.

Bates, A. (1942). Parental role in courtship. *Social Forces, 20*, 482-486.

Battiselli, P. & Farneti, A. (1991). Grandchildren's images of grandparents: A psychodynamic perspective. In: P.K. Smith (Ed.), *The psychology of grandparenthood. An international perspective*, (pp. 143-156) London and New York: Routledge.

Baumrind, D. (1968). Authoritarian vs. authoritative parental control. *Adolescence, 3*, 255-272.

Baumrind, D. (1989). Rearing competent children. In: W. Damon (Ed.), *Child development today and tomorrow* (pp. 349-378). San Francisco: Jossey-Bass.

Bean, J. A., Leeper, J. D., Wallace, R. B., Sherman, B. M. & Jagger, H. J. (1979). Variations in the reporting of menstrual histories. *American Journal of Epidemiology, 109*, 181-185.

Bell, D. C. & Bell, L. G. (1983). Parent validation and support in the development of adolescent daughters. In: H.D. Grotevant & C.R. Cooper (Eds.), *Adolescent development in the family*. San Francisco: Jossey-Bass.

Bell, L. G., Cornwell, C. S. & Bell, D. C. (1988). Peer relationships of adolescent daughters: a reflection of family relationship patterns. *Family Relations, 37*, 171-174.

Belle, D. E. (1981). *The social network as a source of both stress and support to low-income mothers*. Paper presented at the Biennial Meeting of the Society for Research in Child Development, Boston.

Belsky, J., Lerner, R. & Spanier, G. (1984). *The child in the family*. London: Addison-Wesley.

Belsky, J., Steinberg, L.D. & Draper, P. (1991a). Childhood experience, interpersonal development and reproductive strategy: an evolutionary theory of socialisation. *Child Development, 62*, 647-670.

Belsky, J., Steinberg, L.D. & Draper, P. (1991b). Further reflections on an evolutionary theory of socialization. *Child Development, 62*, 682-685.

Berndt, T.J. (1982). The features and effects of friendships in early adolescence. *Child Development, 53*, 1447-1460.

Berndt, T.J. (1989). Friendship in childhood and adolescence. In: W. Damon (Ed.), *Child Development, today and tomorrow* (pp. 332-348). San Francisco: Jossey-Bass.

Berndt, T.J. & Perry, T.B. (1986). Childrens' perception of friendship as supportive relationships. *Developmental Psychology, 22*, 640-648.

Berti, A.E. & Bombi, A.S. (1988). *The child's construction of economics*. Cambridge: Cambridge University Press.

Berti Ceroni, C., Bonini, C., Cerchierini, L. & Zani, B. (1987). *La prima volta. Un'indagine sulla scoperta della sessualità nell'adolescenza*. Milano: Angeli.

Bijstra, J.O., Bosma, H.A., & Jackson, A.E. (in press). The relationship between social skills and psychosocial functioning in early adolescence. *Personality and Individual Differences*.

Bijttebier, P. (1991). *Loneliness and social discrepancy: A review of the literature and empirical research on children and young adolescents*. Unpublished Master's thesis, Catholic University of Louvain, Leuven, Belgium. (In Dutch)

Black, D. (1983). Crime as social control. *American Sociological Review, 48*, 34-45.

Blanchard-Fields, F. & Irion, J. C. (1987). Coping strategies from the perspective of two developmental markers: Age and social reasoning. *Journal of Genetic Psychology, 149*, 141-151.

Blos, P. (1962). *On adolescence*. New York: The Free Press.

Blos, P. (1964). *On adolescence: a psycho-analytic interpretation*. New York: Free Press of Glencoe.

Blos, P. (1967). The second individuation process of adolescence. *Psychoanalytic Study of the Child, 22*, 162-168.

Bonini, M.C. & Zani, B. (Eds.) (1991). *Dire e non dire. Modelli educativi e comunicazione sulla sessualità nella famiglia con adolescenti*. Milano: Giuffré Editore.

Borys, S. & Perlman, D. (1985). Gender differences in loneliness. *Personality and Social Psychology Bulletin, 11*, 63-74.

Bosma, H.A. (1985). *Identity development in adolescence: Coping with commitments*. State University. of Groningen.

Bosma, H.A. & Jackson, A.E. (Eds.) (1990). *Coping and self-concept in adolescence*. Heidelberg: Springer-Verlag.

Boszormenyi-Nagy, I. & Spark, G.M. (1973). *Invisible loyalties: Reciprocity in intergenerational family therapy*. New York: Harper and Row.

Bowlby, J. (1969). *Attachment and loss: Vol. I. Attachment*. New York: Basic Books.

Bowlby, J. (1973). *Attachment and loss: Vol. II. Separation: Anxiety and anger*. New York: Basic Books.

Bowlby, J. (1980). *Attachment and loss: Vol. III. Loss: Sadness and depression*. New York: Basic Books.

Brennan, T. (1982). Loneliness at adolescence. In: L.A. Peplau & D. Perlman (Eds.), *Loneliness: A sourcebook of current theory, research and therapy* (pp. 269-290). New York: Wiley.

Bronfenbrenner, U. (1974). The origins of alienation. *Scientific American, 231*, 53-61.

Bronfenbrenner, U. (1979a). *The ecology of human development: Experiments by nature and design*. Cambridge, Mass: Harvard University Press.

Bronfenbrenner, U. (1979b). Contexts of child rearing: Problems and prospects. *American Psychologist*, Special Issue Psychology and Children: Current Research and Practice, *10*, 844-850.

Bronfenbrenner, U. (1986). Ecology of the family as a context for human development: research perspectives. *Developmental Psychology, 22*, 723-742.

Bronfenbrenner, U. (1989). Ecological systems theory. In: R. Vasta (Ed.), *Six theories of child development: Revised formulations and current issues*. (Annals of Child Development, Vol. 6, pp. 187-249). Greenwich, CO: JAI Press.

Brooks-Gunn, J., Petersen, A.C. & Eichhorn, D. (1985). The study of maturational timing effects in adolescence. *Journal of Youth and Adolescence, 14*, 149-161.

Brooks-Gunn, J. & Warren, M.P. (1988). Mother-daughter differences in menarcheal age in adolescent dancers and non-dancers. *Annals of Human Biology, 15*, 35-43.

Brooks-Gunn, J. & Warren, M.P. (1989). Biological and social contributions to negative affect in young adolescent girls. *Child Development, 60*, 40-55.

Brooks-Gunn, J., Warren, M.P., Rosso, J. & Gargiulo, J. (1987). Validity of self-report measures of girls' pubertal status. *Child Development, 58*, 829-841.

Brown, B.B. (1982). The extent and effects of peer pressure among high school students: a retrospective analysis. *Journal of Youth and Adolescence, 11*, 121-133.

Brown, B.B., Eicher, S.A. & Petrie, S. (1986). The importance of peer-group (crowd) affiliation in adolescence. *Journal of Adolescence, 9*, 73-95.

Brown, D. (1974). Adolescent attitudes and lawful behaviour. *Public Opinion Quarterly, 38*, 96-106.

Brown, R. (1988). *Group processes: Dynamics within- and between-groups.* Worcester: Billing and Sons.

Buhrmester, D. (1990). Intimacy of friendship, interpersonal competence and adjustment during pre-adolescence and adolescence. *Child Development, 61*, 1101-1111.

Buhrmester, D. & Furman, W. (1987). The development of companionship and intimacy. *Child Development, 58*, 1101-1113.

Burke, R.J. & Weir, T. (1978). Benefits to adolescents of informal helping relationships with parents and peers. *Psychological Reports, 42*, 1175-1184.

Bush, D.M. (1987). Changing definitions of self for young women. In: T. Honess & K. Yardley (Eds.), *Self and identity perspectives across the life-span.* London: Routledge and Kegan Paul.

Campbell, E., Adams, G.R. & Dobson, W.R. (1984). Familial correlates of identity formation in late adolescence: a study of the predicative utility of connectedness and individuality in family relations. *Journal of Youth and Adolescence, 13*, 509-525.

Cantor, N. (1981). A cognitive-social approach to personality. In: N. Cantor & J.F. Kihlstrom (Eds.), *Personality, cognition and social interaction.* Hillsdale, NJ: Lawrence Erlbaum Associates Inc.

Cantor, N. & Kihlstrom, J.F. (Eds.) (1981). *Personality, cognition and social interaction.* Hillsdale, NJ: Lawrence Erlbaum Associates Inc.

Caplow, T., Bahr, H.M., Chadwick, B.A., Hill, R. & Williamson, M.H. (1982). *Middletown families.* Minneapolis: University of Minnesota Press.

Caspi, A. & Moffitt, T.E. (1991). *Individual differences during periods of social change: The sample case of girls at puberty.* Unpublished manuscript, University of Wisconsin, Madison.

Cate, R.M. & Koval, J.E. (1983). Heterosexual relationship development: Is it really a sequential process? *Adolescence, 18* (71), 507-514.

Cavallero, P., Battiselli, P. & Farneti, A. (1981). Attegiamento dei nonni confronti del proprio ruolo e del nuovo nucleo familiare, *Atti XVIII Congresso degli Psicologi Italiani, Acireale 1979, 4*, p. 257-64. Palermo, Edikronos.

Chodorow, N. (1979). *The reproduction of mothering: psychoanalysis and the sociology of gender.* Berkeley: University of California Press.

Clark, J.P. & Wenninger, E.P. (1964). The attitude of juveniles toward the legal institution. *Journal of Criminal Law, Criminology and Police Science, 55*, 482-489.

Coffield, F., Borrill, C. & Marshall, S. (1986). *Growing up at the margins.* Milton Keynes, UK: Open University Press.

Cohen, L., Burt, C.E. & Bjorck, J.P. (1987). Life stress and adjustment: Effects of life events experienced by young adolescents and their parents. *Developmental Psychology, 23*, 583-592.

Cohen, S. & Wills, T.A. (1985). Stress, social support and the buffering hypothesis. *Psychological Bulletin, 98*, 310-357.

Cohler, S.J. & Grunebaum, H.U. (1980). *Mothers, grandmothers and daughters: Personality and child-care in three-generation families.* New York: Wiley.

Colby, A. & Kohlberg, L. (1987). *The measurement of moral judgement. Vol. 1: Theoretical foundations and research validation*. Cambridge: Cambridge University Press.

Colby, A., Kohlberg, L., Candee, D., Gibbs, J.C., Hewer, A., Kaufman, K., Power, C. & Speicher-Dubin, B. (1986). *Assessing moral judgements: A manual*. New York: Cambridge University Press.

Coleman, J.C. (1974). *Relationships in Adolescence*. London: Routledge.

Coleman, J.C. (1978). Current contradictions in adolescent theory. *Journal of Youth and Adolescence, 7*, 1-11.

Coleman, J.C. (1980). Friendship and the peer group in adolescence. In: J. Adelson (Ed.), *Handbook of adolescent psychology*. New York: Wiley.

Coleman, J.C. (1991). *Teenagers and step-parents*. Brighton, UK: Trust for the Study of Adolescence.

Coleman, J.C. & Hendry, L. (1989). *The nature of adolescence*. London: Routledge.

Coleman, J.C. & Hendry, L. (1990). *The nature of adolescence*. (Second Edition) London: Routledge.

Coleman, J.S. (1972). Youth: Transition to adulthood. *Report of the Panel on Youth of the President's Science Advisory Committee*. Chicago and London: University of Chicago Press.

Collins, W.A. (1990). Parent-child relationships in the transition to adolescence. In: R. Montemayor, G. Adams & T. Gullotta (Eds.), *From childhood to adolescence: a transitional period?* London: Sage.

Compas, B.E. (1987). Stress and life events during childhood and adolescence. *Clinical Psychology Review, 7*, 275-302.

Compas, B.E., Davis, G.E. & Forsythe, C.J. (1985). Characteristics of life-events during adolescence. *American Journal of Community Psychology, 13*, 677-691.

Compas, B.E., Davis, G.E., Forsythe, C.J. & Wagner, B.M. (1987). Assessment of major and daily life events during adolescence. The Adolescent Perceived Events Scale. *Journal of Consulting and Clinical Psychology, 55*, 534-541.

Compas, B.E. & Phares, B. (1986). Stress during childhood and adolescence: Sources of risk and vulnerability. In: A.L. Greene, J.J Conger & A.C. Petersen (Eds.), *Adolescence and youth*. New York: Harper & Row.

Condon, S.M., Cooper, C.R. & Grotevant, H.D. (1984). *Manual for analysis of family discourse*. Psychological Documents, 14:8, MS Number: 2616

Conger, J.J. & Peterson, A.C. (1984). *Adolescence and youth*. New York: Harper Row.

Constantine, L.L. (1987). Adolescent process and family organization: A model of development as a function of family paradigm. *Journal of Adolescent Research, 2*, 349-366.

Cooley, C.H. (1909). *Social organisation*. New York: Scribners.

Cooper, C.R. (1987). Conceptualizing research on adolescent development in the family: four root metaphors. *Journal of Adolescent Research, 2*, 321-330.

Cooper, C.R. & Ayers-Lopez, S. (1985). Family and peer systems in early adolescence: new models of the role of relationships in development. *Journal of Early Adolescence, 5*, 9-21.

Cooper, C.R. & Grotevant, H.D. (1979). *Manual for the role-taking task*. Family Process Project, University of Texas at Austin. Unpublished manuscript.

Cooper, C.R., Grotevant, H.D. & Condon, S.M. (1982). Methodological challenges of selectivity in family interaction: Assessing temporal patterns of individuation. *Journal of Marriage and the Family, 44*, 749-754.

Cooper, C.R., Grotevant, H.D. & Condon, S.M. (1983). Individuation and connectedness in the family as a context for adolescent identity formation and role taking skill. In: H.D. Grotevant & C.R. Cooper (Eds.), *Adolescent development in the family*. San Francisco: Jossey Bass.

Costell, R.M. & Reiss, D. (1982). The family meets the hospital: a clinical presentation of a laboratory-based family typology. *Archives of General Psychiatry, 39*, 433-438.

Craig-Bray, L., Adams, G.R. & Dobson, W.R. (1988). Identity formation and social relations during late adolescence. *Journal of Youth and Adolescence, 17*, 173-187

Crockett, L.J., Silbereisen, R.K. & Kracke, B. (1990). *Timing of maturation and adolescent substance use*. Paper presented at the Third Biennial Meeting of the Society for Research on Adolescence, March 22-25, Atlanta, GA.

Csikszentmihalyi, M. & Larson, R. (1984). *Being adolescent*. New York: Basic Books.

Csikszentmihalyi, M. & Larson, R. (1987). Validity and reliability of the Experience-Sampling Method. *Journal of Nervous and Mental Disease, 175*, 526-536.

Csikszentmihalyi, M., Larson, R. & Prescott, S. (1977). The ecology of adolescent activity and experience. *Journal of Youth and Adolescence, 6*, 281-294.

Cutrona, C.E. (1982). Transition to college: Loneliness and the process of social adjustment. In: L.A. Peplau & D. Perlman (Eds.), *Loneliness: A sourcebook of current theory, research and therapy* (pp. 291-309). New York: Wiley.

Damon, W. (1983). *Social and personality development*. New York: Norton.

Daniels, D. & Moos, R. (1990). Assessing life stressors and social resources among adolescents. *Journal of Adolescent Research, 5*, 268-290.

Danziger, K. (1971). *Socialization*. Harmondsworth: Penguin.

de Armas, A. & Kelly, J.A. (1989). Social relationships in adolescence: skill development and training. In: J. Worrell & F. Danner (Eds.), *The adolescent as decision-maker: Applications to development and education*. New York: Academic Press.

De Jong-Gierveld, J. & Raadschelders, J. (1982). Types of loneliness. In: L.A. Peplau & D. Perlman (Eds.), *Loneliness: A sourcebook of current theory, research and therapy* (pp. 105-119). New York: Wiley.

Delestre, A. (1991). *Grandparents et petits-enfants aujourdhui*. Nancy: Presses Universitaires de Nancy.

De Saeger, I. (1991). *Affinity for aloneness and privacy preferences in adolescence: empirical research on 15- and 17-year-olds*. Unpublished Master's thesis, Catholic University of Louvain, Leuven, Belgium. (In Dutch)

De Wuffel, F.J. (1986). *Attachment beyond childhood: individual and developmental differences in parent-adolescent attachment relationships*. Unpublished Doctoral dissertation, Catholic University of Nijmegen, the Netherlands.

Dodge, K.A. (1986). A social information processing model of social competence in children. In: M. Perlmutter (Ed.), *Minnesota Symposium on Child Psychology*. (pp. 77-125). Hillsdale, NJ: Lawrence Erlbaum Associates Inc.

Dohrenwend, B.S. & Dohrenwend, B.P. (Eds.) (1974). *Stressful life events: Their nature and effects*. New York: Wiley.

Dornbusch, S.M., Carlsmith, J.M., Duncan, P.D., Gross, R.T., Martin, J.A., Ritter, P.L. & Siegel-Gorelick, B. (1984). Sexual maturation, social class and the desire to be thin among adolescent females. *Developmental and Behavioral Pediatrics, 5*, 308-314.

Dornbusch, S.M., Carlsmith, J.M., Gross, R.T., Martin, J.A., Jennings, D., Rosenberg, A. & Duke, P. (1981). Sexual development, age and dating: A comparison of biological and social influences upon one set of behaviors. *Child Development, 52*, 179-185.

Douvan, E. & Adelson, J. (1966). *The adolescent experience*. New York: Wiley.

Draper, P. & Harpending, H. (1982). Father absence and reproductive strategy: an evolutionary perspective. *Journal of Anthropological Research, 38*, 255-273.

Dreher, E. & Dreher, M. (1985). Entwicklungsaufgaben im Jugendalter: Bedeutsamkeit und bewèltigungskonzepte. In: D. Liepmann & A. Stiksrud (Eds.), *Entwicklungsaufgaben und Bewèltigungprobleme in der Adoleszenz*. Güttingen: Hogrefe.

Driscoll, R., Davis, K. & Lipetz, M. (1972). Parental interference and romantic love: The Romeo and Juliet effect. *Journal of Personality and Social Psychology, 24*, 1-10.

Dubas, J.S., Graber, J.A. & Petersen, A.C. (1991). A longitudinal investigation of adolescents' changing perceptions of pubertal timing. *Developmental Psychology, 27*, 580-586.

Duke, P.M., Carlsmith, J.M., Jennings, D., Martin, J.A., Dornbusch, S.M., Gross, R.T. & Siegel-Gorelick, B. (1982). Educational correlates of early and late sexual maturation in adolescence. *Adolescent Medicine, 100*, 633-637.

Duke, P.M., Litt, I.F. & Gross, R.T. (1980). Adolescents' self-assessment of sexual maturation. *Pediatrics, 66*, 918-920.

Duke-Duncan, P., Mendoza, F., Varenhorts, B. & Carey, R. (1984). *Young adolescents' concerns about pubertal growth and development: What the pediatrician should know*. Unpublished manuscript.

Duke-Duncan, P., Morgan, L., Jones, L. & Hole, W. (1985). *Evaluation of an alternative pedriatric approach to puberty education*. Paper presented at the Ambulatory Pediatric Association Meeting, Washington, DC.

Duncan, P.D., Ritter, P., Dornbusch, S.M., Gross, R.T. & Carlsmith, J.M. (1985). The effects of pubertal timing on body image, school behavior and deviance. *Journal of Youth and Adolescence, 14*, 227-235.

Dunphy, D.C. (1963). The social structure of urban adolescent peer groups. *Sociometry, 26*, 230-246.

Dunphy, D.C. (1972). Peer group socialisation. In: F.J. Hunt (Ed.), *Socialisation in Australia*. Sydney: Angus & Robertson.

Durkin, D. (1959). Children's concepts of justice: A comparison with the Piaget data. *Child Development, 30*, 59-67.

Dyk, P.H. & Adams, G.R. (1990). Identity and intimacy: An initial investigation of three theoretical models using cross-lag panel correlations. *Journal of Youth and Adolescence, 19*, 91-110.

Ebata, A. & Moos, R. (1989). *Coping and adjustment in distressed and healthy adolescents*. Palo Alto, CA: Stanford University and Department of Veteran Affairs Medical Centers.

Eisenberg, A.R. (1988). Grandchildren's perspectives on relationships with grandparents: the influence of gender across generations. *Sex Roles, 19*, 205-219.

Elder, G.H. (1974). *Children of the Great Depression*. Chicago: University of Chicago Press.

Elder, G.H. (1986). Military times and turning points in men's lives. *Developmental Psychology, 22*, 233-245.

Elkind, D. (1974). *Children and adolescents: Interpretative essays on Jean Piaget*. London: Oxford University Press.

Ellis, N.B. (1991). An extension of the Steinberg acceleration hypothesis. *Journal of Early Adolescence, 11*, 221-235.

Emler, N. (1984). Differential involvement in delinquency: toward an interpretation in terms of reputation management. In: B.A. Maher & W.B. Maher (Eds.), *Progress in experimental personality research. Vol. 13*. New York: Academic Press.

Emler, N. & Hogan, R. (1991). Moral Psychology and public policy. In: W. Kurtines & J. Gewirtz (Eds.), *Handbook of moral behaviour and development, III*. Hillsdale, NJ: Lawrence Erlbaum Associates Inc.

Emler, N. & Ohana, J. (1992). Réponses au préjudice: représentations sociales enfantines. *Bulletin de Psychologie, 45*, 223-231.

Emler, N., Ohana, J. & Dickinson, J. (1990). Children's representations of social relations. In: G. Duveen, & B. Lloyd (Eds.), *Social representations and the development of knowledge* (pp. 47–69). Cambridge: Cambridge University Press.

Emler, N., Ohana, J. & Moscovici, S. (1987). Children's beliefs about institutional roles: A cross-national study of representations of the teacher's role. *British Journal of Educational Psychology, 57*, 26-37.

Emler, N. & Reicher, S. (1987). Orientations to institutional authority in adolescence. *Journal of Moral Education, 16*, 108-116.

Emler, N. & Reicher, S. (in press). *A social psychology of adolescent delinquency*. Oxford: Blackwell.

Emler, N., Reicher, S. & Ronson, B. (1987). *Young people's perceptions of the personal attributes of rule breakers and rule followers*. Unpublished Manuscript, University of Dundee, UK.

Emler, N., Reicher, S. & Ross, A. (1987). The social context of delinquent conduct. *Journal of Child Psychology and Psychiatry, 28*, 99-109.

Emler, N. & St. James, A. (1990). Staying on at school after sixteen: Social and psychological correlates. *British Journal of Education and Work, 3*, 61-70.

Emmerich, W., Goldman, K.S. & Shore, R.E. (1971). Differentiation and development of social norms. *Journal of Personality and Social Psychology, 18*, 323-353.

Engel, U. & Hurrelmann, K. (1989). *Psychosoziale Belastung im Jugendalter*. Berlin: de Gruyter & Co.

Erikson, E.H. (1953). *Childhood and society*. New York: Longman Green & Co.

Erikson, E. H. (1968). *Identity: Youth and crisis*, New York: W. W. Norton.

Erikson, E. H. (1980). *Identity: Youth and crisis*. New York: W. W. Norton.

Eveleth, P.B. & Tanner, J.M. (1976). *Worldwide variation in human growth*. Cambridge: Cambridge University Press.

Ewert, O.M. (1984). Psychische Begleiterscheinungen des puberalen Wachstumsschubs bei maennlichen Jugendlichen—eine retrospektive Untersuchung. *Zeitschrift fuer Entwicklungspsychologie und Paedagogische Psychologie, 26*, 1-11.

Eysenck, H.J. (1977). *Crime and personality (3rd Edition)*. London: Routledge & Kegan Paul.

Farrell, C. (1978). *My mother said*. London: Routledge.

Farrington, D.P., Biron, L. & LeBlanc, M. (1982). Personality and delinquency in London and Montreal. In: J. Gunn & D.P. Farrington (Eds.), *Abnormal offenders, delinquency and the criminal justice system*. New York: Wiley.

Feehan, M., McGee, R., Stanton, W.R. & Silva, P.A. (1991). Strict and inconsistent discipline in childhood: Consequences for adolescent mental health. *British Journal of Clinical Psychology*, 325-332.

Feffer, M.H. (1959a). The cognitive implications of role taking behaviour. *Journal of Personality, 27*, 152-168.

Feffer, M.H. (1959b). *Role-taking task: criteria for scoring*. (ADI Document No. 5844), The Library of Congress Photoduplication Service, Washington, DC 20540.

Feinstein, S.C. & Ardon, M.S. (1973). Trends in dating patterns and adolescent development. *Journal of Youth and Adolescence, 2*, 157-166.

Feldman, S. & Elliott, G. (Eds). (1990). *At the threshold: The developing adolescent*. London: Harvard University Press.

Feldman, S., Mont-Reynaud, R. & Rosenthal, D. (1992). When East meets West: The acculturation of values of Chinese adolescents in the U.S. and Australia. *Journal of Research in Adolescence, 2*, 147-174.

Feldman, S.S. & Rosenthal, D.A. (1991). Age expectations of behavioural autonomy in Hong Kong, Australian and American youths: The influence of family variables and adolescent values. *International Journal of Psychology, 26*, 1-23.

Felner, R., Aber, M., Primavera, J. & Cauce, A. (1985). Adaptation and vulnerability in high-risk adolescents: An examination of environmental mediators. *American Journal of Community Psychology, 13*, 365-379.

Felner, R.D., Farber, S.S. & Primavera, J. (1983). Transitions and stressful life-events: a model for primary prevention. In: R.D. Felner, L.A. Jason, J.N. Morisugu & S.S. Farber (Eds.), *Preventative psychology: Theory research and practice*. New York: Pergamon.

Felson, B. (1981). An interactionist approach to aggression. In: J. Tedeschi (Ed.), *Impression management theory and social psychological research*. New York: Academic Press.

Felson, R. (1978). Aggression as impression management. *Social Psychology, 41*, 205-213.

Fend, H. (1990). Ego-strength development and pattern of social relationships. In: H.A. Bosma & A.E. Jackson (Eds.), *Coping and self-concept in adolescence*. Heidelberg: Springer-Verlag.

Fiske, S.T. & Taylor, S.E. (1984). *Social cognition*. Reading, Mass.: Addison-Wesley.

Folkman, S. & Lazarus, R.S. (1980). An analysis of coping in a middle-aged sample. *Journal of Health and Social Behaviour, 21*, 219-239.

Folkman, S. & Lazarus, R.S. (1985). If it changes it must be a process: A study of emotion and coping during three stages of a college examination. *Journal of Personality and Social Psychology, 48*, 150-170.

Ford, M.E. (1985). Social cognition and social competence in adolescence. *Developmental Psychology, 18*, 323-340.

Franz, C. and White, K. (1985). Individuation and attachment in personality development. Extending Erikson's theory. In: A. Stewart & B. Lykes (Eds.), *Gender and personality*. Durham, NC: Duke University Press.

Freedman, B.J., Rosenthal, L., Donahoe, C.P. Schlundt, D.G. & McFall, R.M. (1978). A social-behavioral analysis of skills deficits in delinquent and non-delinquent adolescent boys. *Journal of Consulting and Clinical Psychology, 46*, 1448-1462.

Freud, S. (1973). 1. *Introductory Lectures on Psychoanalysis*. Harmondsworth: Penguin Books. (First published 1915.)

Friday, N. (1979). *My mother, myself*. London: Fontana.

Fromm, E. (1956). *The art of loving*. London: Allen & Unwin.

Furnham, A. (1986). Social skills training with adolescents and young adults. In: C.R. Hollin & P. Trower (Eds.), *Handbook of social skills training: Applications across the life-span*, 33-57. Oxford: Pergamon Press.

Furnham, A. & Stacey, B. (1991). *Young people's understanding of society*. London: Routledge.

Furstenberg, F. (1990). Coming of age in a changing family system. In: S.S. Feldman & G.R. Elliott (Eds.), *At the threshold: The developing adolescent*. London: Harvard University Press.

Furth, H. (1978). Young children's understanding of society. In: H. McGurk (Ed.), *Issues in childhood social development*. London: Methuen.

Galligan, R.J. (1989). Theory has arrived, will real dynamic variables be far behind? *Journal of Family Psychology, 3*, 206-210.

Garbarino, J. & Gilliam, G. (1980). *Understanding abusive families*. Lexington, MA: Lexington Books.

Garbarino, J., Sebes, J. & Schellenbach, C. (1984). Families at risk for destructive parent-child relations in adolescence. *Child Development, 55*, 174-183.

Gilligan, C. (1982). *In a different voice*. Cambridge, Mass.: Harvard University Press.

Giordano, P.C., Cernovich, S.A. & Pugh, M.D. (1986). Friendships and delinquency. *American Journal of Sociology, 91*, 1170-1202.

Glynn, T. (1981). From family to peer: A review of transitions of influence among drug using youth. *Journal of Youth and Adolescence, 10*, 363-377.

Goldstein, A.P. (1981). Social skill training. In: A.P. Goldstein, E.G. Carr, W.S. Davidson & P. Wehr (Eds.), *In response to aggression*. Oxford: Pergamon.

Goodyer, I.M. (1990a). Family relationships, life events and childhood psychopathology. *Journal of Child Psychology and Psychiatry, 31*, 161-192.

Goodyer, I.M. (1990b). Recent life events and psychiatric disorder in school-age children. *Journal of Child Psychology and Psychiatry, 31*, 839-848.

Goor-Lambo, G. van, Orley, J., Poustka, F. & Rutter, M. (1990). Classification of abnormal psychosocial situations: Preliminary report of a WHO scheme. *Journal of Child Psychology and Psychiatry, 31*, 229-242.

Goossens, L. (1984). Imaginary audience behavior as a function of age, sex and formal operational thinking. *International Journal of Behavioral Development, 7*, 77-93.

Goossens, L., Marcoen, A. & De Smedt, C. (1989). *Adolescent self-consciousness: The role of parent- and peer-related loneliness and subjects' views on being alone*. Unpublished manuscript, Catholic University of Louvain (K.U. Leuven), Center for Developmental Psychology, Belgium.

Gottlieb, G. (1991). Experiential canalisation of behavioral development: Theory. *Developmental Psychology, 27,* 1-13.

Graham, C.A. & McGrew, W.C. (1980). Menstrual synchrony in female undergraduates living on a co-educational campus. *Psychoendocrinology, 5,* 245-252.

Greenberg, M.T., Siegel, J.M. & Leitch, C.J. (1983). The nature and importance of attachment relationships to parents and peers during adolescence. *Journal of Youth and Adolescence, 12,* 373-383.

Grietens, H. (1988). *Loneliness and identity formation in adolescence: An empirical study.* Unpublished Master's thesis, Catholic University of Louvain (K. U. Leuven), Belgium. (In Dutch)

Grotevant, H.D. (1983). The contribution of the family to the facilitation of identity formation in early adolescence. *Journal of Early Adolescence, 3,* 225-237.

Grotevant, H.D. (1989). Theory in guiding family assessment. *Journal of Family Psychology, 3,* 104-117.

Grotevant, H.D. & Adams, G.R. (1984). Development of an objective measure to assess ego identity in adolescence: Validation and replication. *Journal of Youth and Adolescence, 13,* 419-438.

Grotevant, H.D. & Cooper, C.R. (Eds.) (1983). *Adolescent development in the family,* San Francisco: Jossey-Bass.

Grotevant, H.D. & Cooper, C.R. (1985). Patterns of interaction in family relationships and the development of identity exploration in adolescence. *Child Development, 56,* 415-428.

Grotevant, H.D. & Cooper, C.R. (1986). Individuation in family relationships: A perspective on individual differences in the development of identity and role-taking skills in adolescence. *Human Development, 29,* 82-100.

Haan, N. (1974). The adolescents ego model of coping and defense and comparisons with Q-sorted ideal personalities. *Genetic Psychology Monographs, 89,* 273-306.

Haan, N., Smith, B. & Block, J. (1968). The moral reasoning of young adults. *Journal of Personality and Social Psychology, 10,* 183-201.

Hall, G.S. (1904). *Adolescence. Vol. I and II.* New York: Appleton.

Hamburg, B.A. (1974). Early adolescence: A specific and stressful stage of the life cycle. In: G.V. Coelho, D.A. Hamburg & J.A. Adams (Eds.), *Coping and adaptation* (pp. 101-124). New York: Basic Books.

Hamilton, L.H., Brooks-Gunn, J., Warren, M. & Hamilton, W.G. (1988). The role of selectivity in the pathogenesis of eating problems in ballet dancers. *Medicine and Science in Sports and Exercise, 20,* 560-565.

Hansen, S.L. (1977). Dating choices of high school students. *The Family Coordinator, 26,* 133-138.

Hare-Mustin, R. & Maracek, J. (1986). Autonomy and gender: Some questions for therapists. *Psychotherapy, 23,* 205-212.

Hargreaves, D.H. (1967). *Social relations in a secondary school.* London: Routledge & Kegan Paul.

Hartog, J., Audy, J.R. & Cohen, Y.A. (Eds.) (1980). *The anatomy of loneliness.* New York: International Universities Press.

Hartshorne, T.S. & Manaster, G.J. (1982). The relationship with grandparents: Contact, importance, role conception. *International Journal of Aging and Human Development, 15,* 233-245

Hartup, W.W. (1983). Peer relations. In: P.H. Mussen & M. Hetherington (Eds.), *Carmichael's manual of child psychology, (4th Edition)*. New York: Wiley.

Hastie, R. & Carlston, D. (1980). Theoretical issues in person memory. In: R. Hastie, T.M. Ostrom, E.R. Ebbesen, R.S. Wyer Jr., D.L. Hamilton & D.E. Carlston (Eds.), *Person memory: The cognitive basis of social perception*. Hillsdale, NJ: Lawrence Erlbaum Associates Inc.

Haswell, D. (1991). *Adolescent's perceptions of character as a function of target's behaviour*. Unpublished MA Thesis, University of Dundee, UK.

Hathaway, S.R., Reynolds, P.C. & Monachesi, E.D. (1969). Follow-up of the later career and lives of 1,000 boys who dropped out of high school. *Journal of Consulting and Clinical Psychology, 33*, 370-380.

Hauser, S.T., Book, B., Houlihan, J., Powers, S., Weiss-Perry, B., Follansbee, D., Jacobson, A. & Noam, G. (1987). Sex differences within the family: Studies of adolescents and parent family interactions. *Journal of Youth and Adolescence, 16*, 199-220.

Hauser, S.T., Powers, S., Jacobson, A. M. & Noam, G. G. (1986). *Family interiors of adolescent development*. New York: Free Press.

Hauser, S.T., Powers, S., Noam, G., Jacobson, A., Weiss-Perry, B. & Follansbee, D. (1984). Familial contexts of adolescent ego development. *Child Development, 55*, 195-213.

Havighurst, R.J. (1948). *Developmental tasks and education*. New York: Plenum Press.

Havighurst, R.J. (1953). *Human development and education*. New York: Davis McKay.

Havighurst, R.J. (1972). *Developmental tasks and education*. New York: Davis McKay.

Hayden Thomson, L.K. (1989). *Children's loneliness*. Unpublished Doctoral dissertation, University of Waterloo, Canada.

Hendry, L., Shucksmith, J., Love, J. & Glendinning, A. (1992). *Young people's leisure and lifestyles*. London: Routledge.

Hetherington, E.M. & Clingempeel, W.G. (1992). Coping with marital transitions. *Monographs of the Society for Research in Child Development, Vol. 57*, Nos. 2-3.

Higgins, E.T. & King, G.A. (1981). Accessibility of social constructs: Information processing consequences of individual and contextual variability. In: N. Cantor & J.F. Kihlstrom (Eds.), *Personality, cognition and social interaction* (pp. 69-122). Hillsdale, NJ: Lawrence Erlbaum Associates Inc.

Hill, J.P. (1987). Research on adolescents and their families: Past and prospect. In: Irwin, C.E. (Ed.), *Adolescent social behaviour and health* (pp. 13-31). San Francisco: Jossey-Bass.

Hill, J.P. & Holmbeck, G.N. (1986). Attachment and autonomy. *Annals of Child Development, 3*, 145-189.

Hill, J.P., Holmbeck, G.N., Marlow, L., Green, T. & Lynch, M. (1985). Menarcheal status and parent-child relations in families of seventh-grade girls. *Journal of Youth and Adolescence, 14*, 301-316.

Hill, J.P. & Palmquist, W. (1978). Social cognition and social relations in early adolescence. *International Journal of Behavioral Development, 1*, 1-36.

Hill, P. (1993). Recent advances in selected aspects of adolescent development. *Journal of Child Psychology and Psychiatry, 34*, 69-100.

Hinde, R.A. (1979). *Towards understanding relationships.* London: Academic Press.

Hinde, R.A. (1988). Introduction. In: R.A. Hinde & J. Stevenson-Hinde (Eds.), *Relationships within families.* Oxford: Clarendon Press.

Hinde, R.A. (1991). When is an evolutionary approach useful? *Child Development, 62,* 671-675.

Hindelang, M., Hirschi, T. & Weiss, J. (1981). *Measuring delinquency.* Beverly Hills: Sage.

Hirschi, T. (1969). *Causes of delinquency.* Berkeley, California: University of California Press.

Hirschi, T. & Gottfredson, M. (1983). Age and the explanation of crime. *American Journal of Sociology, 89,* 552-584.

Hoffman, M. (1977). Moral internalization: Current theory and research. In: L. Berkowitz (Ed.), *Advances in experimental social psychology, Vol. 10.* New York: Academic Press.

Hogan, R. (1983). A socioanalytic theory of personality. In: M. M. Page (Ed.), *Personality, current theory and research: Nebraska symposium on motivation, (1982).* Lincoln, Nebraska: University of Nebraska Press.

Hojat, M. & Crandall, R. (Eds.) (1987). Loneliness: theory, research and applications. *Journal of Social Behavior and Personality, 2(2).*

Hollin, C.R. & Trower, P. (1986). *Handbook of social skills training. Volumes I & II.* Oxford: Pergamon Press.

Holmes, S.J. & Robins, L.N. (1987). The influence of child disciplinary experience on the development of alcoholism and depression. *Journal of Child Psychology and Psychiatry, 28,* 399-415.

Honess, T. (1979). Children's implicit theories of their peers: A developmental analysis. *British Journal of Psychology, 72,* 485-497.

Honess, T. (1981). Girls' and boys' perception of their peers: Peripheral vs. central and objective vs. interpretative aspects of free descriptions. *British Journal of Psychology, 70,* 417-424.

Honess, T. & Edwards, A. (1990). Selves-in-relation: School-leavers' accommodation to different interpersonal and situational demands. In: H.A. Bosma & A.E. Jackson (Eds.) *Coping and self-concept in adolescence* (pp. 69–86). Heidelberg: Springer-Verlag.

Honess, T. & Lintern, F. (1990). Relational and systems methodologies for analysing parent-child relationships: An exploration of conflict, support and independence in adolescence and post-adolescence. *British Journal of Social Psychology, 29,* 331-347.

Houston, B.K. (1977). *An open-ended structural questionnaire to elicit information concerning coping behaviour.* Unpublished manuscript, University of Kansas.

Hunter, F.T. (1985). Adolescent's perception of discussions with parents and friends. *Developmental Psychology, 21,* 433-440.

Hurme, H. (1986). *Attachment and intergenerational relations.* Paper presented at the Second European Conference on Developmental Psychology, Rome, 10th-13th September.

Hurme, H. (1988). *Child, mother and grandmother.* Jyvaskyla: University of Jyvaskyla Press

Hurme, H. (1989). Intergenerational interactions in the family. *Czlowiek i Spoleczenstwo, Vol. 4,* Poznan, Wyd. UAM.

Iacovetta, R.G. (1975). Adolescent-adult interaction and peer-group involvement. *Adolescence, 10*, 327-336.

Ilfeld, F.W. (1980). Coping styles of Chicago adults: description. *Journal of Human Stress, 6*, 2-10.

Inhelder, B. & Piaget, J. (1970). *Od logiki dziecka do logiki mlodziezy.* Warszawa: PWN.

Jackson, A.E. (1987). *Perceptions of a new acquaintance in adolescence.* Groningen: Stichting Kinderstudies.

Jackson, A.E. (in press). Socialisation, social support and social competence in adolescence: the individual in perspective. In: F. Nestmann & K. Hurrelmann (Eds.), *Social networks and social support in childhood and adolescence.* Berlin: de Gruyter.

Jackson, A.E. & Bosma, H.A. (1990). Coping and self-concept in adolescence. In: H.A. Bosma & A.E. Jackson (Eds.), *Coping and self-concept in adolescence.* Heidelberg: Springer-Verlag.

Jackson, A.E. & Elzen, R. (1990). *Difficult social situations in adolescence: An examination of response strategies.* Paper presented at Second European Workshop on Adolescence, Groningen, NL, April.

Jencks, C. (1972). *Inequality: a reassessment of the effect of family and schooling in America.* New York: Basic Books.

Jennings, W.S., Kilkenny, R. & Kohlberg, L. (1983). Moral development: theory and practice for youthful and adult offenders. In: W. Laufer & J.M. Day (Eds.), *Personality theory, moral development and criminal behavior.* Toronto: Lexington Books.

Jensen, G.F. (1976). Race, achievement and delinquency: A further look at delinquency in a birth cohort. *American Journal of Sociology, 82*, 379-387.

Jessor, R. (1986). Adolescent problem drinking: Psychosocial aspects and developmental outcomes. In: R.K. Silbereisen, K. Eyferth & G. Rudinger (Eds.), *Development as action in context* (pp. 241-264). Berlin: Springer-Verlag.

Johnson, B.M. & Collins, W.A. (1988). Perceived maturity as a function of appearance cues in early adolescence: Ratings by unacquainted adults, parents and teachers. *Journal of Early Adolescence, 8*, 357-372.

Jones, W.H. (1981). Loneliness and social contact. *Journal of Social Psychology, 113*, 295-296.

Josselson, R. (1987). *Finding herself: Pathways to identity development in women.* San Francisco: Jossey-Bass.

Juhasz, A. & Sonnenshein-Schneider, M. (1987). Adolescent sexuality: Values, morality and decision making. *Adolescence, 22* (87), 579-590.

Jurkovic, G.J. (1980). The juvenile delinquent as a moral philosopher: A structural developmental approach. *Psychological Bulletin, 88*, 709-727.

Kahana, B. & Kahana, E. (1970). Grandparenthood from the perspective of the developing grandchild, *Developmental Psychology, 3*, 98-105.

Kandel, D.B. (1986). Processes in peer influence in adolescence. In: R. K. Silbereisen, K. Eyferth & G. Rudinger (Eds.), *Development as action in context* (pp. 203-228). Berlin: Springer-Verlag.

Kandel, D.B. & Lesser, G.S. (1969). Parental and peer influence on educational plans of adolescents. *American Sociological Review, 34*, 212-223.

Kandel, D.B. & Lesser, G.S. (1972). *Youth in two worlds.* San Francisco: Jossey-Bass.

Kanner, A.D., Coyne, J.C., Schaefer, C. & Lazarus, R.S. (1981). Comparison of two modes of stress measurement: daily hassles and uplifts versus major life events. *Journal of Behavioural Medicine, 4*, 1-19.

Kaplan, H.B. (1978). Deviant behavior and self-enhancement in adolescence. *Journal of Youth and Adolescence, 7*, 253-277.

Kaplan, H.B. (1980). *Deviant behavior in the defense of self*. New York: Academic Press.

Kelly, D.H. (1975). Status origin, track position and delinquent involvement: A self-report analysis. *Sociological Quarterly, 16*, 264-271.

Kimmel, D.C. & Weiner, I.B. (1985). *Adolescence—a developmental transition*. Hillsdale, NJ: Lawrence Erlbaum Associates Inc.

Kirchler, E., Pombeni, M.L. & Palmonari, A. (1991). Sweet sixteen: adolescents' problems and the peer-group as source of support. *European Journal of Psychology of Education, 6*.

Kivett, V.R. (1985). Grandfathers and grandchildren: patterns of association, helping and psychological closeness. *Family Relations, 34*, 565-571.

Kivnick, H.Q. (1982). *The meaning of grandparenthood*. Ann Arbor: Michigan University Press.

Knox, D. & Wilson, K. (1981). Dating behaviors of university students. *Family Relations, 30*, 255-258.

Kohlberg, L. (1976). Moral stages and moralization: the cognitive developmental approach. In: T. Lickona (Ed.), *Moral development and behaviour: Theory, research and social issues*. New York: Holt, Rinehart & Winston.

Kölbel, G. (1960). *Über die Einsamkeit: Vom Ursprung, Gestaltwandel und Sinn des Einsamkeitserlebnis* [On loneliness: origin, development and meaning of the experience of loneliness]. München/Basel: Reinholt.

Kornhaber, A. & Woodward, K. (1985). *Grandparent/grandchild: The vital connection*. Oxford: Transaction Books.

Kracke, B. & Silbereisen, R.K. (1990). *On the interaction between maturational timing and social factors in the development of problem behavior*. Paper presented at the Second European Workshop on Adolescence, April 6-10, Groningen, Netherlands.

Kreutz, H. (1988). Çnderungen der politischen und gesellschaftlichen Wertvorstellungen. In: H. Kreutz (Ed.), *Pragmatische Soziologie*. Opladen: Leske & Budrich.

Kroger, J. (1985). Relationships during adolescence: A cross-national comparison of New Zealand and United States teenagers. *Journal of Adolescence, 8*, 47-56.

Labouvie, E.W. (1986). The coping function of adolescent alcohol and drug use. In: R.K. Silbereisen, K. Eyferth & G. Rudinger (Eds.), *Development as action in context* (pp. 229-240). Berlin: Springer-Verlag.

Larsen, L.E. (1972). The influence of parents and peers during adolescence: The situation hypothesis revisited. *Journal of Marriage and the Family, 34*, 67-74.

Larson, R.W. (1989). Beeping children and adolescents: A method for studying time use and daily experience. *Journal of Youth and Adolescence, 18*, 511-530.

Larson, R.W. (1990). The solitary side of life: An examination of the time people spend alone from childhood to old age. *Developmental Review, 10*, 155-183.

Larson, R. & Csikszentmihalyi, M. (1978). Experiential correlates of time alone in adolescence. *Journal of Personality, 46*, 677-693.

Larson, R., Csikszentmihalyi, M. & Graef, R. (1982). Time alone in daily experience: Loneliness or renewal? In: L. A. Peplau & D. Perlman (Eds.), *Loneliness: A sourcebook of current theory, research and therapy*. New York: Wiley.

Larson, R. & Richards, M.H. (1991) Daily companionship in late childhood and early adolescence: Changing developmental contexts. *Child Development, Vol. 62*, No. 2, 284-300.

Latane, B. & Darley, J. (1970). *The unresponsive bystander: Why doesn't he help*. New York: Appleton-Century-Crofts.

Lazarus, R.S. (1984). Puzzles in the study of daily hassles. *Journal of Behavioral Medicine, 7*, 375-389.

Lazarus, R.S., Averill, J. & Opton, E. (1974). The psychology of coping. In: G.V. Coelho, D.A. Hamburg & J.E. Adams (Eds.), *Coping and adaptation* (pp. 249-315). New York: Basic Books.

Lazarus, R.S. & Folkman, S. (1984). *Stress, appraisal and coping*. New York: Springer-Verlag.

Leahy, R.L. (1981). Parental practices and the development of moral judgment and self-image disparity during adolescence. *Developmental Psychology, 17*, 580-594.

Leaper, C., Hauser, S.T., Kremen, A., Powers, S.I., Jacobson, A. M., Noam, G.G., Weiss-Perry, B. & Follansbee, D. (1989). Adolescent-parent interactions in relation to adolescents' gender and ego development pathways: A longitudinal Study. *Journal of Early Adolescence, 9*, 335- 361.

Le Bon, G. (1896). *The crowd: A study of the popular mind*. London: Unwin.

Lerner, R.M. (1985). Adolescent maturational changes and psycho-social development: A dynamic interactional perspective. *Journal of Youth and Adolescence, 14*, 355-372.

Leslie, L.A., Huston, T.L. & Johnson M.P. (1986). Parental reactions to dating relationships: Do they make a difference? *Journal of Marriage and the Family, 48*, 57-66.

Levine, R.A. & Campbell, D.T. (1973). *Ethnocentrism*. New York: Wiley.

Lewin, K. (1954). Behaviour and development as a function of total situation. In: L. Carmichael (Ed.), *Manual of Child Psychology*, New York, Wiley.

Lewis, R. (1973). Social reaction and the formation of dyads: An interactionist approach to mate selection. *Sociometry, 36*, 409-418.

Liska, A.E. & Reed, M.D. (1985). Ties to conventional institutions and delinquency: Estimating reciprocal effects. *American Sociological Review, 50*, 547-560.

Livesley, W.J. & Bromley, D.B. (1973). *Person perception in childhood and adolescence*. Chichester: Wiley.

Loevinger, J. & Wessler, R. (1970). *Measuring ego development, Vol. 1: Construction and use of a Sentence Completion Test*. San Francisco, Jossey-Bass.

Long, B.H. (1983). A steady boyfriend: A step toward resolution of the intimacy crisis for American college women. Journal of Psychology, 115, 275-280.

Long, B.H. (1989). Heterosexual involvement of unmarried undergraduate females in relation to self-evaluations. *Journal of Youth and Adolescence, 18*, 489-500.

Lynd, R.S. & Lynd, H.M. (1929). *Middletown*. New York: Harcourt Brace Jovanovich.

Maccoby, E. & Jacklin, C. (1975). *The Psychology of Sex Differences*. London: Oxford University Press.

Maccoby, E.E. (1991). Different reproductive strategies in males and females. *Child Development, 62*, 676-681.

Maccoby, E.E. & Martin, J.A. (1983). Socialisation in the context of the family: Parent-child interaction. In: E.M. Hetherington & P.H. Mussen (Eds.), *Carmichael's Manual of Child Psychology: Vol. 4. Socialisation, personality and social development*. New York: Wiley.

Maddock, J.W. (1973). Sex in adolescence: Its meaning and its future. *Adolescence, 8*(31), 325-342.

Maggs, J.L. & Galambos, N.L. (1990). *A comparison of alternative structural models for understanding adolescent problem behavior*. Unpublished manuscript, University of Victoria, Canada.

Magnusson, D., Stattin, H. & Allen, V. (1985). Biological maturation and social development: A longitudinal study of some adjustment processes from mid-adolescence to adulthood. *Journal of Youth and Adolescence, 14*(4), 267-283.

Magnusson, D., Stattin, H. & Allen, V.A. (1986). Differential maturation among girls and its relevance to social adjustment: A longitudinal perspective. In: D.L. Featherman & R.M. Lerner (Eds.), *Life-span Development and Behavior* (Vol. 7, pp. 135-172). New York: Academic Press.

Main, M., Kaplan, N. & Cassidy, J. (1985). Security in infancy, childhood and adulthood: A move to the level of representation. In: I. Bretherton & E. Waters (Eds.), Growing points of attachment theory and research. *Monographs of the Society for Research in Child Development, 50*, 1-2, Serial No. 209, pp. 66-104.

Marangoni, C. & Ickes, W. (1989). Loneliness: A theoretical review with implications for measurement. *Journal of Social and Personal Relationships, 6*, 93-128.

Marcia, J. (1966). Development and validation of ego-identity status. *Journal of Personality and Social Psychology, 3*(5), 551-558.

Marcia, J. E. (1980). Identity in adolescence. In: J. Adelson (Ed.), *Handbook of adolescent psychology* (pp. 158-178). New York: Wiley.

Marcoen, A. & Brumagne, M. (1985). Loneliness among children and young adolescents. *Developmental Psychology, 21*, 1025-1031.

Marcoen, A. & Goossens, L. (1989). *Adolescent feelings of loneliness and aloneness: Relationships with ideological identity, interpersonal identity and intimacy*. Paper presented at the Tenth Biennial Meetings of the International Society for the Study of Behavioural Development, Jyväskylä, Finland.

Marcoen, A., Goossens, L. & Caes, P. (1987). Loneliness in pre- through late adolescence: Exploring the contributions of a multi-dimensional approach. *Journal of Youth and Adolescence, 16*, 561-577.

Markus, H. & Sentis, K. (1982): The self in information processing. In: J. Suls (Ed.), *Psychological perspectives on the self. Vol.1*. Hillsdale, NJ: Lawrence Erlbaum Associates Inc.

Marshall, N.J. (1974). Dimensions of privacy preferences. *Multivariate Behavioral Research, 9*, 255-272.

Marshall, W.A. & Tanner, J.M. (1969). Variations in the pattern of pubertal changes in girls. *Archives of Disease in Childhood, 44*, 291-303.

Marshall, W.A. & Tanner, J.M. (1970). Variations in the pattern of pubertal changes in boys. *Archives of Disease in Childhood, 45*, 13-23.

Mathes, E.W., Adams, H.E. & Davis, R.M. (1985). Jealousy: Loss of relationship rewards, loss of self-esteem, depression, anxiety and anger. *Journal of Personality and Social Psychology, 48*, 1552-1561.

Matthews, S.H. & Sprey, J. (1985). Adolescents' relationships with grandparents: An empirical contribution to conceptual clarification. *Journal of Gerontology, 40*, 621-626.

McCabe, M.P. (1984). Toward a theory of adolescent dating. *Adolescence, 19* (73), 159-170.

McCabe, M.P. & Collins, J.K. (1979). Sex role and dating orientation. *Journal of Youth and Adolescence, 8*, 407-425.

McCandless, B.R. (1970). *Adolescents: Behavior and development.* Hinsdale, Illinois: Dryden Press.

McCrae, R.R. (1982). Age differences in the use of coping mechanisms. *Journal of Gerontology, 37*, 454-460.

McCubbin, H.L., Larson, A. & Olson, D.H. (1981). *F-copes, copes, family crisis oriented personal evaluation scales.* Family & Social Sciences, University of Minnesota, St. Paul, MN.

Mead, G.H. (1934). *Mind, Self and Society.* Chicago: University of Chicago Press.

Mekos, D. (1991). *Changes in puberty and parent-child distance: A reciprocal process?* Paper presented at the SRCD Biennial Meetings, April 18-20, Seattle, WA.

Meltzer, D. (1981). Teoria psicoanalitica dell'adolescenza. *Quaderni di Psicoterapia Infantile, 1.*

Menard, S. & Morse, B.J. (1984). A structuralist critique of the IQ-delinquency hypothesis: Theory and evidence. *American Journal of Sociology, 89*, 1347-1378.

Merton, R.K. (1969). Social structure and anomie. In: D.R. Cressey & D.A. Ward (Eds), *Delinquency, crime and social process.* New York: Harper.

Milgram, S. (1974). *Obedience to authority.* New York: Harper & Row.

Miller, K.E. (1990). Adolescents' same-sex and opposite-sex peer relations: Sex differences in popularity, perceived social competence and social cognitive skills. *Journal of Adolescent Research, 5*, 222-241.

Miller, P.H. (1989). Theories of Adolescent Development. In: J. Worrell & F. Danner (Eds.), *The adolescent as decision-maker: Applications to development and education.* New York: Academic Press.

Miller, P.Y. & Simon, W. (1980). The development of sexuality in adolescence. In: J. Adelson (Ed.), *Handbook of adolescent psychology.* New York: Wiley.

Minuchin, P. (1988). Relationships within the family: A systems perspective on development. In: R.A. Hinde, J. Stevenson-Hinde (Eds.), *Relationships within families: Mutual influences.* Oxford: Clarendon Press.

Minuchin, P. & Shapiro, E. (1983). The school as a context for social development. In: E.M. Hetherington (Ed.), *Handbook of Child Psychology: Vol. 4. Socialization, personality and social development,* (pp. 197-274). New York: Wiley.

Mitchell, J.C. (1969). *Social networks in urban situations.* Manchester: Manchester University Press.

Mitchell, J.J. (1976). Adolescent intimacy. *Adolescence, 11*, 275-280.

Moffitt, T. E., Caspi, A., Belsky, J. & Silva, P.A. (1990). *Childhood experience and the onset of menarche: A test of a socio-biological model.* Unpublished manuscript.

Monroe, S.M. (1983). Social support and disorder: Toward an untangling of cause and effect. *American Journal of Community Psychology, 11*, 81-97.

Montemayor, R. (1982). The relationship between parent-adolescent conflict and the amount of time adolescents spend alone and with parents and peers. *Child Development, 53*, 1512-1519.

Montemayor, R. (1983). Parents and adolescents in conflict: All families some of the time and some families most of the time. *Journal of Early Adolescence, 3*, 83-103.

Montemayor, R. (1984). Picking up the pieces: The effects of parental divorce on adolescents, with some suggestions for school-based intervention programmes. *Journal of Early Adolescence, 4*, 289-314.

Montemayor, R. (1986). Family variation in parent-adolescent storm and stress. *Journal of Adolescent Research, 1*, 15-31.

Montemayor, R. & Hanson, E. (1985). A naturalistic view of conflict between adolescents and their parents and siblings. *Journal of Early Adolescence, 5*, 23-30.

Moos, R.H. (1989). *Coping response inventory: Manual.* Department of Psychiatry, Stanford University, Palo Alto.

Moos, R.H. & Moos, B.S. (1981). *Family environment scale: Manual.* Palo Alto: Consulting Psychologists Press.

Morash, M. (1983). Gangs, groups and delinquency. *British Journal of Criminology, 32*, 309-331.

Murphy, L.B. & Moriarty, A.E. (1976). *Vulnerability, coping and growth from infancy to adolescence.* New Haven: Yale University Press.

Mussen, P., Sullivan, L.B. & Eisenberg-Berg, N. (1977). Changes in political-economic attitudes during adolescence. *Journal of Genetic Psychology, 130*, 69-76.

Newtson, D. (1973). Attribution and the unit of perception of ongoing behaviour. *Journal of Personality and Social Psychology, 28*, 28-38.

Nisbett, R.E. & Wilson, T.C. (1977). Telling more than we can know: Verbal reports on mental processes. *Psychological Review, 84*, 231-259.

Noller, P. & Callan, V. (1991). *The adolescent in the family.* London: Routledge.

Offer, D. (1969). *The Psychological world of teenagers.* New York: Basic Books.

Offer, D. & Offer, J.B. (1975). *From teenage to young manhood.* New York: Basic Books.

Offer, D., Ostrov, E. & Howard, K.J. (1981). *The adolescent: A psychological self-portrait.* New York: Basic Books.

Olbrich, E. (1984). Jugendalter Zeit der Krise oder der Produktiven Anparsung? In: E. Olbrich & E. Todt (Eds.), *Probleme des Jugendalters.* Berlin, Springer-Verlag.

Olbrich, E. (1985). Konstruktive Auseinandersetzung im Jugendalter: Entwicklung, Fürderung und Verhaltenseffekte. In: R. Oerter (Ed.), *Lebensbewèltigung im Jugendalter.* Weinheim: VCH.

Olbrich, E. (1990). Coping and development. In: H.A. Bosma & A.E. Jackson (Eds.), *Coping and self concept in adolescence.* Heidelberg: Springer-Verlag.

Oliveri, M.E. & Reiss, D. (1981). The structure of families' ties to their kin: The shaping role of social constructions. *Journal of Marriage and the Family, 43*, 391–407.

Olson, D.H., Portner, J. & Bell, R. (1984). Family adaptability and cohesion evaluation scales. In: D.H. Olson, et al. (Eds.), *Family inventories: Inventories used in a national survey of families across the family life cycle.* St Paul: Family Social Science, University of Minnesota.

O'Mahony, J.F. (1986). Development of person description over adolescence. *Journal of Youth and Adolescence, 15*, 389-404.

Orlofsky, J. & Ginsburg, S.D. (1981). Intimacy status: Relationship to affect cognition. *Adolescence, 16*, 91-100

Orlofsky, J.L., Marcia, J.E. & Lesser, I.M. (1973). Ego identity status and the intimacy versus isolation crisis of young adulthood. *Journal of Personality and Social Psychology, 27*, 221-219.

Palmonari, A., Kirchler, E. & Pombeni M.L. (1991). Differential effects of identification with family and peers on coping with developmental tasks in adolescence. *European Journal of Social Psychology, 21*, 381-402.

Palmonari, A., Pombeni, M.L. and Kirchler, E. (1989). Peer-groups and evolution of the self-system in adolescence. *European Journal of Psychology of Education, 4*, 3-15.

Palmonari, A., Pombeni, M.L. & Kirchler, E. (1990). Adolescents and their peer groups: A study on the significance of peers, social categorization processes and coping with developmental tasks. *Social Behaviour, 5*, 33-48.

Parks, M., Stan, C. & Eggert, L. (1983). Romantic involvement and social network involvement. *Social Psychology Quarterly, 46*, 116-131.

Patterson, G.P., DeBaryshe, B.D. & Ramsey, E. (1989). A developmental perspective on anti-social behavior. *American Psychologist, 44*, 329-335.

Patterson, G.P. & Stouthamer-Loeber, M. (1984). The correlation of family management practices and delinquency. *Child Development, 55*, 1299-1307.

Patterson, J. & McCubbin, H. (1987). Adolescent coping style and behaviours: Conceptualization and measurement. *Journal of Adolescence, 10*, 163-186.

Paul, E.L. & White, K.M. (1990). The development of intimate relationships in late adolescence. *Adolescence, 25*, 375-400.

Pedersen, D.L. (1979). Dimensions of privacy. *Perceptual and Motor Skills, 48*, 1291-1297.

Peeters, A. (1986). *Boredom in adolescence: A review of the literature and an exploratory study*. Unpublished Master's thesis, Catholic University of Louvain, Leuven, Belgium. (In Dutch)

Peevers, B.H. & Secord, P.F. (1973). Developmental changes in attribution of descriptive concepts to persons. *Journal of Personality and Social Psychology, 27*, 120-128.

Peplau, L.A. & Perlman, D. (Eds.) (1982). *Loneliness: A sourcebook of current theory, research and therapy*. New York: Wiley.

Peplau, L.A., Rubin, Z. & Hill, C.T. (1977). Sexual intimacy in dating relationships. *Journal of Social Issues, 33*, 86-109.

Perlman, D. (1988). Loneliness: A life-span, family perspective. In: R. Milardo (Ed.), *Families and social networks* (pp. 190-220). Newbury Park, CA: Sage.

Perlman, D. & Peplau, L.A. (1981). Toward a social psychology of loneliness. In: R. Gilmour & S. Duck (Eds.), *Personal relationships: Vol. 3. Relationships in disorder* (pp. 31-56). London: Academic Press.

Petersen, A.C. (1986). *Early adolescence: A critical developmental transition?* Paper presented at the annual meeting of the American Educational Research Association, San Francisco.

Petersen, A.C. (1988). Adolescent development. *Annual Review of Psychology, 39*, 593-607.

Petersen, A.C. & Crockett, L.J. (1985). Pubertal timing and grade effects on adjustment. *Journal of Youth and Adolescence, 14*, 191-206.

Petersen, A.C., Crockett, L.J., Richards, M. & Boxer, A.M. (1988). A self-report measure of pubertal status: Reliability, validity and initial norms. *Journal of Youth and Adolescence, 17*, 117-133.

Petersen, A.C., Graber, J.A. & Sullivan, P. (1990). *Pubertal timing and problem behavior: Variations in effects*. Paper presented at Biennial Meetings of SRA, March 22-25, Atlanta, GA.

Petersen, A.C. & Spiga, R. (1982). Adolescence and stress. In: L. Goldberger & S. Breznitz (Eds.), *Handbook of stress* (pp. 515-528). London: Free Press.

Piaget, J. (1932). *The moral judgment of the child*. London: Routledge & Kegan Paul.

Piliavin, I. & Briar, S. (1964). Police encounters with juveniles. *American Journal of Sociology, 70*, 206-214.

Pombeni, M.L., Kirchler. E. & Palmonari, A. (1990). Identification with peers as a strategy to muddle through the troubles of adolescent years. *Journal of Adolescence, 13*, 351-369.

Powers, S.I. (1989). Theory and assessment in family psychology: Weak links. *Journal of Family Psychology, 3*, 222-228.

Powers, S.I., Hauser, S.T., Schwartz, J.M., Noam, G.G. & Jacobson, A.M. (1983). Adolescent ego development and family interaction: A structural developmental perspective. In: H.D. Grotevant & C.R. Cooper (Eds.), *Adolescent development in the family*. San Francisco: Jossey-Bass.

Raviv, A., Weitzman, E. & Raviv, A. (1992). Parents of adolescents: Help-seeking intentions as a function of help sources and parenting issues. *Journal of Adolescence*.

Reicher, S. & Emler, N. (1985). Delinquent behaviour and attitudes to formal authority. *British Journal of Social Psychology, 3*, 161-168.

Reiss, D. (1971). Varieties of consensual experience. I. A theory for relating family interaction to individual thinking. *Family Process, 10*, 1-28.

Reiss, D. & Oliveri, M.E. (1987). *Developing a clear image of the family. The card sort procedure as an easy and precise method for measuring family process in the rehabilitation setting*. A pre-publication report on current rehabilitation research. George Washington University Medical Center.

Reiss, D., Oliveri, M.E. & Curd, K. (1983). Family paradigm and adolescent social behaviour. In: H.D. Grotevant & C.R. Cooper (Eds.), *Adolescent development in the family*. San Francisco: Jossey-Bass.

Remmers, H.H. & Radler, D.H. (1962). *The American teenager*. Indianapolis: Bobbs-Merrill.

Renwick, S. & Emler, N. (1991). The relationship between social skills deficits and juvenile delinquency. *British Journal of Clinical Psychology, 30*, 61-71.

Rhodes, A.L. & Reiss, A.J. (1970). Apathy, truancy and delinquency as adaptations to school failure. *Social Forces, 48*, 12-22.

Rice, F.P. (1984). *The adolescent: development, relations and culture*. Boston: Allyn and Bacon.

Rice, K. (1990). Attachment in adolescence. *Journal of Youth and Adolescence, 19*, 511-538.

Rigby, K. & Rump, E.E. (1979). The generality of attitude to authority. *Human Relations, 32*, 469-487.

Rivenbark, W. (1971). Self-disclosure among adolescents. *Psychological Reports,* *28,* 35-42.

Robertson, J.F. (1975). Interaction in three-generation families parents as mediators: Towards a theoretical perspective. *International Journal of Aging and Human Development, 6,* 103-110.

Robertson, J. F. (1976). Significance of grandparents: Perceptions of young adult grandchildren. *The Gerontologist, 16,* 137-140

Roche, J. P. (1986). Premarital sex: Attitudes and behavior by dating stage. *Adolescence, 21,* 107-121.

Rodriguez-Tomé, H. & Bariaud, F. (1990). Anxiety in adolescence: Sources and reactions. In: H.A. Bosma & A.E. Jackson (Eds.), *Coping and self-concept in adolescence.* Heidelberg: Springer-Verlag.

Rodriguez-Tomé, H., Bariaud, F., Cohen-Zardi, M.F., Delmas, C., Jeanvoine, B. & Szylagyi, F. (in press). The effects of pubertal change on body image and relations with peers of the opposite sex in adolescence. *Journal of Adolescence.*

Rook, K.S. (1988). Toward a more differentiated view of loneliness. In: S.W. Duck (Ed.), *Handbook of social relationships* (pp. 571-589). Chichester: Wiley.

Roscoe, B., Diana, M.S. & Brooks, R.H. (1987). Early, middle and late adolescents' views on dating and factors influencing partner selection. *Adolescence, 22,* 59-68.

Roscoe, B. Kennedy, D. & Pope, T. (1987). Adolescents' view of intimacy: distinguishing intimate from non-intimate relationships. *Adolescence, 22,* 511-516.

Rosenthal, D.A., Gurney, R.M. & Moore, S.M. (1981). From trust to intimacy: A new inventory for examining Erikson's stages of psychosocial development. *Journal of Youth and Adolescence, 10,* 523-537.

Rowlinson, R.T. & Felner, R.D. (1988). Major life-events, hassles and adaptation in adolescence: Confounding in the conceptualization and measurement of life stress and adjustment revisited. *Journal of Personality and Social Psychology, 55,* 432-444.

Rubenstein, C. & Shaver, P. (1982). *In search of intimacy.* New York: Delacorte Press.

Rump, E.E., Rigby, K. & Walters, L. (1985). The generality of attitudes to authority: Cross-cultural comparisons. *Journal of Social Psychology, 125,* 307-312.

Russell, D. (1982). The measurement of loneliness. In: L.A. Peplau & D. Perlman (Eds.), *Loneliness: A sourcebook of current theory, research and therapy.* New York: Wiley.

Russell, D., Peplau, L.A. & Cutrona, C.E. (1980). The revised UCLA Loneliness Scale: Concurrent and discriminant validity evidence. *Journal of Personality and Social Psychology, 46,* 1313-1321.

Rutter, M. (1983). Stress, coping and development. In: N. Garmezy & M. Rutter (Eds.), *Stress, coping & development in children.* New York: McGraw-Hill.

Rutter, M. (1989). Pathways from childhood to adult life. *Journal of Child Psychology and Psychiatry, 30,* 23-52.

Sabatelli, R.M. & Mazor, A. (1985). Differentiation, individuation and identity formation: The integration of family systems and individual development perspectives. *Adolescence, 20,* 619-633.

Sachs, J. & Levy, S. (1952). The sentence completion test. In: L.E. Abt & L. Bellak (Eds.), *Projective psychology*. New York: Knopf.

Salmon, P. (1979). The role of the peer group. In: J.C. Coleman (Ed.), *The School Years*. London: Methuen.

Samet, N. & Kelly, E.W. (1987). The relationship of steady dating to self-esteem and sex role identity among adolescents. *Adolescence, 22*(85), 231-245.

Santili, N. & Furth, H. (1987). Adolescent work perception: A developmental approach. In: J. Lewko (Ed.), *How children and adolescents view the world of work*. San Francisco: Jossey-Bass.

Savin-Williams, R.C. & Small, S.A. (1986). The timing of puberty and its relationship to adolescent and parent perceptions of family interaction. *Developmental Psychology, 22*, 342-347.

Schaie K.W. (1984). Historical time and cohort effects. In: K.W. Schaie (Ed.), *Life-span Developmental Psychology*, New York: Academic Press.

Schmidt, N. & Sermat, V. (1983). Measuring loneliness in different relationships. *Journal of Personality and Social Psychology, 44*, 1038-1047.

Schulz, B., Bohrnstedt, G.W., Borgatta, E.F. & Evans, R.R. (1977). Explaining premarital sexual intercourse among college students: A causal model. *Social Forces, 56*, 148-165.

Schultz, N.W. (1980). A cognitive-developmental study of the grandchild-grandparent bond, *Child Study Journal, 10*, p. 7-26

Schün, B. (1990). *Jugendliche und ihre Problemwelt: Sozialer Kontext und Bewèltigungsstrategien*. Unpublished Master's Thesis, University of Linz, Austria.

Segers, E. (1985). *An exploratory study on the relationship between adolescent loneliness and the quality of interpersonal relationships*. Unpublished Master's Thesis, State University of Ghent, Belgium. (In Dutch)

Seiffge-Krenke, I. (1984). *Problembewältigung im Jugendalter*. Unpublished Habilitation Thesis, University of Giessen [Habilitationsschrift, Universität Gießen].

Seiffge-Krenke, I. (1985). Die Funktion des Tagebuches bei der Bewèltigung alterstypischer Probleme in der Adoleszenz. In: R. Oerter (Ed.), *Lebensbewèltigung im Jugendalter*. Weinheim: VCH.

Seiffge-Krenke, I. (1986). Problembewältigung im Jugendalter. *Zeitschrift für Entwicklungspsychologie und Pädagogische Psychologie, 2*, 122-152.

Seiffge-Krenke, I. (1989a). Problem intensity and the disposition of adolescents to take therapeutic advice. In: M. Brambring, F. Lösel & H. Skowronek (Eds.), Children at risk: assessment and longitudinal research. Berlin, New York: de Gruyter.

Seiffge-Krenke, I. (1989b). Bewältigung alltäglicher Problemsituationen: Ein Coping-Fragebogen für Jugendliche. *Zeitschrift für Differentielle & Diagnostische Psychologie, 10*, 201-220.

Seiffge-Krenke, I. (1990a). Health related behaviour and coping with illness in adolescence: a cross cultural perspective. In: L.R. Schmidt, P. Schwenkmezger, J. Weinman & S. Maes (Eds.), *Health psychology: Theoretical and applied aspects* (pp. 267-280). London: Harwood Academic Publishers.

Seiffge-Krenke, I. (1991a). *Coping behaviour of Finnish adolescents: Remarks on a cross-cultural comparison*. Unpublished article.

Seiffge-Krenke, I. (1992). *Stress, coping and relationships*. Hillsdale, NJ: Lawrence Erlbaum Associates Inc.

Seiffge-Krenke, I. & Brath, K. (1980). Krankheitsverarbeitung bei Kindern und Jugenlichen: In: I. Seiffge-Krenke (Ed.), *Jahrbuch der Medizinischen Psychologie*, Berlin: Springer-Verlag.

Seiffge-Krenke, I. & Brath, K. (1990). Krankheitsverarbeitung bei Kindern und Jugendlichen: Forschungstrends und Ergebnisse. In: I. Seiffge-Krenke (Ed.), *Jahrbuch für Medizinische Psychologie, Vol. IV Krankheitsbewältigung bei Kindern und Jugendlichen* (pp. 3-22). Heidelberg, New York: Springer-Verlag.

Seiffge-Krenke, I. & Olbrich, E. (1982). Psychosoziale Entwicklung im Jugendalter. In: W. Wieczerkowski and H. zur Oeveste (Eds.), *Lehrbuch der Entwicklungspsychologie*. Dusseldorf: Schwann.

Seiffge-Krenke, I. & Shulman, S. (1990). Coping styles in adolescence: A cross-cultural study. *International Journal of Cross-Cultural Psychology, 21*, 351-377.

Selman, R.L. (1980). *The growth of interpersonal understanding*. New York: Academic Press.

Semin, G. (1986). Editorial: The individual, the social and the social individual. *British Journal of Social Psychology*, (Special Issue), *25*, 177-180.

Shell-Studie 1981 (1981). Jugend '81—Lebensentwürfe, Alltagskulturen, Zukunftsbilder. Jugendwerk der Deutschen Shell.

Sherif, M. & Sherif, C.W. (1964). *Reference Groups*. New York: Harper & Row.

Sherif, M. & Sherif, C.W. (1965a). The adolescent in his group in its setting. Vol. I. Theoretical approach and methodology required. In: M. Sherif & C.W. Sherif (Eds.) *Problems of youth: Transition to adulthood in a changing world*. Chicago: Aldine Publishing Company.

Sherif, M. & Sherif, C.W. (1965b). The adolescent in his group in its setting. Vol. II. Research procedures and findings. In: M. Sherif & C.W. Sherif (Eds.), *Problems of youth: Transition to adulthood in a changing world*. Chicago: Aldine Publishing Company.

Shulman, S., Carlton-Ford, S., Levian, R. & Hed, S. (submitted). *Coping styles of learning disabled adolescents and their parents*.

Shulman, S. & Klein, M.M. (1982). The family and adolescence: A conceptual and experimental approach. *Journal of Adolescence, 5*, 219-234.

Shulman, S., Seiffge-Krenke, I. & Samet, N. (1987). Adolescent coping style as a function of perceived family climate. *Journal of Adolescent Research, 2*, 367-381.

Siddique, C. & D'Arcy, C. (1984). Adolescence, stress and psychological well-being. *Journal of Youth and Adolescence, 13*, 459-473.

Silbereisen, R.K. & Kracke, B. (1990). *The impact of maturational timing and parental support on contacts with deviant peers*. Unpublished paper presented at a Colloquium at the Academy of Sciences, July, 3-4, Prague, Czechoslovakia.

Silbereisen, R.K. & Noack, P. (1988). Adolescence and environment. In: D. Canter, M. Krampen & D. Stea (Eds.), *Ethnoscapes: Transcultural studies in action and place*. Guildford: Gower.

Silbereisen, R.K. & Noack, P. (1990). Adolescents' orientations for development. In: H.A. Bosma & A.E. Jackson (Eds.), *Coping and self-concept in adolescence*. Heidelberg: Springer-Verlag.

Silbereisen, R.K., Noack, P. & Eyferth, K. (1986). Place for development: adolescents, leisure settings & developmental tasks. In: R.K. Silbereisen, K. Eyferth & G. Rudinger (Eds.) *Development as action in context*. Berlin: Springer-Verlag.

Silbereisen, R.K., Noack, P.D. & Schönpflug, U. (in press). Comparative analysis of beliefs, leisure contexts and substance use in West Berlin and Warsaw. In: R.K. Silbereisen & E. Todt (Eds.), *Adolescence in context: The interplay of family, school peers and work in adjustment.* New York: Springer.

Silbereisen, R.K., Petersen, A.C., Albrecht, H.T. & Kracke, B. (1989). Maturational timing and the development of problem behavior: Longitudinal studies in adolescence. *Journal of Early Adolescence, 9,* 247-268.

Silbereisen, R.K. & Schmitt-Rodermund, E. (1991). *Wir haben befuerchtet, die Familie wuerde auseinanderreissen. Veraenderungen der Familienbeziehungen: Folgen fuer Jugendliche in Aussiedlerfamilien. In Berichte der Arbeits- gruppe, Erfolg und Verlauf der Aneignung neuer Umwelten durch Aussiedler. Phase 1, Pilotstudie.* Unpublished manuscript, University of Giessen, Germany.

Simmons, R. & Blyth, D. (1987). Moving into adolescence. New York: Aldine de Gruyter.

Simmons, R.G., Blyth, D.A., van Claeve, E.F. & Bush, D.E. (1979). Entry into early adolescence: The impact of school structure, puberty and early dating on self-esteem. *American Sociological Review, 44,* 948-967.

Simmons, R.G., Burgeson, R. & Reef, M.J. (1988). Cumulative change at entry to adolescence. In: M.R. Gunnar & W.A. Collins (Eds.), *Development during the transition to adolescence. The Minnesota Symposium on Child Psychology, Vol. 21.* Hillsdale, NJ: Lawrence Erlbaum Associates Inc.

Skipper, J.K. & Nass, G. (1966). Dating behaviour: A framework for analysis and an illustration. *Journal of Marriage and the Family, 28,* 412-420.

Slavin, A.L. & Compas, B.E. (1989). The problem of confounding social support and depressive symptoms: A brief report on a college sample. *American Journal of Community Psychology, 17,* 57-65.

Small, F. & Eastman, G. (1991). Rearing adolescents in contemporary society. *Family Relations, 40,* 455-462.

Smetana, J. G. (1988). Concepts of self and social convention: Adolescents' and parents' reasoning about hypothetical and actual family conflicts. In: M.R. Gunnar & W.A. Collins (Eds.), *Development during the transition to adolescence. The Minnesota Symposium on Child Psychology* (Vol. 21, pp. 79-122). Hillsdale, NJ: Lawrence Erlbaum Associates Inc.

Smith, P.K. (1991). Introduction: The study of grandparenthood. In: Smith P.K. (Ed.), *The psychology of grandparenthood: An international perspective.* London: Routledge.

Smith, T.E. (1976). Push versus pull—intra-family versus peer group variables as possible determinants of adolescent orientation toward parents. *Youth and Society, 8,* 5-26.

Spence, S.H. (1981). Differences in social skills performance between institutionalised juvenile male offenders and a comparable group of boys without offence records. *British Journal of Clinical Psychology, 20,* 163-171.

Sroufe, L.A. (1979). The coherence of individual development. *American Psychologist, 34,* 834-841.

Sroufe, L.A. & Fleeson, J. (1986). Attachment and the construction of relationships. In: W.W. Hartup & Z. Rubin (Eds.), *Relationships and development.* Hillsdale, NJ: Lawrence Erlbaum Assoociates Inc.

Statistisches Bundesamt (1984). *Die situation der jugend in der Bundesrepublik Deutschland* (The situation of youth in the Federal Republic of Germany). Mainz: Kohlhammer.

Stattin, H. & Magnusson, D. (1990). *Pubertal maturation in female development*. Hillsdale, NJ: Lawrence Erlbaum Associates Inc.

Steinberg, L. (1985). *Adolescence*. New York: Knopf.

Steinberg, L. (1987). The impact of puberty on family relations: Effects of pubertal status and pubertal timing. *Developmental Psychology, 23,* 451-460.

Steinberg, L. (1990). Autonomy, conflict and harmony in the family relationship. In: S.S. Feldman & G.R. Elliott (Eds), *At the threshold: The developing adolescent*. London: Harvard University Press.

Steinberg, L. & Silverberg, S.B. (1986). The vicissitudes of autonomy in early adolescence. *Child Development, 57,* 841-851.

Steinberg, L.D. (1981). Transformations in family relations at puberty. *Developmental Psychology, 17,* 833-840.

Steinberg, L.D. (1989). Pubertal maturation and parent-adolescent distance: An evolutionary perspective. In: G. Adams, R. Montemayor, & T. Gullotta (Eds.), *Advances in adolescent development, Vol. 1* (pp. 71-97). Beverly Hills, CA: Sage.

Stern, M. & Zevon, M.A. (1990). Stress, coping & family environment: The adolescent's response to naturally occurring stressors. *Journal of Adolescent Research, 5,* 290-305.

Sticker, E. J. (1991). The importance of grandparenthood during the life cycle in Germany. In: P.K. Smith (Ed.), *The psychology of grandparenthood: An international perspective*. London: Routledge.

Stone, G. & Farberman, H. (Eds.) (1970). *Social psychology through symbolic interaction*. Waltham, Mass.: Ginn-Blaisdell

Storr, A. (1990). *Solitude: A return to the self*. London: Fontana.

Strodbeck, F.L. (1951). Husband-wife interactions over revealed differences. *American Sociological Review, 16,* 468-473.

Stueve, A. (1982). The elderly as network members. *Marriage and the Family Review, 5,* 59-87

Suedfeld, P. (1982). Aloneness as a healing experience. In: L.A. Peplau & D. Perlman (Eds.), *Loneliness: A sourcebook of current theory, research and therapy* (pp. 54-67). New York: Wiley.

Sugarman, L. (1986). *Life-span development: Concepts, theories and interventions*. London: Methuen.

Sullivan, H.S. (1953). *The interpersonal theory of psychiatry*. New York: Norton.

Sullivan, K. & Sullivan, A. (1980). Adolescent-parent separation. *Developmental Psychology, 16,* 91-99.

Surbey, M.K. (1990). Family composition, stress and human menarche. In: T.E. Ziegler & F.B. Bercovitch (Eds.), *Socioendocrinology of primate reproduction* (pp. 11-32). New York: Wiley-Liss.

Sutherland, E.H. & Cressy, D.R. (1970). *Principles of criminology*. (8th Edition). Chicago: Lippincott.

Swearingen, E.M. & Cohen, L.H. (1985). Life events and psychological distress: A prospective study of young adolescents. *Developmental Psychology, 21,* 1045-1054.

Tardiff, S. (1984). Social influences on sexual maturation of female Saguinus Oedipus. *American Journal of Primatology, 6,* 199-209.

Terrell-Deutsch, B. (1990). *Assessing loneliness in children.* Paper presented at the Biennial University of Waterloo Conference on Child Development, Waterloo, Ontario, Canada.

Tesch, S.A. & Whitbourne, S.K. (1982). Intimacy and identity status in young adults. *Journal of Personality and Social Psychology, 43,* 1041-1051.

Troll, L.E. (1980). Grandparenting. In: L.W. Poon (Ed.), *Aging in the 1980s: Psychological issues.* Washington, DC: American Psychological Association.

Troll, L.E., Bengtson, V. & McFerland, D. (1979). Generations in the family. In: R. Hill, F.I. Nye & I.L. Reiss (Eds.), *Contemporary theories about the family: Research-based theories.* London: Free Press.

Tuma, E. & Livson, N. (1960). Family socio-economic status and adolescent attitudes to authority. *Child Development, 31,* 387-399.

Turiel, E. (1976). A comparative analysis of moral knowledge and moral judgment in males and females. *Journal of Personality, 44,* 195-208.

Turner, J.C. (1982). Towards a cognitive redefinition of the social group. In: H. Tajfel (Ed.), *Social identity and intergroup relations.* Cambridge: Cambridge University Press.

Turner, J.C., Hogg, M.A., Oakes, P.J., Reicher, S.D. & Wetherell, M.S. (Eds.) (1987). *Re-discovering the social group: A self-categorization theory.* Oxford: Blackwell.

Tyler, F. (1978). Individual psychosocial competence: A personality configuration. *Educational and Psychological Measurement, 38,* 309-323.

Tyszkowa, M. (1986a). Psychic development of the individual: A process of structuring and re-structuring experience. In: P. van Geert (Ed.), *Theory-building in developmental psychology.* Amsterdam: North Holland

Tyszkowa, M. (1986b). Cyklzycia rodziny a rozwoj indywidualny [Family life cycle and the development of the individual]. In: M. Ziemska (Ed.), *Spoleczne konsekwencje integracji i dezintegracji rodziny.* Warszawa: TWWP.

Tyszkowa, M. (1990a). Coping with difficult school situations and stress resistance. In: H. A. Bosma and A. E. Jackson (Eds.), *Coping and self-concept in adolescence.* Heidelberg: Springer-Verlag.

Tyszkowa, M. (Ed.) (1990b). *Rodzina a rozwoj jednostki* [Family and the development of the individual]. Poznan: CPBP.

Tyszkowa, M. (1991). The role of grandparents in the development of grandchildren as perceived by adolescents and young adults in Poland. In: P.K. Smith (Ed.), *The psychology of grandparenthood: An international perspective.* London: Routledge.

Van Hees, S. (1990). *Adolescent loneliness, aloneness and internal working models of attachment.* Unpublished Master's Thesis, Catholic University of Louvain, Leuven, Belgium. (In Dutch)

Vunchinich, S. (1987). Starting and stopping spontaneous family conflicts. *Journal of Marriage and the Family, 79,* 591-601.

Wagner, B.M., Compas, B.E. & Howell, D.C. (1988). Daily and major life events: A test of an integrative model of psychosocial stress. *American Journal of Community Psychology, 16,* 189-205.

Wahler, R.G. (1980). The insular mother: her problems in parent-child treatment. *Journal of Applied Behaviour Analysis, 13,* 207-219.

Walker, L.S. & Greene, J.W. (1987). Negative life events, psychological sources and psychophysiological symptoms in adolescents. *Journal of Clinical Child Psychology, 16,* 29-36.

Wallach, M., Kogan, N. & Bem, D. (1962). Group influence on individual risk-taking. *Journal of Abnormal Psychology, 68*, 263-274.

Wallerstein, J.S. (1985). Children of divorce: Preliminary report of a ten-year follow-up of older children and adolescents. *Journal of the American Academy of Child Psychiatry, 24*, 518-530.

Waters, E. & Sroufe, L.A. (1983). Social competence as a developmental construct. *Developmental Review, 3*, 79-97.

Weber, M. (1947). *The theory of social and economic organisations.* (A.M. Henderson & T. Parsons, translators). New York: Free Press.

Weinstein, E. A. (1973). The development of interpersonal competence. In: D.A. Goslin (Ed.), *Handbook of socialization theory and research.* New York: Rand-McNally.

Weiss, R.S. (1973). *Loneliness: The experience of emotional and social isolation.* Cambridge, MA: MIT Press.

Wellman, B. (1979). The community question: The intimate networks of East Yorkers. *American Journal of Sociology, 84*, 1201-1231.

Werner, E.E. (1991). Grandparent-grandchildren relationships amongst US ethnic group. In: P.K. Smith (Ed.), *The psychology of grandparenthood: An international perspective.* London: Routledge.

West, D.J. & Farrington, D.P. (1973). *Who becomes delinquent?* London: Heinemann.

West, D.J. & Farrington, D.P. (1977). *The delinquent way of life.* London: Heinemann.

White, K.M., Speisman, J.C. & Costos, D. (1983). Young adults and their parents: Individuation to mutuality. In: H.D. Grotevant & C.R. Cooper (Eds.), *New directions for child development: Adolescent development in the family.* San Francisco: Jossey-Bass.

White, K.M., Speisman, J.C., Costos, D. & Smith, A. (1987). Relationship maturity: A conceptual and empirical approach. In: J. Meacham (Ed.), *Interpersonal relations: Family, peers, friends.* Basel, Switzerland: Karger.

White, K.M., Speisman, J.C., Jackson, D., Bartis, S. & Costos, D. (1986). Intimacy maturity and its correlates in young married couples. *Journal of Personality and Social Psychology, 50*, 152-162.

Whiting, J.W.M. (1965). Menarcheal age and infant stress in humans. In: F.A. Beach (Ed.), *Sex and behavior.* New York: John Wiley & Sons.

Willis, P. (1977). *Learning to Labour.* Farnborough, UK: Saxon House.

Winefield, A.H. (1992). *Growing up with unemployment.* London: Routledge.

Winnicott, D.W. (1958). The capacity to be alone. *International Journal of Psychoanalysis, 39*, 416-420.

Wish, M., Deutsch, M. & Kaplan, S.J. (1976). Perceived dimensions of interpersonal relationships. *Journal of Personality and Social Psychology, 33*, 409-420.

Wong, M.M. & Csikszentmihalyi, M. (1991). Affiliation motivation and daily experience: Some issues on gender differences. *Journal of Personality and Social Psychology, 60*, 154-164.

Wyer, R.S. & Gordon, S.E. (1984). The cognitive representation of social information. In: R.S. Wyer, Jr. & T.K. Srull (Eds.), *Handbook of social cognition* (I–III). Hillsdale, NJ: Lawrence Erlbaum Associates Inc.

Wyer, R.S. & Srull, T.K. (1980). The processing of social stimulus information: A conceptual integration. In: R. Hastie, E.B. Ebbesen, D. Hamilton & D.E. Carlston (Eds.), *Person memory: The cognitive basis of social perception.* Hillsdale, NJ: Lawrence Erlbaum Associates Inc.

Wyer, R.S. & Srull, T.K. (Eds.) (1984). *Handbook of social cognition* (Vol II). Hillsdale, NJ: Lawrence Erlbaum Associates Inc.

Wyer, R.S. & Srull, T.K. (1986). Human cognition in its social context. *Psychological Review, 93,* 322-359.

Youniss, J. (1980). *Parents and Peers in Social Development: A Sullivan-Piaget perspective.* Chicago: The University of Chicago Press.

Youniss, J. (1983). Social construction of adolescence by adolescents and parents. In: H.D. Grotevant & C.R. Cooper (Eds.), *Adolescent development in the family.* San Francisco: Jossey-Bass.

Youniss, J. & Ketterlinus, R.D. (1987). Communication and connectedness in mother-father-adolescent relationships. *Journal of Youth and Adolescence, 16,* 265-280.

Youniss, J. & Smollar, J. (1985). *Adolescent relations with mothers, fathers and friends.* London: University of Chicago Press.

Youniss, J. & Smollar, J. (1990). Self through relationship development. In: H.A. Bosma & A.E. Jackson (Eds.), *Coping and self-concept in adolescence.* Heidelberg: Springer-Verlag.

Zani, B. (1991). Male and female patterns in the discovery of sexuality during adolescence. *Journal of Adolescence, 14,* 163-178.

Zani, B., Altieri, L. & Signani, F. (1991). *Amore giovane: Una ricerca sugli adolescenti a Ferrara.* Ferrara: CDS Edizioni

Zimbardo, P. (1970). The human choice: Individuation, reason and order versus deindividuation, impulse and chaos. In: W.J. Arnold & D. Levine (Eds.), *Nebraska symposium on motivation,* Lincoln, Nebraska: University of Nebraska Press.

Zimbardo, P. G. (1977). *Shyness.* Reading, MA : Addison Wesley.

Zinnecker, J. (1990). Sportives Kind und jugendliches Koerperkapital. *Neue Sammlung, 30,* 645-653.

Ziolkowski, M. (1981). *Znaczenie, interakcja, rozumienie* (Meaning, Interaction, Understanding). Warszawa: PWN.

Author Index

Houlihan, J., 51–52
Houston, B.K., 171
Howard, K.J., 109
Howell, D.C., 171, 173, 177, 194
Huh, K., 52, 62
Hunter, F.T., 158
Hurme, H., 122, 123, 126, 131, 143
Hurrelmann, K., 146, 147, 148, 149,
    151, 165
Huston, T.L., 104–105
Hymel, S., 200, 208

Iacovetta, R.G., 166
Ickes, W., 199
Ilfeld, F.W., 180, 196
Inhelder, B., 124
Irion, J.C., 190

Jacklin, C., 59
Jackson, A.E., 5, 7, 12–13, 20, 124,
    135, 141, 146, 261–262
Jackson, D., 115
Jackson, S., *see Jackson, A.E.*
Jacobson, A.M., 51–52, 58, 172, 184
Jagger, H.J., 70
Jamieson, L., 1, 13, 233, 239
Jeanvoine, B., 3
Jencks, C., 246
Jennings, D., 68, 85–86
Jennings, W.S., 236
Jensen, G.F., 246
Jessor, R., 193
Johnson, B.M., 76
Johnson M.P., 104–105
Jones, L., 77
Jones, R.M., 53
Jones, W.H., 148
Josselson, R., 114
Juhasz, A., 110
Jurkovic, G.J., 236

Kahana, B., 122, 123, 124, 140
Kahana, E., 122, 123, 124, 140
Kandel, D.B., 158, 192–193, 195, 196
Kanner, A.D., 173
Kaplan, H.B., 77
Kaplan, N., 219
Kaplan, S.J., 211
Kaufman, K., 51

Kelly, D.H., 245, 246
Kelly, E.W., 96, 108
Kelly, J.A., 146, 148
Kennedy, D., 112, 114
Ketterlinus, R.D., 58
Kihlstrom, J.F., 20
Kilkenny, R., 236
Kimmel, D.C., 92
King, G.A., 21, 43
Kirchler, E., 8–9, 21, 98, 103, 147,
    148–150, 150–152, 154–155,
    157–158, 159–164, 165, 259
Kivett, V.R., 122
Kivnick, H.Q., 125
Klein, M.M., 195
Knox, D., 109
Kogan, N., 238
Kohlberg, L., 51, 236–237, 238, 245
Kölbel, G., 199
Kornhaber, A., 125
Koval, J.E., 116
Kracke, B., 6, 43, 68, 77, 78–79, 80,
    81, 83, 119, 262
Kremen, A., 52
Kreutz, H., 147
Kroger, J., 204, 267

Labouvie, E.W., 192
Laron, Z., 75
Larsen, L.E., 158
Larson, A., 191
Larson, R., 1, 124, 135, 136, 141, 201,
    204
Larson, R.W., 201, 204, 205
Latane, B., 238
Lazarus, R.S., 44, 169, 171, 172, 173,
    176–177, 187, 193–194
Le Bon, G., 237
Leahy, R.L., 195
Leaper, C., 52
LeBlanc, M., 242
Lee, T.R., 52, 53–54, 58
Leeper, J.D., 70
Leitch, C.J., 164, 166
Lerner, R.M., 42, 92, 263, 264–265,
    267
Leslie, L.A., 104–105
Lesser, G.S., 158, 192, 195
Lesser, I.M., 113

Subject Index